Diagnosis and Treatment of Small Bowel Disorders

Diagnosis and Treatment of Small Bowel Disorders

Editors

Anastasios Koulaouzidis
Wojciech Marlicz

MDPI • Basel • Beijing • Wuhan • Barcelona • Belgrade • Manchester • Tokyo • Cluj • Tianjin

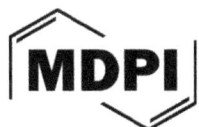

Editors
Anastasios Koulaouzidis
The Royal Infirmary of Edinburgh
UK

Wojciech Marlicz
Pomeranian Medical University
Poland

Editorial Office
MDPI
St. Alban-Anlage 66
4052 Basel, Switzerland

This is a reprint of articles from the Special Issue published online in the open access journal *Journal of Clinical Medicine* (ISSN 2077-0383) (available at: https://www.mdpi.com/journal/jcm/special_issues/small_bowel_disorder).

For citation purposes, cite each article independently as indicated on the article page online and as indicated below:

LastName, A.A.; LastName, B.B.; LastName, C.C. Article Title. *Journal Name* **Year**, *Volume Number*, Page Range.

ISBN 978-3-03943-873-0 (Hbk)
ISBN 978-3-03943-874-7 (PDF)

© 2020 by the authors. Articles in this book are Open Access and distributed under the Creative Commons Attribution (CC BY) license, which allows users to download, copy and build upon published articles, as long as the author and publisher are properly credited, which ensures maximum dissemination and a wider impact of our publications.

The book as a whole is distributed by MDPI under the terms and conditions of the Creative Commons license CC BY-NC-ND.

Contents

About the Editors vii

Wojciech Marlicz and Anastasios Koulaouzidis
Small Bowel—Key Player in Health and Disease
Reprinted from: *J. Clin. Med.* **2019**, *8*, 1748, doi:10.3390/jcm8101748 1

Johanna K. Larsson, Konstantinos J. Dabos, Peter Höglund, Johan Bohr, Andreas Münch, Andry Giannakou, Artur Nemeth, Gabriele Wurm-Johansson, Ervin Toth, John N. Plevris, Paul Fineron, Anastasios Koulaouzidis and Klas Sjöberg
Cancer Risk in Collagenous Colitis
Reprinted from: *J. Clin. Med.* **2019**, *8*, 1942, doi:10.3390/jcm8111942 7

Raphaël Enaud, Katarzyna B. Hooks, Aurélien Barre, Thomas Barnetche, Christophe Hubert, Marie Massot, Thomas Bazin, Haude Clouzeau, Stéphanie Bui, Michael Fayon, Patrick Berger, Philippe Lehours, Cécile Bébéar, Macha Nikolski, Thierry Lamireau, Laurence Delhaes and Thierry Schaeverbeke
Intestinal Inflammation in Children with Cystic Fibrosis Is Associated with Crohn's-Like Microbiota Disturbances
Reprinted from: *J. Clin. Med.* **2019**, *8*, 645, doi:10.3390/jcm8050645 17

May Min, Michael G. Noujaim, Jonathan Green, Christopher R. Schlieve, Aditya Vaze, Mitchell A. Cahan and David R. Cave
Role of Mucosal Protrusion Angle in Discriminating between True and False Masses of the Small Bowel on Video Capsule Endoscopy
Reprinted from: *J. Clin. Med.* **2019**, *8*, 418, doi:10.3390/jcm8040418 31

Karolina Skonieczna-Żydecka, Mariusz Kaczmarczyk, Igor Łoniewski, Luis F. Lara, Anastasios Koulaouzidis, Agata Misera, Dominika Maciejewska and Wojciech Marlicz
A Systematic Review, Meta-Analysis, and Meta-Regression Evaluating the Efficacy and Mechanisms of Action of Probiotics and Synbiotics in the Prevention of Surgical Site Infections and Surgery-Related Complications
Reprinted from: *J. Clin. Med.* **2018**, *7*, 556, doi:10.3390/jcm7120556 39

Masanao Nakamura, Takeshi Yamamura, Keiko Maeda, Tsunaki Sawada, Yasuyuki Mizutani, Takuya Ishikawa, Kazuhiro Furukawa, Eizaburo Ohno, Hiroki Kawashima, Ryoji Miyahara, Anastasios Koulaouzidis, Yoshiki Hirooka and the Nagoya University Crohn's Disease Study Group
Validity of Capsule Endoscopy in Monitoring Therapeutic Interventions in Patients with Crohn's Disease
Reprinted from: *J. Clin. Med.* **2018**, *7*, 311, doi:10.3390/jcm7100311 67

Alka Singh, Atreyi Pramanik, Pragyan Acharya and Govind K. Makharia
Non-Invasive Biomarkers for Celiac Disease
Reprinted from: *J. Clin. Med.* **2019**, *8*, 885, doi:10.3390/jcm8060885 79

Samuel Ortega, Himar Fabelo, Dimitris K. Iakovidis, Anastasios Koulaouzidis and Gustavo M. Callico
Use of Hyperspectral/Multispectral Imaging in Gastroenterology. Shedding Some–Different–Light into the Dark
Reprinted from: *J. Clin. Med.* **2019**, *8*, 36, doi:10.3390/jcm8010036 97

Karolina Skonieczna-Żydecka, Wojciech Marlicz, Agata Misera, Anastasios Koulaouzidis and Igor Łoniewski
Microbiome—The Missing Link in the Gut-Brain Axis: Focus on Its Role in Gastrointestinal and Mental Health
Reprinted from: *J. Clin. Med.* **2018**, *7*, 521, doi:10.3390/jcm7120521 . . . . **119**

About the Editors

Anastasios Koulaouzidis MD, DM, Ph.D., FASGE: Dr Koulaouzidis is currently with the Centre for Liver and Digestive Disorders at the Royal Infirmary of Edinburgh, Scotland. He was also Affiliate Professor to the Department of Social Medicine and Public Health, Faculty of Health Sciences, Pomeranian Medical University. He obtained his MD from the Medical School of the Aristotle University of Thessaloniki (Greece), in 1995. His Doctorate in Medicine (DM) is from the University of Edinburgh, UK; his second, a Doctorate in Philosophy (Ph.D.), is from Lunds Universitet, Sweden. He became a Member of the Royal College of Physicians of Edinburgh (UK) in 2004 and a Fellow of the same College (2013). He is also a Fellow of the European Board of Gastroenterology (2009), and the American Society for Gastrointestinal Endoscopy (2017). His was recognized by WEO with the WEO Emerging Star Award (2017) Dr Koulaouzidis has published extensively on capsule endoscopy and has co-authored several relevant book chapters. He is the (co)author of >210 PubMed-indexed articles, out of which at least 115 are on capsule endoscopy. His research interests include clinical applications of capsule endoscopy, quality improvement and software diagnostics as well as hardware and concept development in capsule a minimally invasive endoscopy. He is also interested in colonoscopy, colorectal cancer, and microscopic colitis. He is an active member of the editorial board of several specialty journals, Editor-in-Chief of the World Journal of Gastrointestinal Endoscopy, and has won numerous research grants.

Wojciech Marlicz, MD, Ph.D., FACG, FRCPE: Wojciech Marlicz is a consultant in gastroenterology and internal medicine at the Department of Gastroenterology, Pomeranian Medical University, and also holds his practice at The Centre for Digestive Diseases, Endoklinika, in Szczecin, Poland. His interests revolve around diagnostic and therapeutic gastrointestinal endoscopy as well as scientific basic and clinical research themes focused on the role of adult stem cells, gut barrier, small bowel microbiome, and probiotics in human gastrointestinal diseases. Dr Marlicz is also involved in teaching and educational activities highlighting the importance of healthy lifestyle and nutrition to promote wellbeing and longevity. Dr Marlicz is a member of World Gastroenterology Organisation (WGO) Foundation and Train the Trainers Committees, European Society of Neurogastroenterology and Motility (ESNM), Polish Society of Gastroenterology PTG-E (Head of West Pomeranian Division of PTG-E 2012-2016), European Lifestyle Medicine Organization (ELMO—Country Representative for Poland), and Polish Coeliac Society (Honorary Member). He is also a member of European Microscopic Colitis Group (EMCG) and European Colonoscopy Quality Investigation Group (ECQI). Fellow of American College of Gastroenterology (FACG) and Fellow of the Royal College of Physicians (Edinburgh).

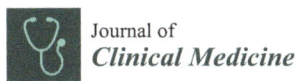 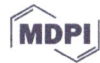

Editorial

Small Bowel—Key Player in Health and Disease

Wojciech Marlicz [1,*] and Anastasios Koulaouzidis [2]

1. Department of Gastroenterology, Pomeranian Medical University, 71-252 Szczecin, Poland
2. Centre for Liver & Digestive Disorders, Royal Infirmary of Edinburgh, Edinburgh EH16 4SA, UK; akoulaouzidis@hotmail.com
* Correspondance: marlicz@hotmail.com

Received: 7 October 2019; Accepted: 14 October 2019; Published: 21 October 2019

Over the last two decades, remarkable progress has been made in understanding the etiology and pathophysiology of diseases. New discoveries emphasize the importance of the small bowel (SB) 'ecosystem' in the pathogenesis of acute and chronic illness alike. Emerging factors, such as microbiome, stem and progenitor cells, innate intestinal immunity, and the enteric nervous system, along with mucosal and endothelial barriers, play a key role in the development of gastrointestinal (GI) and extra-GI diseases. The results of other studies point also towards a link between the digestive tract and common non-communicable diseases, such as obesity and cancer. These discoveries unravel novel dimensions of uncertainty in the area of clinical decision-making motivating researchers to search for novel diagnostic and therapeutic solutions.

Recent studies unravel the role of the poorly-understood complexity of the SB. Insights into its critical physiologic and pathophysiologic role in metabolic homeostasis and its potential role as a driver of obesity, insulin resistance, and subsequent type 2 diabetes mellitus (T2DM) have been revealed [1]. For example, bypassing the proximal small intestine by means of bariatric surgery results in a significant metabolic benefit to an individual undergoing such a procedure. Moreover, endoscopic procedures aimed at placing devices separating luminal contents from the duodenal mucosa result in modest weight loss and improvement in glucose homeostasis [1].

Another endoscopic treatment which aims at resurfacing duodenal mucosa (DMR, duodenal mucosal resurfacing), leads to improvement in glycemia and insulin resistance in patients with T2DM [2]. It is not surprising when we recall that SB endocrine cells secrete glycemia-regulating incretin hormones (e.g., glucagon-like peptide, GLP-1), and this process is dependent on food content in the intestinal lumen. Moreover, bile acids with various targets in the liver and small intestine (e.g., farnesoid receptor, FXR) together with a plethora of other small signaling molecules act in concert in regulating metabolic and digestive GI function.

The human digestive tract and enteric nervous system (ENS) communicate with the central nervous system (CNS) through the gut-brain axis (GBA). This bidirectional communication involves diverse neural networks through the X cranial vagal nerve—dorsal roots of the sympathetic/ parasympathetic nervous system. Important roles in the regulation of the gut-brain axis are played by: (i) the hypothalamus-pituitary-adrenal axis (HPA), (ii) the stress hormones (cortisol), (iii) the short-chain fatty acids (SCFAs), and (iv) the gut microbiota. The intestinal barrier, another important part of GBA, is composed of: (i) goblet cells derived mucus, (ii) microbiota, (iii) epithelial cells, (iv) endothelial cells, (v) lymphatic vessels, and v) enterocytes' tight cellular junctions. Of interest, the structure and function of the intestinal barrier resemble that of the blood-brain barrier (BBB). The gut-brain communication is mediated via blood, portal/hepatic circulation, and the bone marrow [3].

Recently, it has been described that the alterations of the intestinal barrier play a crucial role in the pathology of several human inflammatory and autoimmune diseases. Mohanan et al. documented the crucial role of the C1orf106 inflammatory bowel disease (IBD) susceptibility gene in stabilizing intestinal barrier function and intestinal inflammation [4]. Manfredo Vieira et al. evidenced the role of pathobionts in the process of intestinal barrier alterations, which were followed by their translocation to lymph nodes and the hepatic portal system, triggering systemic lupus erythematosus (SLE) [5]. Thaiss et al. reported that hyperglycemia leads to disruption of the intestinal barrier followed by intestinal inflammation and systemic infection [6]. Spadoni et al. recently documented that the presence of the gut-vascular barrier (GVB) in the small intestine controls the dissemination of bacteria into the bloodstream [7]. The authors reported a decrease of the wnt/beta catenin-inducible gene Axin2 (a marker of stem cell renewal) in gut endothelium under the presence of *Salmonella typhimirum* in the SB. The GVB was modified in patients with coeliac disease (CD) with altered serum transaminases, which suggests that GVB deterioration may be responsible for liver damage in CD patients [7]. It has been shown that disruption of epithelial and vascular barriers in the intestine were early events in non-alcoholic steatohepatitis (NASH), and GVB leakage marker could be identified in colonic biopsies in patients with NASH [8]. Of importance, SB epithelial and vascular barriers are FXR-controlled, which opens avenues to clinical trials aimed at investigation of novel FXR-agonists as future therapeutics [9]. Of interest, intestinal barriers could be monitored in vivo with the aid of confocal laser endomicroscopy (CLE) [10,11].

Therefore, the SB is considered a key player in metabolic disease development [12], including diabetes mellitus and NASH, and other diet-related disorders such as coeliac and non-coeliac enteropathies. Another major field is drug metabolism and its interaction with small bowel microbiome [13]. Moreover, the emergence of gut-brain, gut-liver, and gut-blood barriers point towards the important role of the SB in the pathogenesis of previously unthought and GI-unrelated conditions such as neurodegenerative and cardiovascular disease [14,15]. The SB remains an organ that is difficult to fully access and assess and accurate diagnosis often poses a clinical challenge. Undoubtedly, the therapeutic potential remains untapped. Therefore, it is now time to direct more of our interest towards the SB and unravel the interplay between the SB and other GI and non-GI related diseases.

In this Journal of Clinical Medicine Special Issue, "Diagnosis and Treatment of Small Bowel Disorders", several groups of investigators contributed their knowledge to the field of SB research by presenting original papers and reviews.

Enaud et al. [16] describe original observations by utilizing next-generation sequencing (NGS), that intestinal inflammation in children with Cystic Fibrosis (CF) was associated with alterations of microbiota similar to those observed in Crohn's disease (CrDs). Authors for the first time applied novel CrDs Microbial-Dysbiosis index in CF patients and pointed towards the importance of gut-lung axis in CF prognosis [16]. Of interest, intestinal inflammation was associated with previous intravenous antibiotic courses for CF [13]. This observation is important as global awareness of antibiotic resistance rises. Nakamura et al. [17] sought to evaluate the validity of using capsule endoscopy (CE) to monitor the effect of medical treatment on SB mucosal healing in post-operative CrDs patients, regardless of the presence of clinical symptoms. Although the significance of endoscopic monitoring has been widely accepted in CrDs, to date, only a few studies looked at the validity and effectiveness of escalating treatment for patients in clinical remission but with endoscopically visible active mucosal lesion. The authors demonstrated that CrDs patients in clinical remission with ongoing intestinal inflammation at the time of the CE could benefit from additional treatment. This study motivates physicians to optimize treatment plans for asymptomatic CD patients.

Several characteristics of SB lesions (e.g., mucosal disruption, bleeding, irregular surface, polypoid appearance, color, delayed passage, white villi, and invagination) have been described to better predict SB lesions, such as intestinal bulges, masses, and tumors. The lack of precise features in characterizing these lesions places a limitation on the accuracy of CE diagnosis. Therefore, Min et al. [18] in their retrospective study, evaluated the utility of an additional morphologic criterion, the mucosal protrusion angle (MPA), which was defined as the angle between a SB protruding lesion and its surrounding mucosa. The authors documented that MPA was a simple and useful tool for differentiating between intestinal true masses and non-significant bulges [18]. Their observation creates a useful extra tool for those who are faced with the question of 'mass or bulge?'

SB microbiota alterations have also been implicated in the pathogenesis of surgical site infections (SSIs) and surgery-related complications (SRCs). Skonieczna-Żydecka et al. [19] conducted a systematic review with meta-analysis and meta-regression of randomized clinical trials investigating the efficacy of probiotics and synbiotics to counteract SSIs and SRCs in patients under various surgical treatments. The authors aimed to determine the mechanisms behind probiotic/synbiotic action. Their meta-analysis revealed that probiotics/synbiotics administration prior and at a time of major abdominal surgery, leads to a reduction in the incidence of SSIs and SRCs (e.g., abdominal distension, diarrhea, pneumonia, sepsis, urinary tract infection, postoperative pyrexia). Furthermore, probiotics/synbiotics were associated with shortening of the duration of antibiotic therapy and hospital stay. Based on current evidence, the action of probiotics/synbiotics in surgical patients seems to be exerted via modulation of gut-immune response and production of short-chain fatty acids (SCFAs) [19].

Included also in this special issue, Singh et al. [20] comprehensively reviewed the pros and cons of biomarkers in coeliac disease and summarized the current status of coeliac disease screening, diagnosis, and monitoring. The review could guide clinicians in diagnosis and monitoring of patients with coeliac disease. As biomarkers allow for smart targeted-screening, similarly imaging spectroscopy (a combination of digital imaging and spectroscopy, also known as hyperspectral/multispectral (HS/MS) imaging (HSI/MSI) technology) allows for smart tissue visualization beyond the limitations of the human eye. HSI has been utilized for various research purposes including: (i) food quality inspection, (ii) optimization of the recycling process, (iii) art painting renovations, (iv) geology and minerals inspection, (v) soil evaluation and (vi) plant response to stress. HSI has also been evolving in the field of medical research in gastroenterology, pathology, and surgery. This modality was used to generate alternative visualization of tissues, abdominal organ differentiation, identification of surgical site resection, and abdominal ischemia to name a few. Ortega et al. [21] in their thorough review provided a detailed summary of the most relevant research work in the field of gastroenterology using HSI.

Last but not least, Skonieczna-Żydecka et al. [22] in a narrative review published in this issue of Journal of Clinical Medicine, discussed involvements of GBA deregulation in the origin of brain-gut disorders. The authors hypothesized that stem cell-host microbiome cross-talk was potentially involved in GBA disorders. Interestingly, patients with inflammatory bowel disease (IBD) have an elevated risk of mental illness, and depression increases the risk of IBD. Of key interest, are observations that multiple drugs are known to induce metabolic malfunctions, possibly through alterations of SB milieu. These alterations result in body weight gain, metabolic disturbances, and suppression of metabolic resting rate. The authors in their comprehensive review presented the current state of the art knowledge of the role of GBA in GI and psychiatric comorbidities. The current evidence supports the notion that an injury to the intestinal mucosa can result in significant, though delayed, metabolic consequences that may seriously affect the health of an individual. Future investigations [23] into the pathophysiology of host-microbe interactions should focus on the small bowel [24,25], which is still relatively inaccessible. Therefore, the research is challenging but necessary to pave the way to new findings and solutions in the clinical area of the small bowel [26] and beyond [27].

Dr Marlicz and Dr Koulaouzidis are Guest Editors of this Special Issue of the Journal of Clinical Medicine (ISSN 2077-03830), which belongs to the journal's section Gastroenterology and Hepato-Pancreato-Biliary Medicine.

Conflicts of Interest: The authors declare that there is no conflict of interest.

References

1. Van Baar, A.C.G.; Nieuwdorp, M.; Holleman, F.; Soeters, M.R.; Groen, A.K.; Bergman, J.J.G.H.M. The Duodenum harbors a Broad Untapped Therapeutic Potential. *Gastroenterology* **2018**, *154*, 773–777. [CrossRef]

2. Van Baar, A.C.G.; Holleman, F.; Crenier, L.; Haidry, R.; Magee, C.; Hopkins, D.; Rodriguez Grunert, L.; Galvao Neto, M.; Vignolo, P.; Hayee, B.; et al. Duodenal mucosal resurfacing for the treatment of type 2 diabetes mellitus: One year results from the first international, open-label, prospective, multicentre study. *Gut* **2019**. [CrossRef]
3. Odenwald, M.A.; Turner, J.R. The intestinal epithelial barrier: A therapeutic target? *Nat. Rev. Gastroenterol. Hepatol.* **2017**, *14*, 9–21. [CrossRef] [PubMed]
4. Mohanan, V.; Nakata, T.; Desch, A.N.; Lévesque, C.; Boroughs, A.; Guzman, G.; Cao, Z.; Creasey, E.; Yao, J.; Boucher, G.; et al. C1orf106 is a colitis risk gene that regulates stability of epithelial adherens junctions. *Science* **2018**, *359*, 1161–1166. [CrossRef] [PubMed]
5. Vieira, S.M.; Hiltensperger, M.; Kumar, V.; Zegarra-Ruiz, D.; Dehner, C.; Khan, N.; Costa, F.R.C.; Tiniakou, E.; Greiling, T.; Ruff, W.; et al. Translocation of a gut pathobiont drives autoimmunity in mice and humans. *Science* **2018**, *359*, 1156–1161. [CrossRef] [PubMed]
6. Thaiss, C.A.; Levy, M.; Grosheva, I.; Zheng, D.; Soffer, E.; Blacher, E.; Braverman, S.; Tengeler, A.C.; Barak, O.; Elazar, M.; et al. Hyperglycemia drives intestinal barrier dysfunction and risk for enteric infection. *Science* **2018**, *359*, 1376–1383. [CrossRef]
7. Spadoni, I.; Zagato, E.; Bertocchi, A.; Paolinelli, R.; Hot, E.; Di Sabatino, A.; Caprioli, F.; Bottiglieri, L.; Oldani, A.; Viale, G.; et al. A gut-vascular barrier controls the systemic dissemination of bacteria. *Science* **2015**, *350*, 830–834. [CrossRef]
8. Mouries, J.; Brescia, P.; Silvestri, A.; Spadoni, I.; Sorribas, M.; Wiest, R.; Mileti, E.; Galbiati, M.; Invernizzi, P.; Adorini, L.; et al. Microbiota-driven gut vascular barrier disruption is a prerequisite for non-alcoholic steatohepatitis development. *J. Hepatol.* **2019**. [CrossRef]
9. Neuschwander-Tetri, B.A.; Loomba, R.; Sanyal, A.J.; Lavine, J.E.; Van Natta, M.L.; Abdelmalek, M.F.; Chalasani, N.; Dasarathy, S.; Diehl, A.M.; Hameed, B.; et al. NASH Clinical Research Network. Farnesoid X nuclear receptor ligand obeticholic acid for non-cirrhotic, non-alcoholic steatohepatitis (FLINT): A multicentre, randomised, placebo-controlled trial. *Lancet* **2015**, *385*, 956–965. [CrossRef]
10. Sorribas, M.; Jakob, M.O.; Yilmaz, B.; Li, H.; Stutz, D.; Noser, Y.; de Gottardi, A.; Moghadamrad, S.; Hassan, M.; Albillos, A.; et al. FXR-modulates the gut-vascular barrier by regulating the entry sites for bacterial translocation in experimental cirrhosis. *J. Hepatol.* **2019**. [CrossRef]
11. Fritscher-Ravens, A.; Pflaum, T.; Mösinger, M.; Ruchay, Z.; Röcken, C.; Milla, P.J.; Das, M.; Böttner, M.; Wedel, T.; Schuppan, D. Many Patients with Irritable Bowel Syndrome Have Atypical Food Allergies Not Associated with Immunoglobulin E. *Gastroenterology* **2019**, *157*, 109–118. [CrossRef] [PubMed]
12. Tilg, H.; Zmora, N.; Adolph, T.E.; Elinav, E. The intestinal microbiota fuelling metabolic inflammation. *Nat. Rev. Immunol.* **2019**. [CrossRef] [PubMed]
13. Skonieczna-Żydecka, K.; Łoniewski, I.; Misera, A.; Stachowska, E.; Maciejewska, D.; Marlicz, W.; Galling, B. Second-generation antipsychotics and metabolism alterations: A systematic review of the role of the gut microbiome. *Psychopharmacology* **2019**, *236*, 1491–1512. [CrossRef] [PubMed]
14. Tanaka, M.; Itoh, H. Hypertension as a Metabolic Disorder and the Novel Role of the Gut. *Curr. Hypertens Rep.* **2019**, *21*, 63. [CrossRef] [PubMed]
15. Kowalski, K.; Mulak, A. Brain-Gut-Microbiota Axis in Alzheimer's Disease. *J. Neurogastroenterol. Motil.* **2019**, *25*, 48–60. [CrossRef]
16. Enaud, R.; Hooks, K.B.; Barre, A.; Barnetche, T.; Hubert, C.; Massot, M.; Bazin, T.; Clouzeau, H.; Bui, S.; Fayon, M.; et al. Intestinal Inflammation in Children with Cystic Fibrosis Is Associated with Crohn's-Like Microbiota Disturbances. *J. Clin. Med.* **2019**, *8*, 645. [CrossRef]
17. Nakamura, M.; Yamamura, T.; Maeda, K.; Sawada, T.; Mizutani, Y.; Ishikawa, T.; Furukawa, K.; Ohno, E.; Kawashima, H.; Miyahara, R.; et al. Nagoya University Crohn's Disease Study Group. Validity of Capsule Endoscopy in Monitoring Therapeutic Interventions in Patients with Crohn's Disease. *J. Clin. Med.* **2018**, *7*, 311. [CrossRef]
18. Min, M.; Noujaim, M.G.; Green, J.; Schlieve, C.R.; Vaze, A.; Cahan, M.A.; Cave, D.R. Role of Mucosal Protrusion Angle in Discriminating between True and False Masses of the Small Bowel on Video Capsule Endoscopy. *J. Clin. Med.* **2019**, *8*, 418. [CrossRef]

19. Skonieczna-Żydecka, K.; Kaczmarczyk, M.; Łoniewski, I.; Lara, L.F.; Koulaouzidis, A.; Misera, A.; Maciejewska, D.; Marlicz, W. A Systematic Review, Meta-Analysis, and Meta-Regression Evaluating the Efficacy and Mechanisms of Action of Probiotics and Synbiotics in the Prevention of Surgical Site Infections and Surgery-Related Complications. *J. Clin. Med.* **2018**, *7*, 556. [CrossRef]
20. Singh, A.; Pramanik, A.; Acharya, P.; Makharia, G.K. Non-Invasive Biomarkers for Celiac Disease. *J. Clin. Med.* **2019**, *8*, 885. [CrossRef]
21. Ortega, S.; Fabelo, H.; Iakovidis, D.K.; Koulaouzidis, A.; Callico, G.M. Use of Hyperspectral/Multispectral Imaging in Gastroenterology. Shedding Some Different Light into the Dark. *J. Clin. Med.* **2019**, *8*, 36. [CrossRef] [PubMed]
22. Skonieczna-Żydecka, K.; Marlicz, W.; Misera, A.; Koulaouzidis, A.; Łoniewski, I. Microbiome—The Missing Link in the Gut-Brain Axis: Focus on Its Role in Gastrointestinal and Mental Health. *J. Clin. Med.* **2018**, *7*, 521. [CrossRef] [PubMed]
23. Pełka-Wysiecka, J.; Kaczmarczyk, M.; Bąba-Kubiś, A.; Liśkiewicz, P.; Wroński, M.; Skonieczna-Żydecka, K.; Marlicz, W.; Misiak, B.; Starzyńska, T.; Kucharska-Mazur, J.; et al. Analysis of Gut Microbiota and Their Metabolic Potential in Patients with Schizophrenia Treated with Olanzapine: Results from a Six-Week Observational Prospective Cohort Study. *J. Clin. Med.* **2019**, *8*, 1605. [CrossRef] [PubMed]
24. Zhong, L.; Shanahan, E.R.; Raj, A.; Koloski, N.A.; Fletcher, L.; Morrison, M.; Walker, M.M.; Talley, N.J.; Holtmann, G. Dyspepsia and the microbiome: Time to focus on the small intestine. *Gut* **2017**, *66*, 1168–1169. [CrossRef] [PubMed]
25. Vuik, F.; Dicksved, J.; Lam, S.Y.; Fuhler, G.M.; van der Laan, L.; van de Winkel, A.; Konstantinov, S.R.; Spaander, M.; Peppelenbosch, M.P.; Engstrand, L.; et al. Composition of the mucosa-associated microbiota along the entire gastrointestinal tract of human individuals. *United Eur. Gastroenterol. J.* **2019**, *7*, 897–907. [CrossRef] [PubMed]
26. Quigley, E.M.M. Symptoms and the small intestinal microbiome—The unknown explored. *Nat. Rev. Gastroenterol. Hepatol.* **2019**, *16*, 457–458. [CrossRef]
27. Lynch, S.V.; Ng, S.C.; Shanahan, F.; Tilg, H. Translating the gut microbiome: Ready for the clinic? *Nat. Rev. Gastroenterol. Hepatol.* **2019**. [CrossRef]

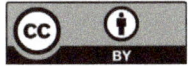

© 2019 by the authors. Licensee MDPI, Basel, Switzerland. This article is an open access article distributed under the terms and conditions of the Creative Commons Attribution (CC BY) license (http://creativecommons.org/licenses/by/4.0/).

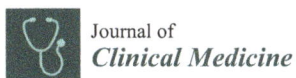 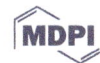

Article
Cancer Risk in Collagenous Colitis

Johanna K. Larsson [1], Konstantinos J. Dabos [2], Peter Höglund [3], Johan Bohr [4], Andreas Münch [5], Andry Giannakou [6], Artur Nemeth [7], Gabriele Wurm-Johansson [7], Ervin Toth [7], John N. Plevris [2], Paul Fineron [8], Anastasios Koulaouzidis [2,†] and Klas Sjöberg [1,*,†]

1. Department of Gastroenterology, Skåne University Hospital, 205 02 Malmö, Sweden; johanna.larsson@med.lu.se
2. Centre for Liver & Digestive Disorders, the Royal Infirmary of Edinburgh, Edinburgh EH16 4SA, Scotland, UK; kostasophia@yahoo.com (K.J.D.); j.plevris@ed.ac.uk (J.N.P.); akoulaouzidis@hotmail.com (A.K.)
3. Department of Laboratory Medicine, Division of Clinical Chemistry and Pharmacology, SUS, Lund University, 221 85 Lund, Sweden; peter.hoglund@med.lu.se
4. Department of Medicine, Division of Gastroenterology, Örebro University Hospital, 702 81 Örebro, Sweden; School of Health and Medical Sciences, Örebro University, 701 85 Örebro, Sweden; johan.bohr@regionorebrolan.se
5. Division of Gastroenterology and Hepatology, Department of Clinical and Experimental Medicine, Faculty of Health Science, Linköpings University, 581 83 Linköping, Sweden; Andreas.Munch@regionostergotland.se
6. Open University of Cyprus, Faculty of Economics and Management, 1678 Nicosia, Cyprus; andry.gianna@gmail.com
7. Department of Medicine, Endoscopy Unit, Skåne University Hospital, 205 02 Malmö, Sweden; artur.nemeth@med.lu.se (A.N.); gabriele-wurm@web.de (G.W.-J.); ervin.toth@med.lu.se (E.T.)
8. Pathology Department, Western General Hospital, Edinburgh EH4 2XU, Scotland, UK; paul.fineron@nhtlothian.scot.nhs.uk
* Correspondence: klas.sjoberg@med.lu.se; Tel.: +464-033-6161
† These authors contributed equally to this work.

Received: 5 September 2019; Accepted: 7 November 2019; Published: 11 November 2019

Abstract: Data on malignancy in patients with collagenous colitis (CC) is scarce. We aimed to determine the incidence of cancers in patients with CC. In a two-stages, observational study, data on cancers in patients diagnosed with CC during 2000–2015, were collected from two cohorts. The risk was calculated according to the age-standardized rate for the first cohort and according to the standardized incidence ratio for the second cohort. The first cohort comprised 738 patients (394 from Scotland and 344 from Sweden; mean age 71 ± 11 and 66 ± 13 years, respectively). The incidence rates for lung cancer (RR 3.9, $p = 0.001$), bladder cancer (RR 9.2, $p = 0.019$), and non-melanoma skin cancer (NMSC) (RR 15, $p = 0.001$) were increased. As the majority of NMSC cases (15/16) came from Sweden, a second Swedish cohort, comprising 1141 patients (863 women, mean age 65 years, range 20–95 years) was collected. There were 93 cancer cases (besides NMSC). The risk for colon cancer was decreased (SIR 0.23, $p = 0.0087$). The risk for cutaneous squamous cell carcinoma was instead markedly increased (SIR 3.27, $p = 0.001$).

Keywords: colon cancer; cancer risk; collagenous colitis; lung cancer; microscopic colitis; skin cancer; squamous cell carcinoma

1. Introduction

Microscopic colitis (MC) is an inflammatory disorder of the colon that causes chronic, watery and non-bloody diarrhoea, occasionally associated with abdominal pain and weight loss. With a predilection for those ≥60 years of age and for females, MC has an incidence rate of approximately 10/100.000 per year [1–3]. Macroscopic findings are rare and the diagnosis is confirmed through histopathology [4–6]. MC comprises two main histologic subtypes; collagenous colitis (CC) and lymphocytic colitis (LC). Histopathological features of CC include a continuous, thickened sub-epithelial fibrous band (>10 µm) and associated chronic mucosal inflammation. The collagen band contains entrapped capillaries, red blood cells, as well as inflammatory cells. Moreover, damaged epithelial cells appear flattened, mucin-depleted, and irregularly-oriented. Focally, small strips of surface epithelium may lift-off the basement membrane [7]. Patients with CC are considered to have a more symptomatic and long-lasting disease course than those with LC [8].

Chronic inflammation is considered a risk factor for cancer development. Moreover, chronic inflammation may result in cancer development in sites other than the affected organ/system. For instance, the risk of lymphoma in rheumatoid arthritis (RA) is increased by 60% [9]. In patients with inflammatory bowel disease (IBD), there is an increased risk of colorectal cancer (CRC), at least in some subgroups, as well as extra-intestinal cancers such as haematological, bladder, lung as well as skin cancers [10–12]. Patients with coeliac disease have a reported increased risk of non-Hodgkin lymphoma, small-bowel cancer, CRC and basal cell carcinoma (BCC) [13]. *Helicobacter pylori* itself contributes to many neoplasias, but studies have shown that the inflammatory response per se contributes to the carcinogenesis as well [14].

Data on the incidence of metachronous cancer(s) in MC is scarce. Although the inflammation is limited as compared to classical IBD the condition may be active for several years; furthermore, it often affects elderly individuals who have already an increased cancer risk. Additionally, many patients with CC smoke [15]. Chan et al described an increased risk of lung cancer in a small cohort of patients with CC with a mean follow-up time of 7 years. The study included 117 patients, and no cases of CRC were described [16]. A negative association has actually been suggested between CRC and MC (including both CC and lymphocytic colitis) in a cohort comprising 647 patients with MC and a mean follow-up time of five years. Twelve MC patients had CRC compared to 27 in a control group of similar size ($p = 0.015$) [17]. Therefore, the aim of the present study was to determine the incidence of metachronous cancer in patients with CC.

2. Patients and Methods

The investigation was carried out as a two-stage, observational, international, multicentre, cohort-study, comprising two sizeable cohorts of patients diagnosed with CC. See Figure 1.

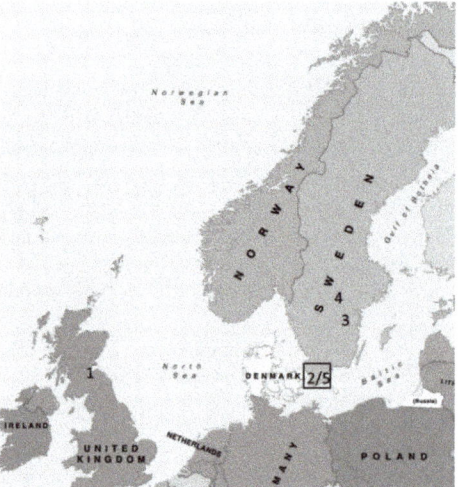

Figure 1. Participating centres: Series 1: 1 = Edinburgh, Scotland, 2 = Malmö; Series 2: 3 = Linköping, 4 = Örebro, 5 = Skåne region.

2.1. First Stage—Scotland and Sweden

In an international, retrospective, two-centre observational study; data on extra-colonic cancer in patients with CC were collected for a 14-year period (2000–2013) from Edinburgh, Scotland and Malmö, Sweden. The CC diagnosis was set according to established criteria i.e., symptoms of chronic, non-bloody diarrhoea and histopathological findings of thickened sub-epithelial collagen layer ≥10 µm, associated with chronic inflammation in the lamina propria and with an increased number of intraepithelial lymphocytes [18]. Data were obtained from the pathology department, Edinburgh and Malmö with a catchment area of 750,000 and 320,000 inhabitants, respectively. The records of those with CC were manually searched for data on metachronous, extra-colonic cancers.

2.2. Second Stage—Sweden

Due to an unexpectedly skewed distribution of cancer cases in the first stage of the study we decided to re-do the study and focus on Swedish data. Patients with CC in three different regions (Skåne, Linköping and Örebro) were included. In Sweden, all patients that are diagnosed with CC according to the established criteria are registered at the Departments of Pathology and are given a specific code number. All specimens taken during colonoscopy in the three regions are regularly sent to specific Pathology Departments. All patients with a CC diagnosis from 2000 in Skåne and Örebro and from 2008 in Linköping until the end of 2015 were included.

For each patient with CC, the follow-up period began at the time of CC diagnosis and continued until whichever of the following occurred first: death or the end of the observation period (31st December, 2015). Patients were not excluded after their first diagnosis of cancer, since we wanted to examine incidence risk for all cancers developed during follow up. The CC cohort was linked up with the National Cancer Register in each region. Cancers preceding the diagnosis of CC were not included in the cancer data.

2.3. Statistical Analysis

2.3.1. First Stage

Person-years at risk was calculated according to age-specific categories up to 85 years. The standard error (Se) was calculated using the Poisson approximation. Confidence interval (CI) of the age-standardised rate (ASR) was compared to public data, available from UK's National Cancer Intelligence Network. The relative risk (RR) for ASR was calculated and compared to ASR in Lothian region, Scotland. The standardised cancer incidence rates (IR) were also compared to the ones of Lothian under the assumption that populations at the same latitude share the same IR.

2.3.2. Second Stage

Person-years at risk were calculated by gender and 5-year age groups, separately for the 3 geographical areas (Skåne, Linköping, and Örebro). Standardized incidence ratios (SIR) were calculated for each of the reported cancers. Because patients in this cohort came from three different Swedish regions and in light of the known national variations of cancer incidence, the expected numbers of cancers were calculated by pooling the patients and linking each area to existing cancer registries. The expected numbers of cases of cancers and specific cancer types were calculated by multiplying the number of person-years for each gender, age and area group by the corresponding specific cancer incidence rates in the respective areas. SIR and their 95% CI were calculated assuming that the observed number of cases followed a Poisson distribution. Mid-P exact test was applied and values below 0.05 were considered significant. For non-melanoma skin cancer (NMSC), both BCC and cutaneous squamous cell carcinoma (cuSCC) that can occur several times in one individual, the number of tumours was recorded—instead of individual cases—in both the CC cohort and in the control group.

This study was approved by the institutional review board at Lund University (The local Ethics Committee at Lund University, date: 6th November 2013; decision LU 2013/650 and date: 27th October, 2016; decision LU 2016/788) and Lothian NHS. Since it was a retrospective registry study the Ethical Board approved that written informed consent was not necessary to obtain prior to the collection of data. The study protocol conforms to the ethical guidelines of the 1975 Declaration of Helsinki as reflected in a priori approval by the institution's human research committee.

3. Results

3.1. First Stage

The demographics of the first cohort can be seen in Table 1. Of the 738 included, 71 (50 women and 21 men) were affected by some form of extra-colonic, metachronous malignancy following the diagnosis of CC. The remainder of this cohort (n = 667) did not develop any extra-colonic cancer during the follow-up period. The average follow-up duration was 7 years (range 2–15 years), while the average time interval between CC and cancer diagnosis was 3 years (range 0–11 years). Of these 71 cases, 14 developed any cancer during the first year, 25 during the following two years and 32 from the third year.

Table 1. Characteristics of the collagenous colitis (CC)-cohort in Scotland and Sweden (Series 1).

	Edinburgh	Malmö	Total
N	394	344	738
Age, median (IQR)	68 (57–76)	69 (59–77)	68 (58–77)
% women (n)	68% (268)	83% (285)	75% (553)

IQR = interquartile range

The RR for all cancers, lung, bladder cancer and NMSC, as well as the ASR in patients with CC were higher compared to those of the general population. The RR for lung cancer was 3.88 (CI: 1.62–9.31), for bladder cancer 9.23 (CI: 1.14–75.03) and for NMSC 14.96 (CI: 2.57–87.08). See Table 2.

Table 2. Observed and expected cancers in the Scottish/Swedish cohort (series 1). RR, relative risk.

Cancer Type	Cases	Exp	RR	P-Value
Skin (NMSC)	16	1	15.0	0.001
Bladder	6	1	9.2	0.019
Lung	18	2	3.9	0.001

NMSC = non-melanoma skin cancer.

The cases with bladder and lung cancer were evenly distributed, but in contrast 15/16 cases with NMSC were addressed from the Malmö cohort. Because of this a decision was taken to proceed to a second stage by including more regions in Sweden. Furthermore, in most countries the number of NMSC is difficult to determine because BCC and cuSCC cases are not reported to national cancer registries, or they are reported as one heterogeneous group [19]. However, in Sweden these cancer types are reported separately and consequently it is possible to obtain data on the occurrence of BCC and cuSCC.

3.2. Second Stage

In this stage, a total of 1141 patients with diagnosis of CC were identified. It should be noted that 344 out of those from Skåne were included also in stage one. The characteristics of the patients are shown in Table 3. The average follow-up duration was 8 years (range 2–15 years), while the average time interval between CC and cancer diagnosis was 4 years (range 0–14 years). Of the 93 solid cancers 17 were diagnosed during the first year, 25 during the following two years and 51 thereafter. The expected and observed cancer cases are presented in Tables 4 and 5. The risk of lung cancer was increased in Skåne (SIR 1.85 CI: 1.053–3.029, $p = 0.034$) but since there were no other cases of lung cancer in the other two Swedish regions, this did not become significant in the whole group. The total number of cancer cases besides NMSC was 98. However, five rare cancer cases were considered not applicable for data calculation and thus excluded, leaving 93 cancer cases (61 women and 32 men). The total number of NMSC was 140. The mean time interval between CC diagnosis and cuSCC was 5.4 years, range 0.6–12.1 years. Of the 46 cases of cuSCC, four developed cuSCC during the first year, eight during the following two years, and 34 after three years or more.

Table 3. Characteristics of the CC-cohort Sweden, three regions (Series 2).

	Linköping	Örebro	Skåne	Total
N	130	133	878	1141
Age, median (IQR)	66 (57–75)	64 (53–74)	68 (58–76)	67 (57–76)
% women (n)	75% (98)	84% (112)	74% (653)	76% (863)

IQR = interquartile range

Table 4. Observed and expected cancers in the Swedish cohort, divided into Skåne, Linköping and Örebro (Series 2).

Cancer site	Skåne			Linköping			Örebro		
	obs	exp	SIR	obs	exp	SIR	obs	exp	SIR
Eye	1	0.13	7.64	0	0.023	0.00	0	0.011	0.00
Oesophagus	3	0.65	4.60	0	0.066	0.00	0	0.068	0.00
Cervix	2	0.46	4.33	0	0.07	0.00	0	0.079	0.00
CuSCC	36	11.58	3.11	6	1.44	4.18	4	1.060	3.78
Vulva	1	0.29	3.46	0	0.033	0.00	0	0.049	0.00
CNS	2	1.29	1.55	2	0.19	10.30	0	0.17	0.00
r	3	1.3	2.31	1	0.19	5.14	0	0.20	0.00
Stomach	1	1.27	0.79	1	0.14	7.14	1	0.14	7.27
Bladder/Ureter	8	4.29	1.87	0	0.5	0.00	2	0.38	5.30
Rectal/Anus	1	3.20	0.31	4	0.39	10.19	2	0.44	4.55
Pancreas	3	1.50	2.00	0	0.25	0.00	0	0.21	0.00
Lung	14	7.57	1.85	0	0.89	0.00	0	0.84	0.00
Prostate	8	7.56	1.06	1	1.56	0.64	1	0.56	1.78
Leukemia/Myeloma	3	2.93	1.02	0	0.37	0.00	1	0.40	2.52
Melanoma	3	3.92	0.76	2	0.63	3.18	0	0.55	0.00
BCC	83	82.08	1.01	7	7.62	0.92	4	6.19	0.65
Breast	11	17.61	0.62	3	1.89	1.59	2	1.98	1.01
r	1	2.47	0.40	0	0.30	0.00	1	0.26	3.78
Uterus	2	2.76	0.72	0	0.38	0.00	0	0.52	0.00
Colon	2	7.11	0.28	0	0.84	0.00	0	0.86	0.00

SIR = Standard Incidence Ratio, BCC = Basal cell carcinoma, cuSCC = Cutaneous squamous cell carcinoma.

Table 5. Observed and expected cancers in the whole Swedish cohort in a forest plot (Series 2).

Cancer site	Observed	Expected	SIR	mid-p
Eye	1	0.16	6.07	0.164
Oesophagus	3	0.79	3.82	0.054
Cervix	2	0.61	3.28	0.15
cuSCC	46	14.08	3.27	0.001
Vulva	1	0.37	2.70	0.364
CNS	4	1.65	2.42	0.113
Kidney	4	1.69	2.37	0.121
Stomach	3	1.54	1.94	0.273
Bladder/Ureter	10	5.16	1.94	0.055
Rectal/Anus	7	4.03	1.74	0.167
Pancreas	3	1.96	1.53	0.449
Lung	14	9.30	1.51	0.142
Prostate	10	9.68	1.03	0.878
Leukemia/Myeloma	4	3.69	1.08	0.816
Melanoma	5	5.10	0.98	1.000
BCC	94	95.89	0.98	0.847
Breast	16	21.48	0.74	0.233
Lymphoma	2	3.03	0.66	0.611
Uterus	2	3.66	0.55	0.411
Colon	2	8.81	0.23	0.009

BCC = Basal cell carcinoma, cuSCC = Cutaneous squamous cell carcinoma.

4. Discussion

This is the largest study published to date on the risk of metachronous malignancies in patients diagnosed with CC. In the first stage, it was noted that the risk for lung and bladder cancer was increased in patients with CC diagnosis. Furthermore, the risk of NMSC was also increased in this cohort. In the second stage of this observational, multicentre study comprising a large Swedish cohort we could confirm the decreased risk of colon cancer in patients with CC, as reported in previous studies [16,17]. However, previous studies either included prevalent cases of CRC (15) or comprised a fairly limited number of CC-patients (14). Analysis of the current large cohort from three counties in Sweden indicated that the risk of getting colon cancer was reduced at least four times (from 8.8 expected cases to two observed). Since we do not have information about previous colonoscopies in this elderly population with gastrointestinal complaints it cannot be excluded that this reduced risk hypothetically could be due to pre-emptive polypectomies preceding the diagnostic endoscopy. However, in patients with longstanding albeit low-grade, inflammatory response in the colon, one would instead expect to observe an increased risk of colon cancer. Nevertheless, not only the inflammation is modest, but it may also be protective. For instance, frequent watery diarrhoea reduces the transit time and likely any potential impact from toxic agents. Yen et al. suggest that elevated intraepithelial lymphocytes in the colonic mucosa in patients with MC may have a protective function against carcinogenesis through recruiting delta-gamma T-cells that kill cells undergoing DNA-damage or cell stress [17].

Data from the second series revealed a more than three-fold increase in cuSCC in patients with CC. Except UV-light exposure and immunosuppressive treatment related to organ transplantation, little is known about risk factors contributing to cuSCC [19–21]. Evidence that glucocorticoids enhance the risk of cuSCC is limited, but has been described previously [22,23]. The incidence of NMSC (both cuSCC and BCC) is increased in patients with IBD, but likely related to the exposure of immunosuppressive treatment (thiopurines and biologics) [24]. However, Singh et al. also described an increased risk of BCC in men with Crohn's disease not treated with immunosuppression [25]. Therefore, not only immunosuppressive treatment is related to an elevated risk of NMSC but also the inflammation per se, probably as a result of dysregulation of the immune system. In CC, Günaltay et al have described a decreased production of IL-37 in such patients, indicating a disturbed immune response [26,27]. Thus, the elevated risk of cuSCC in CC may be related to a malfunctioning immune system caused by the disease itself, medication or other not yet known procarcinogenic factors.

The incidence rate of lung cancer was increased in the first stage cohort but not in the second. However, the incidence was increased also in the second series in Skåne but not for the whole Swedish cohort. In Skåne 878 out of the 1141 cases with CC were identified and 14 cases with lung cancer was found (7.57 expected). In contrast to this large cohort the expected incidence of lung cancer in the cities Örebro and Linköping (based on 150,000 inhabitants in each location) were one case in each location. Consequently, the observed incidence with no cases in these two minor cities must be interpreted with caution. The incidence rate in Skåne with around 1.3 million inhabitants is of course more reliable. The risk of urinary bladder and/or ureteric cancer was increased in the first cohort and showed a positive trend in the second, something that strengthens this observation. The association between CC and smoking habits is already well described [15]. Smoking is related to cancer in both lung and bladder which is probably the reason why these incidence rates are elevated in our CC cohort [28,29].

The risk of cancer in oesophagus also showed a positive trend in the second series. Risk factors of oesophagus cancer are among others, smoking, alcohol, hot liquids and HPV-infection [30]. As can be seen, some of the risk factors are shared with CC such as smoking and alcohol [31]. Furthermore, oesophageal cancer is often of squamous cell origin just as in the skin. In this study we did not get detailed information if the oesophagus cancer cases were of squamous cell or adenomatous origin. However, in view of the low number of cases with oesophageal or bladder cancer, despite a fairly large number of CC patients, a definitive conclusion cannot be drawn regarding putative relationship between CC and cancer in oesophagus or bladder.

Some strengths and limitations should be noted; this is the largest study to date concerning the risk of metachronous cancer in patients with a previous diagnosis of CC. In the second cohort, 1141 patients could be included. The studied regions are well defined, and patients are referred to specific hospitals within these regions. All common cancers types in the western world were represented in the present study. In other words, no common cancer type was totally absent. The control group in the Swedish cohort consisted of all cancer cases in the same regions as our cohorts, adjusted for year of onset, gender and age group. This procedure is necessary in order to obtain more reliable results. Furthermore, the cancer registry at the National Board of Health and Welfare covers more than 96% of the cancer cases in Sweden [32]. Since we wanted to investigate if CC can be considered as a risk factor for cancer, we included only incident cases of cancer diagnosed after the CC diagnosis. The outcome of cancer was assessed from day one after the CC-diagnosis. This may cause a risk of including prevalent cancers, but since we know that the time lapse between disease onset and diagnosis of CC may be long, we believe that these factors level out. A majority of the cancers was diagnosed after more than three years making detection bias less probable.

This study also has some limitations that merit consideration. First, nationwide registers do not contain information about lifestyle habits like smoking, alcohol consumption, family history, exercise or other possible confounding factors. We neither had detailed data of disease severity nor medication in our study population. Information about sun exposure and consequently also about the location of the skin tumours would have been valuable. Furthermore, the associations found are not necessarily causal; one disease could lead to another or a not yet known factor besides the studied could lead to both CC and cancer. The retrospective design also limits the conclusions that can be drawn, although a study with a prospective design would have been difficult to finalize.

Consequently, this study could confirm the previously described negative association between CC and colon cancer, an observation of unknown cause. Even though significance was not achieved for cancers in lung, bladder and oesophagus there was a trend indicating that there could be a correlation anyway. A new, so far, unknown association between CC and cuSCC has also been revealed. There are reports about an increase incidence of BCC in coeliac disease and of NMSC in IBD. Consequently, we have to be extra cautious when examining patients with gastrointestinal inflammation in order to reveal any incident skin cancers.

Author Contributions: Conceptualization, J.K.L., E.T., J.N.P., A.K. and K.S.; methodology, J.K.L., P.H., A.G., A.K., K.S.; software, P.H.; validation and formal analysis, J.K.L., P.H., A.G., A.K., K.S.; investigation, resources and data curation, J.K.L., K.J.D., J.B., A.M., A.G., A.N., G.W.-J., E.T., J.N.P., P.F., A.K. and K.S.; writing- original draft preparation, J.K.L., A.K. and K.S.; writing- review and editing, J.K.L., K.J.D., P.H., J.B., A.M., A.N., G.W.-J., E.T., J.N.P., A.K., K.S.; supervision, P.H., A.K., K.S.; project administration, J.K.L., A.K., K.S.; funding acquisition, J.K.L., K.S.

Funding: This research have got financial support by grants from the Southern Health Care Region in Sweden.

Acknowledgments: We acknowledge the help of Anna Åkesson, statistician at Region Skåne, in designing Table 5.

Conflicts of Interest: The authors declare no conflict of interest.

References

1. Nguyen, G.C.; Smalley, W.E.; Vege, S.S.; Carrasco-Labra, A.; Clinical Guidelines, C. American Gastroenterological Association Institute Guideline on the Medical Management of Microscopic Colitis. *Gastroenterology* **2016**, *150*, 242–246. [CrossRef] [PubMed]
2. Vigren, L.; Olesen, M.; Benoni, C.; Sjoberg, K. An epidemiological study of collagenous colitis in southern Sweden from 2001–2010. *World J. Gastroenterol. WJG* **2012**, *18*, 2821–2826. [CrossRef] [PubMed]
3. Wickbom, A.; Bohr, J.; Eriksson, S.; Udumyan, R.; Nyhlin, N.; Tysk, C. Stable incidence of collagenous colitis and lymphocytic colitis in Orebro, Sweden, 1999–2008: A continuous epidemiologic study. *Inflamm. Bowel Dis.* **2013**, *19*, 2387–2393. [CrossRef] [PubMed]
4. Koulaouzidis, A.; Yung, D.E.; Nemeth, A.; Sjoberg, K.; Giannakou, A.; Qureshi, R.; Bartzis, L.; McNeill, M.; Johansson, G.W.; Lucendo, A.J.; et al. Macroscopic findings in collagenous colitis: A multi-center, retrospective, observational cohort study. *Ann. Gastroenterol.* **2017**, *30*, 309–314. [CrossRef] [PubMed]
5. Langner, C.; Aust, D.; Ensari, A.; Villanacci, V.; Becheanu, G.; Miehlke, S.; Geboes, K.; Munch, A. Histology of microscopic colitis-review with a practical approach for pathologists. *Histopathology* **2015**, *66*, 613–626. [CrossRef] [PubMed]
6. Marlicz, W.; Skonieczna-Zydecka, K.; Yung, D.E.; Loniewski, I.; Koulaouzidis, A. Endoscopic findings and colonic perforation in microscopic colitis: A systematic review. *Dig. Liver Dis.* **2017**, *49*, 1073–1085. [CrossRef] [PubMed]
7. Aust, D.E. Histopathology of microscopic colitis. *Der. Pathol.* **2012**, *33*, 221–224. [CrossRef]
8. Rasmussen, M.A.; Munck, L.K. Systematic review: Are lymphocytic colitis and collagenous colitis two subtypes of the same disease - microscopic colitis? *Aliment. Pharmacol. Ther.* **2012**, *36*, 79–90. [CrossRef] [PubMed]
9. Hellgren, K.; Baecklund, E.; Backlin, C.; Sundstrom, C.; Smedby, K.E.; Askling, J. Rheumatoid Arthritis and Risk of Malignant Lymphoma: Is the Risk Still Increased? *Arthritis Rheumatol.* **2017**, *69*, 700–708. [CrossRef] [PubMed]
10. Pedersen, N.; Duricova, D.; Elkjaer, M.; Gamborg, M.; Munkholm, P.; Jess, T. Risk of extra-intestinal cancer in inflammatory bowel disease: Meta-analysis of population-based cohort studies. *Am. J. Gastroenterol.* **2010**, *105*, 1480–1487. [CrossRef] [PubMed]
11. Kappelman, M.D.; Farkas, D.K.; Long, M.D.; Erichsen, R.; Sandler, R.S.; Sorensen, H.T.; Baron, J.A. Risk of cancer in patients with inflammatory bowel diseases: A nationwide population-based cohort study with 30 years of follow-up evaluation. *Clin. Gastroenterol. Hepatol.* **2014**, *12*, 265–273. [CrossRef] [PubMed]
12. Jess, T.; Simonsen, J.; Jorgensen, K.T.; Pedersen, B.V.; Nielsen, N.M.; Frisch, M. Decreasing risk of colorectal cancer in patients with inflammatory bowel disease over 30 years. *Gastroenterology* **2012**, *143*, 375–381. [CrossRef] [PubMed]
13. Ilus, T.; Kaukinen, K.; Virta, L.J.; Pukkala, E.; Collin, P. Incidence of malignancies in diagnosed celiac patients: A population-based estimate. *Am. J. Gastroenterol.* **2014**, *109*, 1471–1477. [CrossRef] [PubMed]
14. Wang, F.; Meng, W.; Wang, B.; Qiao, L. Helicobacter pylori-induced gastric inflammation and gastric cancer. *Cancer Lett.* **2014**, *345*, 196–202. [CrossRef] [PubMed]
15. Vigren, L.; Sjoberg, K.; Benoni, C.; Tysk, C.; Bohr, J.; Kilander, A.; Larsson, L.; Strom, M.; Hjortswang, H. Is smoking a risk factor for collagenous colitis? *Scand. J. Gastroenterol.* **2011**, *46*, 1334–1339. [CrossRef] [PubMed]

16. Chan, J.L.; Tersmette, A.C.; Offerhaus, G.J.; Gruber, S.B.; Bayless, T.M.; Giardiello, F.M. Cancer risk in collagenous colitis. *Inflamm. Bowel Dis.* **1999**, *5*, 40–43. [CrossRef] [PubMed]
17. Yen, E.F.; Pokhrel, B.; Bianchi, L.K.; Roy, H.K.; Du, H.; Patel, A.; Hall, C.R.; Witt, B.L. Decreased colorectal cancer and adenoma risk in patients with microscopic colitis. *Dig. Dis. Sci.* **2012**, *57*, 161–169. [CrossRef] [PubMed]
18. Warren, B.F.; Edwards, C.M.; Travis, S.P. 'Microscopic colitis': Classification and terminology. *Histopathology* **2002**, *40*, 374–376. [CrossRef] [PubMed]
19. Gordon, R. Skin cancer: An overview of epidemiology and risk factors. *Semin. Oncol. Nurs.* **2013**, *29*, 160–169. [CrossRef] [PubMed]
20. Belbasis, L.; Stefanaki, I.; Stratigos, A.J.; Evangelou, E. Non-genetic risk factors for cutaneous melanoma and keratinocyte skin cancers: An umbrella review of meta-analyses. *J. Dermatol. Sci.* **2016**, *84*, 330–339. [CrossRef] [PubMed]
21. Jensen, P.; Hansen, S.; Moller, B.; Leivestad, T.; Pfeffer, P.; Geiran, O.; Fauchald, P.; Simonsen, S. Skin cancer in kidney and heart transplant recipients and different long-term immunosuppressive therapy regimens. *J. Am. Acad. Dermatol.* **1999**, *40*, 177–186. [CrossRef]
22. Karagas, M.R.; Cushing, G.L., Jr.; Greenberg, E.R.; Mott, L.A.; Spencer, S.K.; Nierenberg, D.W. Non-melanoma skin cancers and glucocorticoid therapy. *Br. J. Cancer* **2001**, *85*, 683–686. [CrossRef] [PubMed]
23. Sorensen, H.T.; Mellemkjaer, L.; Nielsen, G.L.; Baron, J.A.; Olsen, J.H.; Karagas, M.R. Skin cancers and non-hodgkin lymphoma among users of systemic glucocorticoids: A population-based cohort study. *J. Natl. Cancer Inst.* **2004**, *96*, 709–711. [CrossRef] [PubMed]
24. Long, M.D.; Herfarth, H.H.; Pipkin, C.A.; Porter, C.Q.; Sandler, R.S.; Kappelman, M.D. Increased risk for non-melanoma skin cancer in patients with inflammatory bowel disease. *Clin. Gastroenterol. Hepatol.* **2010**, *8*, 268–274. [CrossRef] [PubMed]
25. Singh, H.; Nugent, Z.; Demers, A.A.; Bernstein, C.N. Increased risk of nonmelanoma skin cancers among individuals with inflammatory bowel disease. *Gastroenterology* **2011**, *141*, 1612–1620. [CrossRef] [PubMed]
26. Gunaltay, S.; Ghiboub, M.; Hultgren, O.; Hornquist, E.H. Reduced IL-37 Production Increases Spontaneous Chemokine Expressions in Colon Epithelial Cells. *Dig. Dis. Sci.* **2017**, *62*, 1204–1215. [CrossRef] [PubMed]
27. Gunaltay, S.; Nyhlin, N.; Kumawat, A.K.; Tysk, C.; Bohr, J.; Hultgren, O.; Hultgren Hornquist, E. Differential expression of interleukin-1/Toll-like receptor signaling regulators in microscopic and ulcerative colitis. *World J. Gastroenterol. WJG* **2014**, *20*, 12249–12259. [CrossRef] [PubMed]
28. Burger, M.; Catto, J.W.; Dalbagni, G.; Grossman, H.B.; Herr, H.; Karakiewicz, P.; Kassouf, W.; Kiemeney, L.A.; La Vecchia, C.; Shariat, S.; et al. Epidemiology and risk factors of urothelial bladder cancer. *Eur. Urol.* **2013**, *63*, 234–241. [CrossRef] [PubMed]
29. Dela Cruz, C.S.; Tanoue, L.T.; Matthay, R.A. Lung cancer: Epidemiology, etiology, and prevention. *Clin. Chest Med.* **2011**, *32*, 605–644. [CrossRef] [PubMed]
30. Watanabe, M. Risk factors and molecular mechanisms of esophageal cancer: Differences between the histologic subtype. *J. Cancer Metastasis Treat.* **2015**, *1*, 1–7. [CrossRef]
31. Larsson, J.K.; Sonestedt, E.; Ohlsson, B.; Manjer, J.; Sjoberg, K. The association between the intake of specific dietary components and lifestyle factors and microscopic colitis. *Eur. J. Clin. Nutr.* **2016**, *70*, 1309–1317. [CrossRef] [PubMed]
32. Barlow, L.; Westergren, K.; Holmberg, L.; Talback, M. The completeness of the Swedish Cancer Register: A sample survey for year 1998. *Acta Oncol.* **2009**, *48*, 27–33. [CrossRef] [PubMed]

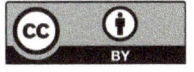

© 2019 by the authors. Licensee MDPI, Basel, Switzerland. This article is an open access article distributed under the terms and conditions of the Creative Commons Attribution (CC BY) license (http://creativecommons.org/licenses/by/4.0/).

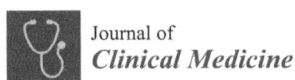

Article

Intestinal Inflammation in Children with Cystic Fibrosis Is Associated with Crohn's-Like Microbiota Disturbances

Raphaël Enaud [1,2,3,*,†], Katarzyna B. Hooks [4,5,*,†], Aurélien Barre [4,5], Thomas Barnetche [3,6], Christophe Hubert [7,8], Marie Massot [9], Thomas Bazin [10], Haude Clouzeau [2], Stéphanie Bui [2], Michael Fayon [1,2,3], Patrick Berger [1,3], Philippe Lehours [11], Cécile Bébéar [3,10], Macha Nikolski [4,5], Thierry Lamireau [2,3], Laurence Delhaes [1,3] and Thierry Schaeverbeke [3,6,10]

1. Centre de Recherche Cardio-Thoracique de Bordeaux, INSERM, University Bordeaux, U1045, F-33000 Bordeaux, France; michael.fayon@chu-bordeaux.fr (M.F.); patrick.berger@u-bordeaux.fr (P.B.); laurence.delhaes@chu-bordeaux.fr (L.D.)
2. CRCM Pédiatrique, CHU Bordeaux, CIC 1401, F-33000 Bordeaux, France; haude.clouzeau@chu-bordeaux.fr (H.C.); stephanie.bui@chu-bordeaux.fr (S.B.); thierry.lamireau@chu-bordeaux.fr (T.L.)
3. Fédération Hospitalo-Universitaire FHU, ACRONIM, F-33000 Bordeaux, France; thomas.barnetche@chu-bordeaux.fr (T.B.); cecile.bebear@u-bordeaux.fr (C.B.); thierry.schaeverbeke@chu-bordeaux.fr (T.S.)
4. Bordeaux Bioinformatics Center, University Bordeaux, F-33000 Bordeaux, France; aurelien.barre@u-bordeaux.fr (A.B.); macha@labri.fr (M.N.)
5. Laboratoire Bordelais de Recherche en Informatique, CNRS, University Bordeaux, UMR 5800, F-33400 Talence, France
6. Service de Rhumatologie, CHU Bordeaux, F-33000 Bordeaux, France
7. INSERM, MRGM, University Bordeaux, U1211, F-33000 Bordeaux, France; christophe.hubert@u-bordeaux.fr
8. PGTB, University Bordeaux, F-33000 Bordeaux, France
9. BIOGECO, INRA, University Bordeaux, F-33610 Cestas, France; marie.massot@inra.fr
10. INRA—Bordeaux Aquitaine Centre, University Bordeaux, USC EA 3671, Infections Humaines à Mycoplasmes et à Chlamydiae, CHU Bordeaux, F-33000 Bordeaux, France; thomasbazin@club-internet.fr
11. BaRITOn, INSERM, University Bordeaux, UMR1053, CHU Bordeaux, F-33000 Bordeaux, France; philippe.lehours@chu-bordeaux.fr
* Correspondence: raphael.enaud@chu-bordeaux.fr (R.E.); katarzyna.hooks@u-bordeaux.fr (K.B.H.); Tel.: +33-556-799-824 (R.E.)
† These authors contributed equally as co-first authors.

Received: 6 April 2019; Accepted: 6 May 2019; Published: 10 May 2019

Abstract: Cystic fibrosis (CF) is a systemic genetic disease that leads to pulmonary and digestive disorders. In the majority of CF patients, the intestine is the site of chronic inflammation and microbiota disturbances. The link between gut inflammation and microbiota dysbiosis is still poorly understood. The main objective of this study was to assess gut microbiota composition in CF children depending on their intestinal inflammation. We collected fecal samples from 20 children with CF. Fecal calprotectin levels were measured and fecal microbiota was analyzed by 16S rRNA sequencing. We observed intestinal inflammation was associated with microbiota disturbances characterized mainly by increased abundances of *Staphylococcus, Streptococcus,* and *Veillonella dispar*, along with decreased abundances of *Bacteroides, Bifidobacterium adolescentis,* and *Faecalibacterium prausnitzii*. Those changes exhibited similarities with that of Crohn's disease (CD), as evidenced by the elevated CD Microbial-Dysbiosis index that we applied for the first time in CF. Furthermore, the significant over-representation of *Streptococcus* in children with intestinal inflammation appears to be specific to CF and raises the issue of gut–lung axis involvement. Taken together, our results provide new arguments to link gut microbiota and intestinal inflammation in CF and suggest the key role of the gut–lung axis in the CF evolution.

Keywords: cystic fibrosis; gut microbiota; intestinal inflammation; fecal calprotectin; dysbiosis index

1. Introduction

Cystic fibrosis (CF) is a genetic disorder caused by mutations in the Cystic Fibrosis Transmembrane Conductance Regulator gene (CFTR), leading to viscous secretions accumulating on epithelial surfaces in both the lungs and the gastrointestinal tract [1]. In recent decades, improved patient care in the management of pulmonary disease has led to an older CF population with new complications, including intestinal disorders [2]. However, some CF gastrointestinal complications such as chronic inflammation, gut microbiota disruption, and increased risk of gastrointestinal malignancies remain poorly understood [3–6].

Gut microbiota has been recently shown to be associated with the human health and diseases including CF [7]. Its composition is clearly different in CF patients, with a decrease in specific bacteria such as *Bifidobacterium* spp., *Eubacterium* spp., *Clostridium* spp., and *Faecalibacterium prausnitzii*, and the emergence of opportunistic pro-inflammatory bacteria such as *Escherichia coli* and *Eubacterium biforme* [4,8–11]. In CF, this disturbed microbiota, usually named "dysbiosis", stems from multiple factors including hydro electrolytic disruptions of the intestinal secretions, slower gastrointestinal transit time [12], drug uses, impaired innate immunity in the gut [13,14], and hypercaloric diet [15,16], and appears to be correlated with the severity of the CFTR mutations [11].

Furthermore, chronic intestinal inflammation is present in the majority of CF patients, even in the absence of digestive symptoms [17]. Inflammation is characterized by an infiltrate of the lamina propria by mononuclear cells expressing inflammation markers (such as ICAM-1, CD-25, IL-2, IFNγ) associated with Crohn's-like endoscopic lesions of the mucosa (edema, erythema, or ulcerations) [3,18,19]. To better assess intestinal inflammation, Bruzzese et al. have adapted in CF the fecal calprotectin measurement, previously used as a non-invasive digestive inflammation biomarker in inflammatory bowel disease (IBD) [20]. Fecal calprotectin level is significantly higher in CF patients compared to healthy subjects [20–22].

The pathophysiology of intestinal inflammation is still unclear in CF. Very few studies have focused on the link between intestinal microbiota composition and inflammation in CF, while this link is well documented in IBD [23]. To our knowledge, only one study using next-generation sequencing (NGS) of microbiota was dedicated to this issue and showed a positive correlation between *E. coli* abundance and intestinal inflammation in CF children [24]. A recent study focused on the evolution of intestinal microbiota and inflammation in CF patients treated with ivacaftor, a CFTR-modifying therapy. An absence of intestinal inflammation was significantly associated with an increased *Akkermansia* abundance [25].

As previous studies focused on mucosal inflammation and microbiota in the gastrointestinal tract of CF patients were highly limited [22,24], our aim was to investigate links between gut microbiome and intestinal inflammation using NGS approach plus fecal calprotectin measurements, in a pediatric CF population.

2. Materials and Methods

2.1. Study Design, Sample Collection, and Ethics Statement

Our observational prospective study took place at the Children's Hospital of Bordeaux from November 2015 to May 2018. The inclusion criteria were patient over 3 years of age with well-documented CF associated with exocrine pancreatic insufficiency. The exclusion criteria were an ongoing enrollment in therapeutic protocols, antibiotics, or probiotics courses during the two months prior the inclusion or patients after organ transplantation.

At the inclusion visit patients' stool samples were collected and stored at −80 °C until use. In parallel, patient clinical status was documented using demographic data, nutritional status assessed by the Body Mass Index expressed as percent of the standard normalized by age (%BMI), respiratory capacity measured by Forced Expiratory Volume in 1s expressed as percent predicted (%FEV$_1$), and microbial pulmonary colonization along with previous intravenous (IV), oral, or inhaled antibiotic courses.

In addition, questionnaires focused on standardized assessments of quality of life (PedsQL™ 4.0 Generic Core Scale) and of digestive symptoms (PedsQL™—Gastrointestinal Symptoms Scales 3.0) were provided at no charge via the ePROVIDE™ online distribution process and filled for each child. These questionnaires, validated for different age groups, include a self-assessment and a parental evaluation. A score negatively correlated with the presence of symptoms was assigned from 0 to 100 to each item based on the collected responses. An average score was calculated for the main questionnaire sections.

Finally, long-term evolution based on clinical monitoring two years after inclusion was recorded for each child, based on %BMI and %FEV$_1$ values at the follow-up visit, plus the corresponding variations (estimated by the difference between %BMI or %FEV$_1$ measures at two years and inclusion), and the number of antibiotic courses during this period (IV, oral, inhaled, or any mode of administration combined) (Table 1 and Supplementary Table S1).

Table 1. Characteristics of patients with and without intestinal inflammation.

	No Inflammatory Group	Inflammatory Group
Patient	13 (65%)	7 (35%)
Fecal calprotectin level	122 (91.0–149.0)	459 (324.5–925.0)
Age in years	9 (7.0–11.0)	8 (7.5-11.5)
Female	7 (53.9%)	3 (43%)
Mutations		
- F508del homozygous	10 (77%)	4 (57%)
- F508del heterozygous	2 (15%)	3 (43%)
- Others	1 (8%)	0
%BMI [†]	97.6 (94.0–108.0)	98.3 (88.5–97.7)
%FEV$_1$ [††]	81 (71.0–91.0)	76 (71.5–93.5)
Chronic pulmonary colonization		
- P. aeruginosa	1 (8%)	0
- S. aureus	11 (85%)	7 (100%)
Previous IV antibiotic courses *	0 (0–2)	5 (0.5–10)
Quality of life		
- Parents' report	81.9 (76.5–88.4)	89.0 (86.7–90.4)
- Child's report	83.9 (71.9–89.2)	85.1 (76.8–88.6)
Digestive symptoms ••		
- Parents' report	83.2 (80.6–90.7)	94.5 (93.6–95.0)
- Child's report	84.5 (79.4–95.1)	91.2 (88.7–98.1)
Follow-up at 2 years		
- %BMI [†]	96.6 (90.6–105.9)	97.6 (92.3–102.6)
- %BMI variation	−0.5 (−3.8–1.5)	−0.3 (-1.0–3.0)
- %FEV$_1$ [††]	84.0 (71.2–95.2)	83.5 (69.5–85.5)
- %FEV$_1$ variation	1 (−21.0–8.5)	9 (-4.7–14.5)
- IV antibiotics	2.5 (0.0–5.2)	6.5 (5.2–9.2)
- Oral antibiotics	1.5 (0.0–3.2)	2 (2.0–2.7)
- Inhaled antibiotics +	1 (1.0–1.2)	2 (2.0–2.7)
- Total antibiotics +	5 (3.7–8.2)	11.5 (10.2–12.7)

Data are presented as n (%) or median (interquartile interval); Abbreviations: BMI, body mass index; FEV$_1$, Forced Expiratory Volume in 1s; IV, intravenous; + $p < 0.05$; [†] expressed as percent of the standard normalized by age; [††] expressed as percent predicted; * Evaluated using PedsQL™ Generic Core Scale 4.0; •• Evaluated using PedsQL™ Gastrointestinal Symptoms Scales 3.0.

The present study was approved by the regional ethical committee "CPP Sud-Ouest et Outremer III" (DC 2015/129). Informed consent was sought from study participants and their parents.

2.2. Measurements of Fecal Calprotectin

The fecal calprotectin assay was carried out using the GHSA kit (Eurobio, Courtabœuf, France). In the absence of a specific threshold in CF, we applied a cut-off of 250 µg/g, recently validated to predict an inflammatory flare associated with endoscopic lesions in IBD [26,27].

2.3. Microbiota Analysis

DNA extraction was performed using DNeasy Blood & Tissue kit (Qiagen, Hilden, Germany) according to the manufacturer's protocol. The DNA samples were the used for V4 region of the 16S rRNA gene sequencing as previously described [28]. For specific analysis of *S. oralis* and total bacteria population, droplet digital PCR (ddPCR) on the fecal DNA was performed, as described in the Supplemental Information.

2.4. Sequencing and Bioinformatics Analysis

Next-generation sequencing was performed using Illumina MiSeq sequencer, and bioinformatic analysis as described previously [28]. Alpha and beta diversity indexes were assessed using raw Operational Taxonomic Unit (OTU) occurrence counts and a Non-Metric Multidimensional Scaling (NMDS) ordination method with Bray-Curtis distance metric implemented by R package phyloseq, respectively. Subsequent OTU filtering and analyses were performed with MicrobiomeAnalyst (http://www.microbiomeanalyst.ca) [29]. OTUs were normalized by total sum scaling. Two groups of patients were defined with low (<250 µg/g) and high (>250 µg/g) fecal calprotectin level and used for DESeq2 [30] (Supplementary Table S2) and LEfSe [31] (Supplementary Table S3) analyses to find differentially present taxa and microbiota markers, respectively. Raw data have been deposited in the European Nucleotide Archive (ENA) sequence read archive (ENA accession number PRJEB28609).

2.5. Microbial Dysbiosis Index Evaluation

We estimated the Microbial Dysbiosis index (MD-index; Supplementary Table S4), a ratio between relative abundance of increased and decreased bacteria recently proposed in Crohn's disease (CD) [32].

2.6. Statistical Analysis

Differentially present taxonomic nodes between groups of patients were calculated using DESeq2 approach and a False Discovery Rate (FDR) < 0.05. LEfSe method was used to identify metagenomic biomarkers [31]. Nonparametric Wilcoxon–Mann–Whitney test was used to compare quantitative variables between groups. Correlations were calculated using Spearman method. Statistical analysis was performed with R studio program (version 1.1.453 for Windows^{TM}); a p-value < 0.05 was considered indicative of statistical significance.

3. Results

Intestinal inflammation is associated with more previous intravenous antibiotic courses in CF. Twenty children with CF between 6 and 14 years of age were included; their main demographic characteristics, clinical and microbiological data are summarized in Table 1. Among them, we identified seven (35%) children (mean of age at 8.0 ± 3.0 years old, Table 1) with significant intestinal inflammation (fecal calprotectin > 250 µg/g, with levels ranged from 300 to 1800 µg/g). Age of patients, mutation severities, %BMI and %FEV$_1$ were not significantly different between children without and with intestinal inflammation (Table 1). In addition, no complaint recorded in questionnaires could discriminate inflammatory status of children (Table 1). However, children with intestinal inflammation have received significantly more intravenous antibiotic courses before inclusion ($p = 0.04$ adjusted with age, Table 1).

CF children with intestinal inflammation are distinguished by their intestinal microbiota composition. The microbiota composition from 20 fecal samples was estimated using targeted 16S rRNA gene sequencing. After bioinformatic analysis, the median number of high-quality reads per patient was 421,720 (from 69,534 to 2,500,796). Taxonomic assignment was used to compare the profiles of patients' microbiota (Figure 1). At the phylum level, the proportion of Firmicutes was significantly higher in microbiota profiles of children with intestinal inflammation (on average 81% vs. 65% respectively for children with and without intestinal inflammation, FDR = 0.0078) (Figure 1A). To evaluate species diversity in patients' microbiome we calculated alpha diversity indices. The Shannon and Simpson indices are two complementary approaches to alpha diversity, sensitive to changes in abundance of the rarest or the most abundant OTUs, respectively. Alpha diversity indexes were not significantly different between children with and without intestinal inflammation (Figure 1B). However, the beta diversity analysis (NMDS) reflecting the variation of microbiome between samples, showed partial separation of the patients with intestinal inflammation (Figure 1C).

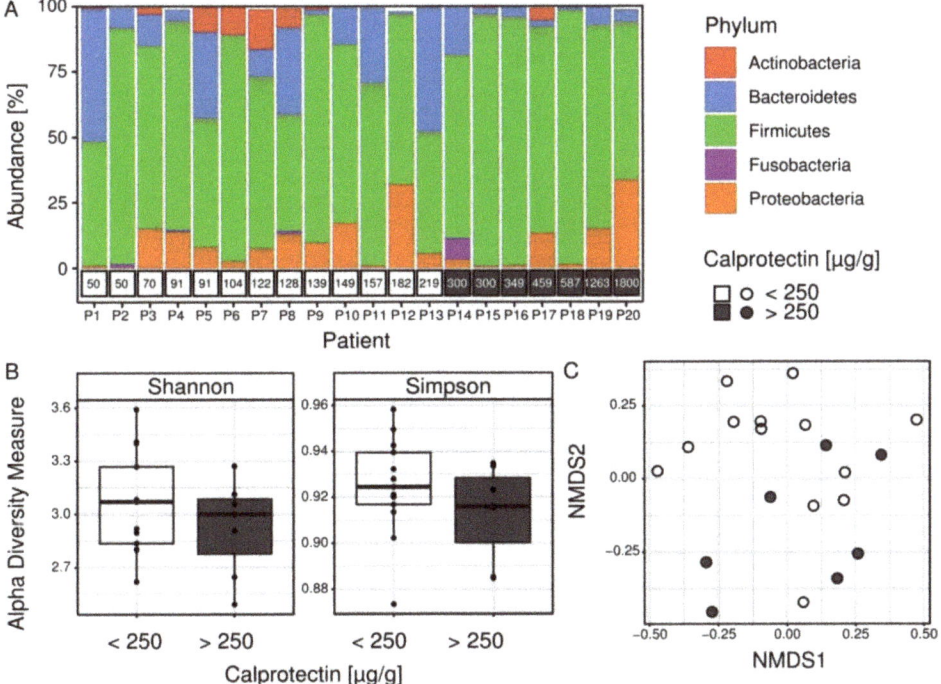

Figure 1. Microbiota composition in the Cystic Fibrosis (CF) cohort. (**A**) Proportions of bacteria from the five most abundant phyla colored according to the legend. Calprotectin measurements per patient are shown in boxes below the bar plot. The proportion of Firmicutes was significantly higher in microbiota profiles of children with intestinal inflammation (gray boxes). (**B**) Alpha diversity values for all patients ($n = 20$) are shown as points and summarized as boxplots for each group. Both Shannon and Simpson alpha indices measure microbial diversity within sample, and they were not significantly different between children with and without intestinal inflammation (Wilcoxon—Mann–Whitney test). (**C**) Beta diversity (NMDS), which assesses differences in microbial composition between samples using a NMDS ordination method with Bray–Curtis distance metric, showed a partial separation of samples of patients with intestinal inflammation.

Differential expression (DESeq2) analysis revealed 80 distinctive OTUs that belonged to 25 unique taxonomic nodes differentially present between patients according to their intestinal inflammation status (Figure 2A, Supplementary Table S2). Among them, increased abundances of *Acidaminococcus* spp., *Staphylococcus* spp., *Streptococcus* spp., and *Veillonella dispar*, along with decreased abundances of *Bacteroides* spp., *Ruminococcus* spp., *Coprococcus* spp., *Dialister* spp., *Parabacteroides* spp., *Bifidobacterium* spp., *Dorea formicigenerans*, and *Faecalibacterium prausnitzii* were observed in children with fecal calprotectin higher than 250 µg/g (Figure 2A).

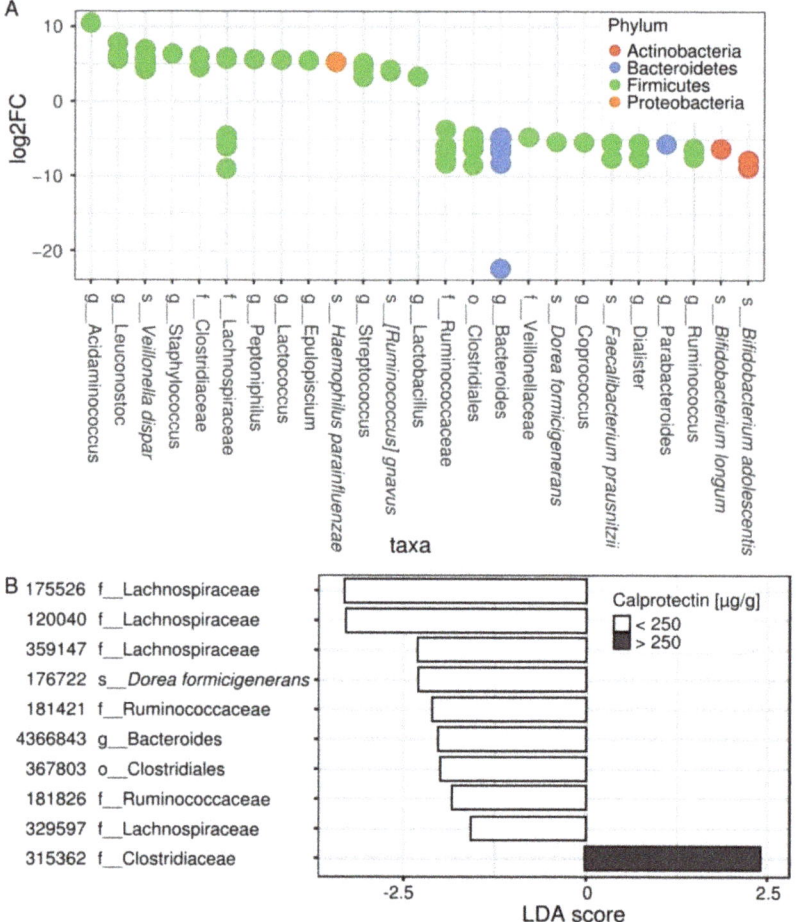

Figure 2. The composition of the microbiota differs according to the inflammation status of CF patients. (**A**) Differential abundance analysis (DESeq) assessing OTU significantly changed in the microbiome of patients with intestinal inflammation, compared with patients without intestinal inflammation. Each circle represents one of 80 significant OTUs colored by a phylum according to the legend. OTUs are collapsed to 25 taxa represented on x axis and ordered by decreasing log of fold change. For full results see Supplementary Table S2. (**B**) LEfSe analysis showing OTUs distinguishing patients without and with intestinal inflammation (*p*-value < 0.01) and confirming DESeq2 results. For full results see Supplementary Table S3.

Using LEfSe analysis (Supplementary Table S3), we identified numerous taxonomic nodes that can predict intestinal inflammation in our young CF population. It confirmed the results of DESeq2 at genus levels regarding *Staphylococcus*, *Streptococcus*, *Bacteroides*, *Ruminococcus*, *Coprococcus*, *Dialister*, and *Parabacteroides*, and at the species level regarding *Veillonella dispar*, *Bifidobacterium adolescentis*, *Dorea formicigenerans*, and *Faecalibacterium prausnitzii*. In addition, some OTUs belonging to the families Lachnospiraceae and Ruminococcaceae appear to be differentially correlated to the inflammatory patient status (Figure 2B, results with *p*-value < 0.01).

CF intestinal inflammation and microbiota exhibit similarities with IBD. In order to analyze deeper the CF intestinal microbiota changes in our cohort, we applied the MD-index, recently designed and validated in CD [32]. This index is based on a ratio between given bacterial taxa known to be increased or decreased in CD listed in Figure 3A. The MD-index was significantly higher in the CF children with intestinal inflammation compared to the group without inflammation ($p = 0.03$) (Figure 3B and Supplementary Table S4). It was not correlated to age, %BMI, or %FEV$_1$ in our cohort.

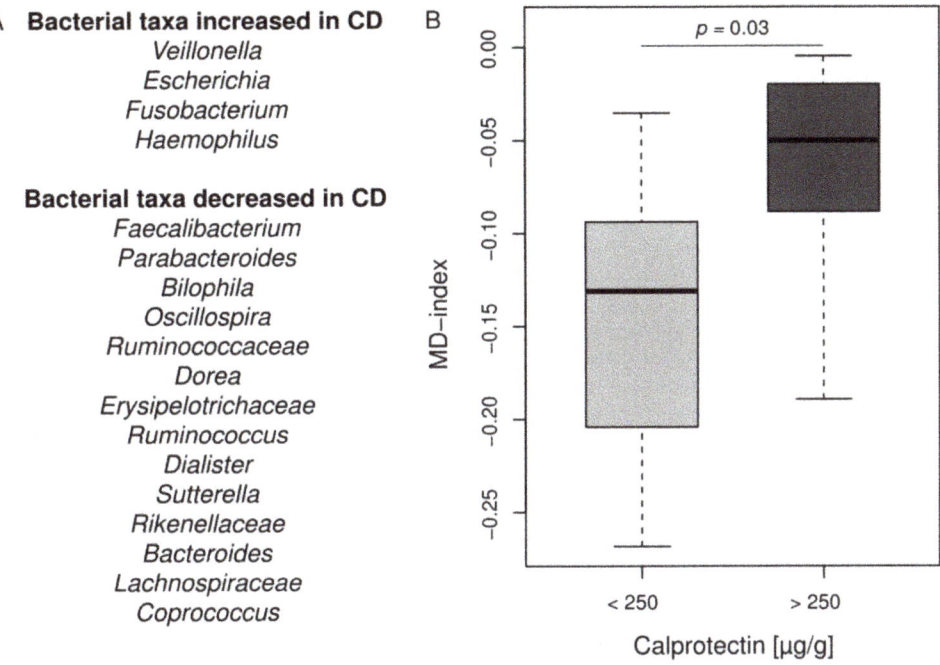

Figure 3. MD-index distribution in CF cohort according to the intestinal inflammation status. (**A**) Bacterial taxa contributing to the MD-index according to [32]. (**B**) Boxplot of MD-index values for patients separated into groups according to calprotectin level. Patients with CF intestinal inflammation have a significant higher MD-index (Wilcoxon–Mann–Whitney test, $p = 0.03$). For full results see Supplementary Table S4.

However, *Streptococcus* genus, increased in our inflammatory patient group, is not usually associated with IBD and is not included in the MD-index. Given the role of *Streptococcus mitis* group in CF lung disease evolution [33,34] and difficulties in distinguishing this group from other *Streptococci* by NGS, we assessed the presence of mitis group species by using ddPCR that specifically targeted *Streptococcus oralis*. We observed a non-significant increase log ratios of *S. oralis* per total bacteria in children with intestinal inflammation, compared to children with low calprotectin levels (ratio median −5.8 and −6.8, respectively, $p = 0.24$) (Figure 4).

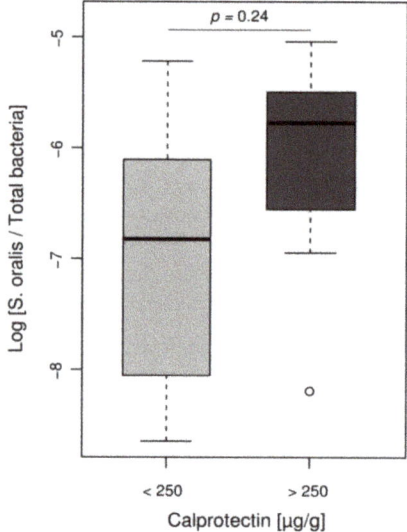

Figure 4. Relative abundance of *S. oralis* assessed by ddPCR according to the inflammation status of CF patients. Boxplot of values representing relative proportion of *S. oralis* in patients' microbiomes, separated into groups according to calprotectin level. Among *Streptococcus* found in CF children, there was a notable proportion of *S. oralis* but without significant difference between children with or without intestinal inflammation (Wilcoxon–Mann–Whitney test, $p = 0.24$).

Intestinal inflammation at the inclusion is associated with increased antibiotic use over the next two years. We compared the clinical evolution at two years between children without and with intestinal inflammation. While intestinal inflammation was not predictive of evolution of %FEV$_1$ or %BMI at two years (Table 1), children with intestinal inflammation at the inclusion had more antibiotic treatments over the next two years, all routes of administration combined ($p = 0.02$). Surprisingly, this discrepancy appears to be more related to inhaled antibiotic courses ($p = 0.02$) than to intravenous ($p = 0.06$) or oral ($p > 0.05$) antibiotic therapies (Table 1).

4. Discussion

Intestinal microbiota disturbances and intestinal inflammation are now widely accepted as an integral part of CF. With the increased life expectancy of patients, the management of these digestive disorders is becoming a topical subject, even if the corresponding physiological mechanisms are not yet well understood. In fact, links between intestinal microbiota and inflammation in CF have been suggested directly or indirectly by a limited number of studies [5]. In one of the few CF studies analyzing gut microbiota by NGS according to inflammation, intestinal inflammation was associated with an increase of *E. coli* abundance [24]. In another study, gastrointestinal mucosal lesions recorded by capsule endoscopy was positively correlated with Firmicutes and negatively correlated with Bacteroidetes [3]. Indirectly, probiotic intake or antibiotic courses in CF patients were able to decrease intestinal inflammation [20,35].

In order to refine the relationships between intestinal microbiota composition and inflammation in the CF, we compared intestinal microbiota profiles from young CF patients, according to their intestinal inflammatory status evaluated by fecal calprotectin. Despite the limited number of children included ($n = 20$) and their young age (mean of age at 8.0 ± 3.0 y.o. in Table 1), we identified a notable proportion of children (35%) with significant intestinal inflammation and microbiota disturbances (Figures 1 and 2). In this group, fecal calprotectin levels ranged from 300 to 1800 µg/g, rates comparable to those seen in IBD [26]. We observed increased abundances of *Staphylococcus* spp., *Streptococcus* spp., and *Veillonella dispar*, along with decreased abundances of *Bacteroides* spp., *Ruminococcus* spp., *Coprococcus* spp., *Dialister* spp., *Parabacteroides* spp., *Bifidobacterium adolescentis*, and *Faecalibacterium prausnitzii* in children with fecal calprotectin higher than 250 µg/g (Figure 3). We did not find significant increased *E. coli* abundances, as previously reported in a cohort of younger CF children (median age at 10 months) [24]. Our results were confirmed using LEfSe (Supplementary Table S3). On the whole, these microbiota disturbances exhibited numerous similarities with the well described IBD microbiota [23,32,36]. Interestingly, the MD-index, which is positively correlated with the clinical disease activity of CD [32], was significantly higher in our group of CF children with high fecal calprotectin levels.

Decrease of *B. adolescentis* and *F. prausnitzii* in group of children with intestinal inflammation confirm the results recently published in CF [22] and are congruent with data exploring in vitro anti-inflammatory proprieties of bacteria. *Bifidobacterium adolescentis* inhibits inflammatory responses in intestinal epithelial cells, by limiting the lipopolysaccharide-induced inflammatory response and the TNF-α production [37]. Furthermore, the intestinal inflammation in our cohort was associated with an under-representation of *F. prausnitzii* (Figure 2B), a strain well investigated in IBD for its anti-inflammatory properties and considered as a viable marker of health [36].

Taken together, these results raise the question of the causal relationship between microbiota composition and inflammation: does a decrease of anti-inflammatory bacteria lead to inflammation or does it result from this inflammation as a basic consequence of anti-inflammatory bacteria decrease? The answer to this question is still a matter of debate in CF as well as IBD [38]. Keeping in mind that the causal relation is probably bidirectional, few published data suggest the existence of a pro-inflammatory microbiota. Experiments using a murine model of colitis showed that disease can be transmitted from a genetically modified mouse to a wild mouse by a microbiota transfer [39]. In CF, oral antibiotic or probiotic exposures were shown to reduce intestinal inflammation [20,35]. A higher MD-index in our inflammatory subpopulation lets us suggest that these patients may have a more pronounced "pro-inflammatory" microbiota (Figures 2A and 3B). This subpopulation exhibited also significantly more Firmicutes and had previously received more IV antibiotics, which is a known factor leading to an increase of Firmicutes (Table 1 and Figure 1A) [8]. Moreover, the young age of our cohort together with the microbiota disturbances observed in CF from the first weeks of life [9,40] seem to indicate that CF gut microbiota changes is inherent to the disease rather than a basic consequence of inflammation and/or antibiotic use.

More recently, the human microbiome (which includes the gut microbiome but also the other body sites) has emerged as a complex interconnected entity leading to the popularization of the concepts of gut–brain and gut–lung axes [41,42]. The gut–lung axis is of major interest in CF, as patients colonize their digestive tract with microorganisms from oral or respiratory tracts by sputum swallowing [43]. Bacteria found in gastric fluid were correlated with CF sputum microbiota composition, especially regarding *Streptococcus* abundance [43]. *Streptococcus* isolates are naturally present in the digestive tract [9] but their proportion seems to be higher in CF patients [9]. We identified a significant over-representation of *Streptococcus* spp. in CF children with intestinal inflammation (Figure 3A), with a notable proportion of *S. oralis* (Figure 4). *Streptococcus* strains may contribute to the inflammatory process by synergistic interactions with other commensal microorganisms such as *Candida albicans* or *Veillonella spp.*, both being increased in IBD flares [23,44,45]. Overall, these data support the relationship between respiratory and digestive microbiomes.

This CF "gut–lung axis" is poorly described. It appears to be bidirectional with intestinal microbiota changes predicting pulmonary colonization of *Pseudomonas aeruginosa* [40] and oral probiotics decreasing pulmonary exacerbations [46]. Interestingly, we found that intestinal inflammation at the inclusion was associated with an increase in short-term antibiotic cures, especially with an increase over the next two years in inhaled antibiotic courses (Table 1). However, in the absence of repeated fecal calprotectin measurement during these two years, we cannot affirm that non-inflammatory patients at baseline remain without intestinal inflammation during this period.

Short-term intestinal inflammation may affect the nutritional status of CF patients, as demonstrated by significant correlations between fecal calprotectin level and both weight z-scores and height z-scores of CF patients [47]. As previously recorded [21], we did not find a significant correlation between intestinal inflammation and BMI. BMI evolution is recognized as multifactorial and is now part of the nutritional management, fully integrated into CF disease treatment [21].

Long-term inflammation could impact morbidity and mortality, especially regarding the increased risk of small intestine and colon cancers in CF patients compared with the general population [48]. The pathogenesis of digestive cancers in CF remains unclear. It has been shown that chronic intestinal inflammation is associated with this malignancy risk [49]. Furthermore in IBD, risk factor for colorectal cancer is correlated with the intensity and duration of the inflammation [50]. CF inflammation is present even at an early age, as well demonstrated in our pediatric cohort than in previous studies [51,52], which may be a key factor in developing digestive malignancy later on.

Microbiota composition has also been associated with digestive cancer, due to a decrease in bacteria protecting against cancer and changes in the corresponding metabolite production, such as a decrease in butyrate production, also observed in CF patients with intestinal inflammation [49,53,54]. We and others [10,22,40,54,55] showed that *Bacteroides*—known as protective bacteria against malignancy [53]—are decreased in CF.

5. Conclusions

To conclude, with more CF patients surviving into advanced adulthood we need to improve our understanding and management of this systemic disease, including the chronic intestinal inflammation. Few studies including ours reinforce the relation between intestinal inflammation and microbiota disturbance. Further in vitro and in vivo studies are warranted given the limited understanding of the CF physiopathology. Even well-documented probiotic strains, such as *Bifidobacterium adolescentis* identified in this study to be significantly decreased—that inhibits inflammatory responses in intestinal epithelial cells [37]—will require further clinical trials to decipher their potential ability to reduce the short-term intestinal inflammation and the long-term cancer risk.

Supplementary Materials: The following are available online at http://www.mdpi.com/2077-0383/8/5/645/s1. Table S1: Clinical information for 20 CF patients; Table S2: Significant differentially present taxa between patients with low and high calprotectin levels. Table S3: Results of LEfSe for patients with low and high calprotectin levels. Table S4: Index of dysbiosis (MD-index) per patient. Supplemental information: Additional informations.

Author Contributions: Conceptualization: R.E., K.B.H., P.B., T.L., L.D. and T.S.; Data curation, A.B., C.H., M.M. and M.N.; Formal analysis, R.E., K.B.H., A.B., T.B. (Thomas Barnetche), M.N. and L.D.; Funding acquisition, R.E. and T.S.; Investigation, R.E., T.B. (Thomas Barnetche), C.H., M.M., H.C., S.B. and P.L.; Methodology, R.E., K.B.H., A.B., T.B. (Thomas Barnetche), M.M., T.B. (Thomas Bazin), M.F., P.B., M.N., L.D. and T.S.; Project administration, M.F., P.B., P.L., T.L., L.D. and T.S.; Supervision, M.F., P.B., T.L., L.D. and T.S.; Validation, K.B.H., C.H., M.M., T.B. (Thomas Bazin), C.B. and T.S.; Visualization, R.E., K.B.H. and C.B.; Writing—original draft, R.E., K.B.H. and L.D.; Writing—review & editing, M.M., T.B. (Thomas Bazin), H.C., S.B., M.F., P.B., P.L., C.B., M.N., T.L., T.S., R.E. and K.B.H. contributed equally to the manuscript. All authors approved the final manuscript as submitted and agree to be accountable for all aspects of the work.

Acknowledgments: We thank Erwan Guichoux from the Genome Transcriptome Facility of Bordeaux, Jessica Latour, Sandrine Lefevre and Caroline Bruneaux from the team of Center for Resources and Skills in Cystic Fibrosis of Bordeaux and Fatima M'Zali from Aquitaine microbiology for their fruitful help and/or discussion. This study was funded by Association Aquitaine pour la Recherche Clinique en Rhumatologie and Biocodex Microbiota Foundation's grant. This study was funded by Association Aquitaine pour la Recherche Clinique en Rhumatologie and Biocodex Microbiota Foundation's award 2017. K.B.H. was supported by the French government via the "Investments for the Future" Programme, IdEx Bordeaux (ANR-10-IDEX-03-02). The funding agency had no role in study design, data collection, or interpretation of the results or submission of the work for publication. The authors declare that they have no competing interests.

Conflicts of Interest: The authors have no conflicts of interest relevant to this article to disclose.

References

1. De Lisle, R.C.; Borowitz, D. The cystic fibrosis intestine. *Cold Spring Harb. Perspect. Med.* **2013**, *3*, a009753. [CrossRef] [PubMed]
2. Parkins, M.D.; Parkins, V.M.; Rendall, J.C.; Elborn, S. Changing epidemiology and clinical issues arising in an ageing cystic fibrosis population. *Ther. Adv. Respir. Dis.* **2011**, *5*, 105–119. [CrossRef]
3. Flass, T.; Tong, S.; Frank, D.N.; Wagner, B.D.; Robertson, C.E.; Kotter, C.V.; Sokol, R.J.; Zemanick, E.; Accurso, F.; Hoffenberg, E.J.; et al. Intestinal lesions are associated with altered intestinal microbiome and are more frequent in children and young adults with cystic fibrosis and cirrhosis. *PLoS ONE* **2015**, *10*, e0116967. [CrossRef] [PubMed]
4. de Freitas, M.B.; Moreira, E.A.M.; Tomio, C.; Moreno, Y.M.F.; Daltoe, F.P.; Barbosa, E.; Ludwig Neto, N.; Buccigrossi, V.; Guarino, A. Altered intestinal microbiota composition, antibiotic therapy and intestinal inflammation in children and adolescents with cystic fibrosis. *PLoS ONE* **2018**, *13*, e0198457. [CrossRef]
5. Garg, M.; Ooi, C.Y. The Enigmatic Gut in Cystic Fibrosis: Linking Inflammation, Dysbiosis, and the Increased Risk of Malignancy. *Curr. Gastroenterol. Rep.* **2017**, *19*, 6. [CrossRef]
6. Yamada, A.; Komaki, Y.; Komaki, F.; Micic, D.; Zullow, S.; Sakuraba, A. Risk of gastrointestinal cancers in patients with cystic fibrosis: A systematic review and meta-analysis. *Lancet Oncol.* **2018**, *19*, 758–767. [CrossRef]
7. Rogers, G.B.; Narkewicz, M.R.; Hoffman, L.R. The CF gastrointestinal microbiome: Structure and clinical impact. *Pediatr. Pulmonol.* **2016**, *51*, S35–S44. [CrossRef] [PubMed]
8. Burke, D.G.; Fouhy, F.; Harrison, M.J.; Rea, M.C.; Cotter, P.D.; O'Sullivan, O.; Stanton, C.; Hill, C.; Shanahan, F.; Plant, B.J.; et al. The altered gut microbiota in adults with cystic fibrosis. *BMC Microbiol.* **2017**, *17*, 58.
9. Nielsen, S.; Needham, B.; Leach, S.T.; Day, A.S.; Jaffe, A.; Thomas, T.; Ooi, C.Y. Disrupted progression of the intestinal microbiota with age in children with cystic fibrosis. *Sci. Rep.* **2016**, *6*, 24857. [CrossRef]
10. Duytschaever, G.; Huys, G.; Bekaert, M.; Boulanger, L.; De Boeck, K.; Vandamme, P. Cross-sectional and longitudinal comparisons of the predominant fecal microbiota compositions of a group of pediatric patients with cystic fibrosis and their healthy siblings. *Appl. Environ. Microbiol.* **2011**, *77*, 8015–8024. [CrossRef]
11. Schippa, S.; Iebba, V.; Santangelo, F.; Gagliardi, A.; De Biase, R.V.; Stamato, A.; Bertasi, S.; Lucarelli, M.; Conte, M.P.; Quattrucci, S. Cystic fibrosis transmembrane conductance regulator (CFTR) allelic variants relate to shifts in faecal microbiota of cystic fibrosis patients. *PLoS ONE* **2013**, *8*, e61176. [CrossRef]
12. De Lisle, R.C. Altered transit and bacterial overgrowth in the cystic fibrosis mouse small intestine. *Am. J. Physiol. Gastrointest. Liver Physiol.* **2007**, *293*, G104–G111. [CrossRef]
13. Clarke, L.L.; Gawenis, L.R.; Bradford, E.M.; Judd, L.M.; Boyle, K.T.; Simpson, J.E.; Shull, G.E.; Tanabe, H.; Ouellette, A.J.; Franklin, C.L.; et al. Abnormal Paneth cell granule dissolution and compromised resistance to bacterial colonization in the intestine of CF mice. *Am. J. Physiol. Gastrointest. Liver Physiol.* **2004**, *286*, G1050–G1058. [CrossRef]
14. Ooi, C.Y.; Pang, T.; Leach, S.T.; Katz, T.; Day, A.S.; Jaffe, A. Fecal Human β-Defensin 2 in Children with Cystic Fibrosis: Is There a Diminished Intestinal Innate Immune Response? *Dig. Dis. Sci.* **2015**, *60*, 2946–2952. [CrossRef]
15. Li, L.; Somerset, S. Associations between Flavonoid Intakes and Gut Microbiota in a Group of Adults with Cystic Fibrosis. *Nutrients* **2018**, *10*, 1264. [CrossRef]
16. Debray, D.; El Mourabit, H.; Merabtene, F.; Brot, L.; Ulveling, D.; Chrétien, Y.; Rainteau, D.; Moszer, I.; Wendum, D.; Sokol, H.; et al. Diet-Induced Dysbiosis and Genetic Background Synergize with Cystic Fibrosis Transmembrane Conductance Regulator Deficiency to Promote Cholangiopathy in Mice. *Hepatol. Commun.* **2018**, *2*, 1533–1549. [CrossRef]
17. Munck, A. Cystic fibrosis: Evidence for gut inflammation. *Int. J. Biochem. Cell Biol.* **2014**, *52*, 180–183. [CrossRef]
18. Raia, V.; Maiuri, L.; de Ritis, G.; de Vizia, B.; Vacca, L.; Conte, R.; Auricchio, S.; Londei, M. Evidence of chronic inflammation in morphologically normal small intestine of cystic fibrosis patients. *Pediatr. Res.* **2000**, *47*, 344–350. [CrossRef]
19. Henker, R.; Oltmanns, A.; Wald, A.; Tuennemann, J.; Opitz, S.; Hoffmeister, A.; Wirtz, H.; Mössner, J.; Jansen-Winkeln, B.; Karlas, T. Severe ileocecal inflammatory syndrome in adult patients with cystic fibrosis. *Z. Gastroenterol.* **2019**, *57*, 312–316. [CrossRef]

20. Bruzzese, E.; Raia, V.; Gaudiello, G.; Polito, G.; Buccigrossi, V.; Formicola, V.; Guarino, A. Intestinal inflammation is a frequent feature of cystic fibrosis and is reduced by probiotic administration. *Aliment. Pharmacol. Ther.* **2004**, *20*, 813–819. [CrossRef]
21. Ellemunter, H.; Engelhardt, A.; Schüller, K.; Steinkamp, G. Fecal Calprotectin in Cystic Fibrosis and Its Relation to Disease Parameters: A Longitudinal Analysis for 12 Years. *J. Pediatr. Gastroenterol. Nutr.* **2017**, *65*, 438–442. [CrossRef]
22. Bruzzese, E.; Callegari, M.L.; Raia, V.; Viscovo, S.; Scotto, R.; Ferrari, S.; Morelli, L.; Buccigrossi, V.; Lo Vecchio, A.; Ruberto, E.; et al. Disrupted intestinal microbiota and intestinal inflammation in children with cystic fibrosis and its restoration with Lactobacillus GG: A randomised clinical trial. *PLoS ONE* **2014**, *9*, e87796. [CrossRef]
23. Sokol, H.; Leducq, V.; Aschard, H.; Pham, H.-P.; Jegou, S.; Landman, C.; Cohen, D.; Liguori, G.; Bourrier, A.; Nion-Larmurier, I.; et al. Fungal microbiota dysbiosis in IBD. *Gut* **2017**, *66*, 1039–1048. [CrossRef]
24. Hoffman, L.R.; Pope, C.E.; Hayden, H.S.; Heltshe, S.; Levy, R.; McNamara, S.; Jacobs, M.A.; Rohmer, L.; Radey, M.; Ramsey, B.W.; et al. Escherichia coli dysbiosis correlates with gastrointestinal dysfunction in children with cystic fibrosis. *Clin. Infect. Dis. Off. Publ. Infect. Dis. Soc. Am.* **2014**, *58*, 396–399. [CrossRef]
25. Ooi, C.Y.; Syed, S.A.; Rossi, L.; Garg, M.; Needham, B.; Avolio, J.; Young, K.; Surette, M.G.; Gonska, T. Impact of CFTR modulation with Ivacaftor on Gut Microbiota and Intestinal Inflammation. *Sci. Rep.* **2018**, *8*, 17834. [CrossRef]
26. Lin, J.-F.; Chen, J.-M.; Zuo, J.-H.; Yu, A.; Xiao, Z.-J.; Deng, F.-H.; Nie, B.; Jiang, B. Meta-analysis: Fecal calprotectin for assessment of inflammatory bowel disease activity. *Inflamm. Bowel Dis.* **2014**, *20*, 1407–1415. [CrossRef]
27. Davidson, F.; Lock, R.J. Paediatric reference ranges for faecal calprotectin: A UK study. *Ann. Clin. Biochem.* **2017**, *54*, 214–218. [CrossRef]
28. Bazin, T.; Hooks, K.B.; Barnetche, T.; Truchetet, M.-E.; Enaud, R.; Richez, C.; Dougados, M.; Hubert, C.; Barré, A.; Nikolski, M.; et al. Microbiota Composition May Predict Anti-Tnf Alpha Response in Spondyloarthritis Patients: An Exploratory Study. *Sci. Rep.* **2018**, *8*, 5446. [CrossRef]
29. Dhariwal, A.; Chong, J.; Habib, S.; King, I.L.; Agellon, L.B.; Xia, J. MicrobiomeAnalyst: A web-based tool for comprehensive statistical, visual and meta-analysis of microbiome data. *Nucleic Acids Res.* **2017**, *45*, W180–W188. [CrossRef]
30. Love, M.I.; Huber, W.; Anders, S. Moderated estimation of fold change and dispersion for RNA-seq data with DESeq2. *Genome Biol.* **2014**, *15*, 550. [CrossRef]
31. Segata, N.; Izard, J.; Waldron, L.; Gevers, D.; Miropolsky, L.; Garrett, W.S.; Huttenhower, C. Metagenomic biomarker discovery and explanation. *Genome Biol.* **2011**, *12*, R60. [CrossRef]
32. Gevers, D.; Kugathasan, S.; Denson, L.A.; Vázquez-Baeza, Y.; Van Treuren, W.; Ren, B.; Schwager, E.; Knights, D.; Song, S.J.; Yassour, M.; et al. The treatment-naive microbiome in new-onset Crohn's disease. *Cell Host Microbe* **2014**, *15*, 382–392. [CrossRef]
33. Kramná, L.; Dřevínek, P.; Lin, J.; Kulich, M.; Cinek, O. Changes in the lung bacteriome in relation to antipseudomonal therapy in children with cystic fibrosis. *Folia Microbiol. (Praha)* **2018**, *63*, 237–248. [CrossRef]
34. Maeda, Y.; Elborn, J.S.; Parkins, M.D.; Reihill, J.; Goldsmith, C.E.; Coulter, W.A.; Mason, C.; Millar, B.C.; Dooley, J.S.G.; Lowery, C.J.; et al. Population structure and characterization of viridans group streptococci (VGS) including Streptococcus pneumoniae isolated from adult patients with cystic fibrosis (CF). *J. Cyst. Fibros. Off. J. Eur. Cyst. Fibros. Soc.* **2011**, *10*, 133–139. [CrossRef]
35. Schnapp, Z.; Hartman, C.; Livnat, G.; Shteinberg, M.; Elenberg, Y. Decreased Fecal Calprotectin Levels in Cystic Fibrosis Patients After Antibiotic Treatment for Respiratory Exacerbation. *J. Pediatr. Gastroenterol. Nutr.* **2019**, *68*, 282–284. [CrossRef]
36. Sokol, H.; Pigneur, B.; Watterlot, L.; Lakhdari, O.; Bermúdez-Humarán, L.G.; Gratadoux, J.-J.; Blugeon, S.; Bridonneau, C.; Furet, J.-P.; Corthier, G.; et al. Faecalibacterium prausnitzii is an anti-inflammatory commensal bacterium identified by gut microbiota analysis of Crohn disease patients. *Proc. Natl. Acad. Sci. USA* **2008**, *105*, 16731–16736. [CrossRef]
37. Khokhlova, E.V.; Smeianov, V.V.; Efimov, B.A.; Kafarskaia, L.I.; Pavlova, S.I.; Shkoporov, A.N. Anti-inflammatory properties of intestinal Bifidobacterium strains isolated from healthy infants. *Microbiol. Immunol.* **2012**, *56*, 27–39. [CrossRef]

38. Ni, J.; Wu, G.D.; Albenberg, L.; Tomov, V.T. Gut microbiota and IBD: Causation or correlation? *Nat. Rev. Gastroenterol. Hepatol.* **2017**, *14*, 573–584. [CrossRef]
39. Garrett, W.S.; Lord, G.M.; Punit, S.; Lugo-Villarino, G.; Mazmanian, S.; Ito, S.; Glickman, J.N.; Glimcher, L.H. Communicable ulcerative colitis induced by T-bet deficiency in the innate immune system. *Cell* **2007**, *131*, 33–45. [CrossRef]
40. Madan, J.C.; Koestler, D.C.; Stanton, B.A.; Davidson, L.; Moulton, L.A.; Housman, M.L.; Moore, J.H.; Guill, M.F.; Morrison, H.G.; Sogin, M.L.; et al. Serial analysis of the gut and respiratory microbiome in cystic fibrosis in infancy: Interaction between intestinal and respiratory tracts and impact of nutritional exposures. *mBio* **2012**, *3*, e00251-12. [CrossRef]
41. Bienenstock, J.; Kunze, W.; Forsythe, P. Microbiota and the gut-brain axis. *Nutr. Rev.* **2015**, *73*, 28–31. [CrossRef]
42. Enaud, R.; Vandenborght, L.-E.; Coron, N.; Bazin, T.; Prevel, R.; Schaeverbeke, T.; Berger, P.; Fayon, M.; Lamireau, T.; Delhaes, L. The Mycobiome: A Neglected Component in the Microbiota-Gut-Brain Axis. *Microorganisms* **2018**, *6*, 22. [CrossRef]
43. Al-Momani, H.; Perry, A.; Stewart, C.J.; Jones, R.; Krishnan, A.; Robertson, A.G.; Bourke, S.; Doe, S.; Cummings, S.P.; Anderson, A.; et al. Microbiological profiles of sputum and gastric juice aspirates in Cystic Fibrosis patients. *Sci. Rep.* **2016**, *6*, 26985. [CrossRef]
44. Xu, H.; Jenkinson, H.F.; Dongari-Bagtzoglou, A. Innocent until proven guilty: Mechanisms and roles of Streptococcus-Candida interactions in oral health and disease. *Mol. Oral Microbiol.* **2014**, *29*, 99–116. [CrossRef]
45. van den Bogert, B.; Erkus, O.; Boekhorst, J.; de Goffau, M.; Smid, E.J.; Zoetendal, E.G.; Kleerebezem, M. Diversity of human small intestinal Streptococcus and Veillonella populations. *FEMS Microbiol. Ecol.* **2013**, *85*, 376–388. [CrossRef]
46. Anderson, J.L.; Miles, C.; Tierney, A.C. Effect of probiotics on respiratory, gastrointestinal and nutritional outcomes in patients with cystic fibrosis: A systematic review. *J. Cyst. Fibros.* **2016**, *16*, 186–197. [CrossRef]
47. Dhaliwal, J.; Leach, S.; Katz, T.; Nahidi, L.; Pang, T.; Lee, J.M.; Strachan, R.; Day, A.S.; Jaffe, A.; Ooi, C.Y. Intestinal Inflammation and Impact on Growth in Children with Cystic Fibrosis. *J. Pediatr. Gastroenterol. Nutr.* **2015**, *60*, 521–526. [CrossRef]
48. Maisonneuve, P.; Marshall, B.C.; Knapp, E.A.; Lowenfels, A.B. Cancer risk in cystic fibrosis: A 20-year nationwide study from the United States. *J. Natl. Cancer Inst.* **2013**, *105*, 122–129. [CrossRef]
49. Arthur, J.C.; Perez-Chanona, E.; Mühlbauer, M.; Tomkovich, S.; Uronis, J.M.; Fan, T.-J.; Campbell, B.J.; Abujamel, T.; Dogan, B.; Rogers, A.B.; et al. Intestinal inflammation targets cancer-inducing activity of the microbiota. *Science* **2012**, *338*, 120–123. [CrossRef]
50. Munkholm, P. Review article: The incidence and prevalence of colorectal cancer in inflammatory bowel disease. *Aliment. Pharmacol. Ther.* **2003**, *18*, 1–5. [CrossRef]
51. Garg, M.; Leach, S.T.; Pang, T.; Needham, B.; Coffey, M.J.; Katz, T.; Strachan, R.; Widger, J.; Field, P.; Belessis, Y.; et al. Age-related levels of fecal M2-pyruvate kinase in children with cystic fibrosis and healthy children 0 to 10years old. *J. Cyst. Fibros. Off. J. Eur. Cyst. Fibros. Soc.* **2018**, *17*, 109–113. [CrossRef]
52. Garg, M.; Leach, S.T.; Coffey, M.J.; Katz, T.; Strachan, R.; Pang, T.; Needham, B.; Lui, K.; Ali, F.; Day, A.S.; et al. Age-dependent variation of fecal calprotectin in cystic fibrosis and healthy children. *J. Cyst. Fibros. Off. J. Eur. Cyst. Fibros. Soc.* **2017**, *16*, 631–636. [CrossRef]
53. Wang, T.; Cai, G.; Qiu, Y.; Fei, N.; Zhang, M.; Pang, X.; Jia, W.; Cai, S.; Zhao, L. Structural segregation of gut microbiota between colorectal cancer patients and healthy volunteers. *ISME J.* **2012**, *6*, 320–329. [CrossRef]
54. Manor, O.; Levy, R.; Pope, C.E.; Hayden, H.S.; Brittnacher, M.J.; Carr, R.; Radey, M.C.; Hager, K.R.; Heltshe, S.L.; Ramsey, B.W.; et al. Metagenomic evidence for taxonomic dysbiosis and functional imbalance in the gastrointestinal tracts of children with cystic fibrosis. *Sci. Rep.* **2016**, *6*, 22493. [CrossRef]
55. del Campo, R.; Garriga, M.; Pérez-Aragón, A.; Guallarte, P.; Lamas, A.; Máiz, L.; Bayón, C.; Roy, G.; Cantón, R.; Zamora, J.; et al. Improvement of digestive health and reduction in proteobacterial populations in the gut microbiota of cystic fibrosis patients using a Lactobacillus reuteri probiotic preparation: A double blind prospective study. *J. Cyst. Fibros. Off. J. Eur. Cyst. Fibros. Soc.* **2014**, *13*, 716–722. [CrossRef]

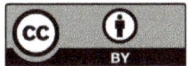

© 2019 by the authors. Licensee MDPI, Basel, Switzerland. This article is an open access article distributed under the terms and conditions of the Creative Commons Attribution (CC BY) license (http://creativecommons.org/licenses/by/4.0/).

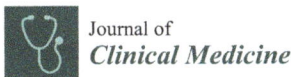

Article

Role of Mucosal Protrusion Angle in Discriminating between True and False Masses of the Small Bowel on Video Capsule Endoscopy

May Min [1,*], Michael G. Noujaim [2], Jonathan Green [3], Christopher R. Schlieve [3], Aditya Vaze [4], Mitchell A. Cahan [3] and David R. Cave [5]

1. Department of Internal Medicine, University of Massachusetts Medical School, 55 Lake Ave N., Worcester, MA 01655, USA
2. Department of Internal Medicine, Duke University School of Medicine, 2301 Erwin Rd, Durham, NC 27705, USA; mgn9@duke.edu
3. Department of Surgery, University of Massachusetts Medical School, 55 Lake Ave N., Worcester, MA 01655, USA; jonathan.green@umassmemorial.org (J.G.); christopher.schlieve@umassmemorial.org (C.R.S.); mitchell.cahan@umassmemorial.org (M.A.C.)
4. Division of Cardiology, University of California Irvine, 333 City Blvd W., Suite 400 Orange, CA 92868, USA; vazea@uci.edu
5. Division of Gastroenterology, University of Massachusetts Medical School, 55 Lake Ave N., Worcester, MA 01655, USA; david.cave@umassmemorial.org
* Correspondence: maym522@gmail.com; Tel.: +1-401-330-9702

Received: 19 January 2019; Accepted: 25 March 2019; Published: 27 March 2019

Abstract: The diagnosis of small-bowel tumors is challenging due to their low incidence, nonspecific presentation, and limitations of traditional endoscopic techniques. In our study, we examined the utility of the mucosal protrusion angle in differentiating between true submucosal masses and bulges of the small bowel on video capsule endoscopy. We retrospectively reviewed video capsule endoscopies of 34 patients who had suspected small-bowel lesions between 2002 and 2017. Mucosal protrusion angles were defined as the angle between the small-bowel protruding lesion and surrounding mucosa and were measured using a protractor placed on a computer screen. We found that 25 patients were found to have true submucosal masses based on pathology and 9 patients had innocent bulges due to extrinsic compression. True submucosal masses had an average measured protrusion angle of 45.7 degrees ± 20.8 whereas innocent bulges had an average protrusion angle of 108.6 degrees ± 16.3 ($p < 0.0001$; unpaired t-test). Acute angle of protrusion accurately discriminated between true submucosal masses and extrinsic compression bulges on Fisher's exact test ($p = 0.0001$). Our findings suggest that mucosal protrusion angle is a simple and useful tool for differentiating between true masses and innocent bulges of the small bowel.

Keywords: small-bowel mass; small-bowel bulge; video capsule endoscopy

1. Introduction

The diagnosis of small-bowel tumors is challenging due to their low incidence, nonspecific clinical presentation, and the limitations of traditional endoscopic techniques. Video capsule endoscopy (VCE) has dramatically improved our ability to detect small-bowel tumors by enabling the visualization of portions of the small-bowel that are not accessible by colonoscopy or upper endoscopy [1]. VCE was able to diagnose small-bowel tumors in 8.9% of the 562 patients in a single-center retrospective study who underwent VCE for occult gastrointestinal bleeding, abdominal pain, and a variety of other indications [2]. Furthermore, VCE missed only 10% of small-bowel tumors compared to a collective miss rate of 73% by double balloon enteroscopy, small-bowel series, colonoscopy, and ileoscopy [3].

One of the major limitations of VCE is its inability to biopsy lesions identified during passage through the small bowel. Though double balloon enteroscopy can potentially be used to visualize the entire small intestine, reported rates for total enteroscopy are widely variable (ranging between 20 and 90%) and are highly user-dependent [1]. A group of experts at the 2006 International Conference on Capsule Endoscopy identified several major and minor characteristics of small-bowel lesions that are predictive of tumors, including mucosal disruption, bleeding, irregular surface, polypoid appearance, color, delayed passage, white villi, and invagination [4]. However, in the absence of these features, it can be challenging to differentiate between true submucosal masses and benign bulges arising from extrinsic compression by adjacent structures.

In order to address this challenge, Girelli et al. developed the "smooth, protruding lesions index at capsule endoscopy" (SPICE) and examined its utility through a single-center, prospective study of 25 patients [5]. SPICE score was calculated by adding one point for each of the following: (1) Well-defined boundary with surrounding mucosa, (2) diameter less than height, (3) visible lumen, and (4) image of lesion lasting more than 10 min. A SPICE score >2 was found to be 83.3% sensitive and 89.4% specific for identifying true submucosal masses, therefore supporting a novel system for differentiating true from false masses on VCE. Through our retrospective study, we will evaluate the utility of an additional morphologic criterion, the mucosal protrusion angle. We have defined this as the angle between the small-bowel protruding lesion and surrounding mucosa. We hypothesize that false masses arising from extrinsic compression will create more obtuse protrusion angles >90° compared with true submucosal masses, <90°. By determining the utility of the mucosal protrusion angle, we hope to increase the specificity and sensitivity of VCE for detecting submucosal masses of the small bowel.

2. Experimental Section

2.1. Study Design

Patient demographics, indication for VCE, findings on VCE, radiographic studies, endoscopic and surgical interventions, pathology results, and survival following VCE were all collected retrospectively. Only those patients who were found to have a small-bowel protruding lesion on VCE were included in the study. Small-bowel protruding lesions were defined as any masses seen on VCE, including suspected submucosal masses and benign bulges. In total, we analyzed the VCEs of 34 patients. All VCEs were performed with the M2 A, PillCam^{TM} SB2 or SB3 (Medtronic, Minneapolis, MN, United States) and were analyzed using RAPID^{TM} version 8.3 (Given Imaging LTD, Yoqneam, Israel). This study was approved by the UMass Medical School Institutional Review board on December 2, 2015.

2.2. Angle Measurement

All angles were obtained through VCE images on RAPID^{TM} software version 8.3 (Given Imaging LTD, Yoqneam, Israel). The mucosal protrusion angle was defined as the angle between the protruding lesion and surrounding mucosa. Mucosal protrusion angles were measured using a protractor placed on the computer screen. We categorized lesions as having a protrusion angle of either >90° or <90° and hypothesized that an angle >90° suggests an external protrusion or bulge while an angle <90° suggests a submucosal mass. The frame for protrusion angle measurement was selected independently at each user's discretion based on the frame in which they felt the protrusion angle could best be measured. A sample image with angle measurement technique was provided to each operator (see Figure 1). Angles were measured independently by two novice users and one expert user to assess for interobserver agreement. Both novice users performed <10 VCEs prior to this study and the expert user performed >1000 VCEs.

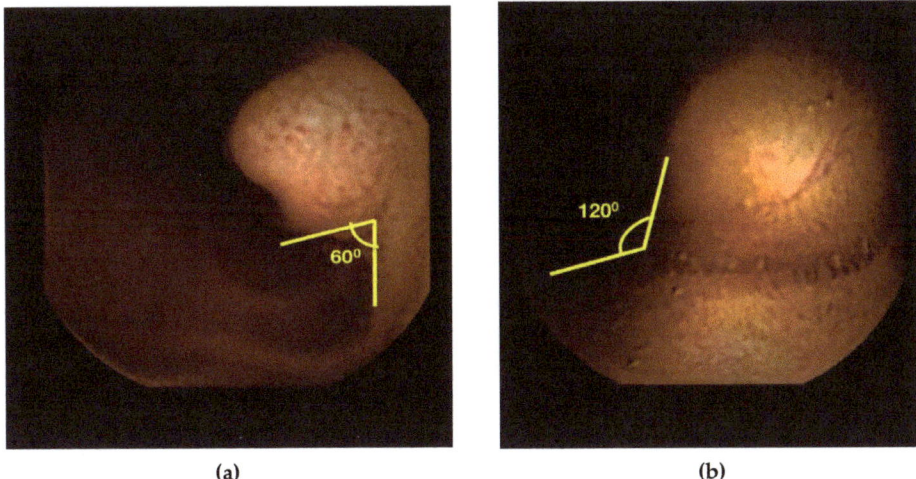

Figure 1. (a) Demonstration of acute angle measurement on RAPID™. (b) Demonstration of obtuse angle measurement on RAPID™.

2.3. SPICE Calculation

SPICE scores were calculated for each patient as outlined in Girelli et al. [5]. Lesions were given 1 point for the following: (1) Sharp boundary with surrounding mucosa, (2) height larger than diameter, (3) visible lumen in the frames in which the lesion appears, and (4) image of the lesion lasting more than 10 min. Any lesion with greater than two of the four SPICE criteria were predicted to be true submucosal masses per the findings in Girelli et al. A ruler placed directly on the computer screen was used to determine exact height and diameter of the small-bowel lesions.

2.4. Statistics

We calculated the sensitivity, specificity, positive predictive value (PPV), and negative predictive value (NPV) of both SPICE and protrusion angle. Fisher's Exact Test was performed to assess the association between protrusion angle and true vs. false submucosal mass. All Fisher's tests were one-tailed and the cutoff for significance was set at a p-value of <0.05. Interobserver agreement (kappa statistic) was assessed by comparing angle measurements of two novice VCE users and an expert user. We ran a logistic regression on capsule angle measurements for expert and novice users combined using a cutoff value of <90 degrees for a true mass and fit the data to a receiver operating characteristic (ROC) curve. We also ran a logistic regression on SPICE scores using a cutoff of >2 for true mass and fit the data to an ROC curve. Statistical analysis was performed using Stata Statistical Software: Release 13 (College Station, TX, USA).

3. Results

3.1. Demographics

We retrospectively reviewed the charts of 289 patients over the age of 18 who had undergone VCE for suspected small-bowel protruding lesions between January 2002 and March 2017. Of the patients, 241 were excluded because no protruding lesion was identified between the pylorus and ileocecal valve. Five patients were excluded because they were later identified as having true submucosal masses but did not have available pathology reports in our medical records. Nine patients were excluded because either the protrusion angle or SPICE score could not be determined due to poor image quality or limited visualization of the protruding lesion. In total, we analyzed the VCEs of

34 patients. The average age was 73.0 ± 16.6 years. There was a larger proportion of female patients (67.6%) compared with male patients (32.4%) (see Table 1)

Table 1. Patient Characteristics.

Gender	Age	Indication	Novice Angle [b]	Expert Angle	Location	Imaging [c]	Endoscopy [c]	Surgery	Final Diagnosis
F	65	OGB	42.5	20.0	Jejunum	CTE +	ASBE +	Yes	GIST
M	52	OGB	16.0	10.0	Ileum	CT +	ASBE +	Yes	GIST
M	81	OGB	50.0	30.0	Ileum	CT −	ASBE −	Yes	Carcinoid
F	56	Carcinoid [a]	20.0	10.0	Ileum	CT ±	Colo +	Yes	Carcinoid
F	77	IDA	27.5	20.0	Ileum	CT −	RSBE +	Yes	Carcinoid
F	56	CD	55.0	50.0	Ileum	CTE ±	RSBE +	Yes	Carcinoid
F	58	AP	10.0	20.0	Ileum	CT ±	Colo +	Yes	Carcinoid
F	62	AP	100.0	10.0	Ileum	CT +	Colo −	Yes	Carcinoid
M	38	AP	72.5	30.0	Jejunum	CT +	ASBE −	Yes	Inflammatory Polyp
F	73	OGB	35.0	110.0	Jejunum	ND	ASBE +	No	Lymphangiectasia
M	53	OGB	25.0	30.0	Ileum	CT −	Colo −	Yes	DLBCL
F	30	Peutz-Jeghers [a]	45.0	30.0	Jejunum	ND	RSBE +	Yes	Peutz-Jeghers
F	39	Peutz-Jeghers [a]	47.5	30.0	Ileum	ND	RSBE +	No	Peutz-Jeghers
F	36	Peutz-Jeghers [a]	45.0	50.0	Duodenum	ND	ASBE +	Yes	Peutz-Jeghers
M	37	IDA	27.5	40.0	Jejunum	ND	ASBE +	Yes	Peutz-Jeghers
F	49	OGB	50.0	20.0	Jejunum	ND	ASBE +	No	Peutz-Jeghers
F	58	OGB	52.5	15.0	Jejunum	CT −	ASBE +	No	Inflammatory Polyp
M	37	Crohn's [a]	65.0	20.0	Jejunum	CT −	ASBE +	No	Inflammatory Polyp
F	76	OGB	40.0	40.0	Jejunum	CTE +	ASBE +	Yes	Hamartoma
F	57	OGB	45.0	10.0	Duodenum	ND	ASBE +	No	Hamartoma
M	78	BO	60.0	20.0	Ileum	MRE ±	ASBE −	Yes	Lipoma
F	83	AP	82.5	>90	Duodenum	ND	ASBE +	No	Tubular Adenoma
F	41	OGB	35.0	10.0	Ileum	ND	Colo −	Yes	Leiomyoma
F	48	OGB	47.5	10.0	Jejunum	ND	ASBE −	Yes	Hemangioma
M	47	AP	30.0	60.0	Duodenum	CT +	ASBE +	No	Hyperplastic Polyp
F	70	AP, OGB	130.0	70.0	Jejunum	CT −	ASBE −	No	Bulge
M	51	Leukemia [a]	95.0	50.0	Jejunum	PET CT +	NA	No	Bulge
F	61	AP/CD	115.0	20.0	Duodenum	ND	ND	No	Bulge
F	29	AP	105.0	110.0	Ileum	CT −	Colo −	No	Bulge
F	55	OGB	75.0	20.0	Jejunum	NA	NA	No	Bulge
M	85	AP	122.5	130.0	Ileum	ND	Colo −	No	Bulge
M	29	AP	105.0	30.0	Ileum	CT −	Colo −	No	Bulge
F	54	OGB	125.0	130.0	Ileum	CT −	Colo −	No	Bulge
F	73	IDA	102.5	130.0	Ileum	CT −	ASBE −	No	Bulge

AP, abdominal pain; ASBE, anterograde small-bowel enteroscopy; BO, bowel obstruction; CD, chronic diarrhea; Colo, colonoscopy; CT, CT abdomen/pelvis; CTE, CT enterography; DLBCL, diffuse large B cell lymphoma; GIST, gastrointestinal stromal tumor; IDA, iron deficiency anemia; MRE, magnetic resonance enterography; NA, not available; ND, not done; OGB, obscure gastrointestinal bleeding; PET CT, positron emission tomography CT; RSBE, retrograde small-bowel enteroscopy. [a] Video capsule endoscopy performed for screening or surveillance. [c] Novice angle represents an average of measurement of 2 novice users. [b] Signs (+), (−), and (±) indicate positive, negative, and equivocal findings, respectively.

3.2. Diagnosis

The most common indication for VCE was obscure gastrointestinal bleeding (41.2%), followed by abdominal pain (29.4.%). Twenty-five patients were found to have true submucosal masses based on pathology report (6 carcinoid, 2 gastrointestinal stromal tumor, 1 diffuse large B-cell lymphoma, 1 leiomyoma, 5 Peutz-Jeghers, 1 tubular adenoma, 1 hyperplastic polyp, 3 inflammatory polyps, 2 hamartomas, 1 lipoma, 1 cavernous hemangioma, 1 lymphangiectasia) and 9 patients had innocent bulges due to extrinsic compression (see Table 1). None of the patients with bulges had available pathology data because no mass was seen on follow-up studies such as enteroscopy or repeat capsule endoscopy.

3.3. Protrusion Angle and SPICE Calculations

True submucosal masses had an average measured angle of protrusion of 45.7° ± 20.80 whereas innocent bulges had an average protrusion angle of 108.6° ± 16.3° ($p < 0.0001$; unpaired t-test). When compared with SPICE scores, a mucosal protrusion angle <90° had a higher sensitivity (92.0% vs. 32.0%), PPV (96.0% vs. 88.9%), and NPV (66.7% vs. 32.0%). Both protrusion angle and SPICE scores had the same specificity of 88.9%. Acute angle of protrusion accurately discriminated between true submucosal masses and extrinsic compression bulges on Fisher's exact test ($p = 0.0001$). Interobserver agreement between the two novice users and the expert user was good ($\kappa = 0.67$; 95% CI, 0.50–0.84). The area under the curve for mass angle using a cutoff value of <90 degrees for true mass was 0.93. The area under the curve for SPICE scores using a cutoff value of >2 for true mass was 0.55 (see Figure 2).

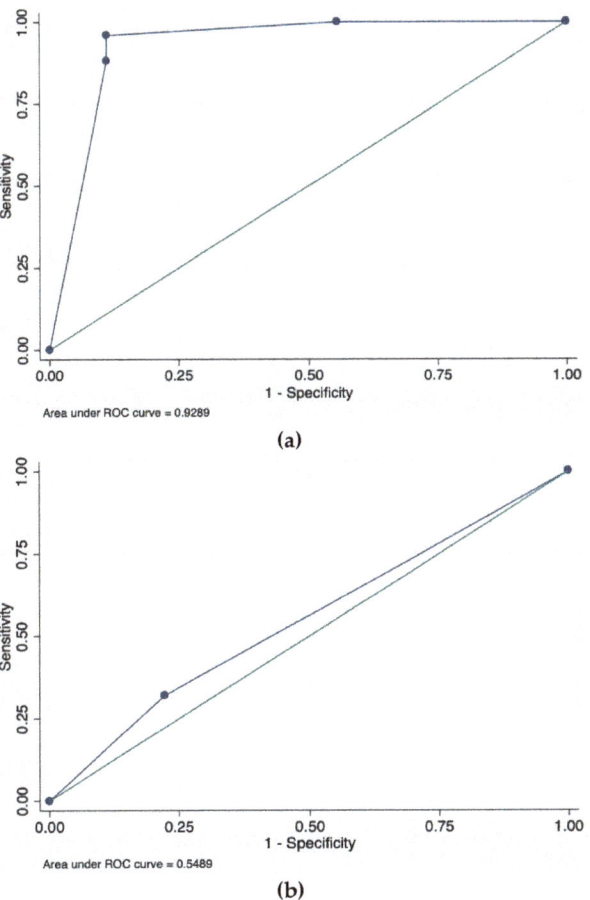

Figure 2. (a) The area under the receiver operating characteristic (ROC) curve for combined expert and novice mucosal protrusion angle using a cutoff of <90° for true mass. (b) The area under the ROC curve for smooth, protruding lesion at capsule endoscopy (SPICE) index using a cutoff of >2 for true mass.

4. Discussion

VCE has emerged as a convenient way to identify small-bowel tumors because it is non-invasive and allows for visualizuation of the entire length of the small bowel. Over the past several decades, its role in detecting malignancies has become more important as the incidence of small-bowel tumors has increased from 11.8 cases per million in 1973 to 22.7 cases per million in 2004. It is unclear how much of this increase can be attributed to improved diagnosis with the advent of VCE, however Bilimora et al. pointed to the rising incidence of carcinoid tumors as a major driving factor [6]. Prior studies have cited VCE malignant tumor detection rates as high as 63–83% [7,8]. In our study, we found a lower but still significant proportion of malignant tumors (45% of true submucosal masses) after excluding patients with Peutz-Jehgers.

Though VCE has significantly improved our ability to detect small-bowel tumors, it has also opened up what Pennazio et al. describes as a "Pandora's box" of findings including both malignant and benign lesions [9]. Bulges are among one of the most problematic benign findings on VCE, as they can often mimic the appearance of small-bowel tumors and contribute to false-positive outcomes [10]. False-positive outcomes may lead to further invasive and costly procedures, therefore highlighting the importance of differentiating bulges from true submucosal masses. Though "alarm" features, including bleeding, mucosal disruption, irregular surface, polypoid appearance, and white villi, have been described based upon expert consensus for malignant small-bowel masses, there are few studies available to support the use of these findings on VCE [4,11]. There have been prior attempts to use of automatic detection methods based on textural alterations on VCE, however none of these methods have been validated in clinical practice for diagnosing submucosal masses [12,13].

The SPICE score described by Girelli et al. was the first scoring system developed to distinguish between submucosal masses and bulges on VCE [5]. This study showed that a SPICE score >2 was highly sensitive (83.3%) and specific (89.4%) for detection of true submucosal masses. A validation study by Rodrigues et al. showed a lower sensitivity (66.7%) but high specificity (100.0%) for the SPICE score [14]. In our study, we found that a SPICE score >2 had an equally high specificity when compared with the mucosal protrusion angle but a significantly lower sensitivity of 32.0%. The discrepancies in our results may in large part be due to differences in study design, as the Girelli et al. study was prospective whereas ours was retrospective. Additionally, we included patients with Peutz-Jehgers and patients with "alarm" features outlined by Shyung et al., all of whom were excluded by Girelli et al. [5,11]. None of our true masses had a length time >10 min, criteria 4 on the SPICE scale, which made SPICE less sensitive in our patient population.

We evaluated the utililty of a new, simpler measure, the mucosal protrusion angle, in differentiating true masses from bulges. We found that an angle <90° accurately discriminated between true masses and extrinsic compression bulges ($p = 0.0001$). Acute protrusion angle also had a high sensitivity (92.0%) and specificity (88.9%) for distinguishing between true masses and bulges. It should be noted that we used both novice and expert users in our study, whereas the Girelli et al. study utilized only expert users. Discrepancies in angle measurements between the novice and expert users in our study were likely due to differences in the frames of the lesion on RAPID^{TM} chosen by each user. Despite these discrepancies, we found that there was good interobserver agreement between the novice and expert users when using mucosal protrusion angle ($\kappa = 0.67$; 95% CI, 0.50–0.84). This suggests that mucosal protrusion angle has the potential to be utilized by a wide range of users regardless of their VCE experience level.

5. Study Limitations

There are several limitations of this study that are important to note. First, this is a retrospective study and therefore is subject to both confounding and selection bias. As mentioned above, one potential source of bias is the variation in frame selection on VCE, as there was no way to ensure that all users would select the same image for angle measurement. In the future, it would be valuable to assess the degree of variability in frame selection between observers as this was not evaluated in our present study. An additional limitation of our study was that none of the bulges had pathologic confirmation due to our inability to visualize these transient lesions on subsequent interventions and the unethical nature of performing surgery or further invasive workup in such patients. We felt that long-term follow up provided an adequate surrogate but recognize this as a limitation. Finally, the number of patients in our study is comparatively small.

6. Conclusions

Mucosal protrusion angle is a novel and simple tool for differentiating between true masses and innocent bulges of the small bowel. To our knowledge, there are no prior studies examining the utility of this index. We found that small-bowel protruding lesions with a protrusion angle >90° are more likely to represent bulges and may not warrant any additional workup, whereas lesions with angle <90° are more likely to be true masses that should be evaluated for malignancy with enteroscopic or surgical interventions. Further prospective studies are still needed to validate our results.

Author Contributions: Conceptualization, D.R.C., M.M. and M.G.N.; methodology, D.R.C., M.M. and M.G.N.; validation, D.R.C., M.M., and M.G.N.; formal analysis, M.M., M.G.N., J.G., and A.V.; investigation, M.M., M.G.N., J.G., and C.R.S.; resources, M.M. and M.G.N.; writing—original draft preparation, M.M.; writing—review and editing, D.R.C., M.M., and M.G.N.; visualization, M.M. and M.G.N.; supervision, D.R.C. and M.A.C.; project administration, D.R.C. and M.M.

Conflicts of Interest: David R. Cave has a research grant with Olympus Corporation and is a clinical trial investigator for Medtronics. Olympus Corporation and Medtronics had no role in the design of the study; in the collection, analyses, or interpretation of data; in the writing of the manuscript, or in the decision to publish the results. The other remaining authors have no conflicts of interest to declare.

References

1. Moglia, A.; Menciassi, A.; Dario, P.; Cuschieri, A. Clinical Update: Endoscopy for small-bowel tumours. *Lancet* **2007**, *370*, 114–116. [CrossRef]
2. Cobrin, G.M.; Pittman, R.H.; Lewis, B.S. Increased diagnostic yield of small bowel tumors with capsule endoscopy. *Cancer* **2006**, *107*, 22–27. [CrossRef] [PubMed]
3. Lewis, B.; Eisen, G.; Friedman, S. A pooled analysis to evaluate results of capsule endoscopy trials. *Endoscopy* **2007**, *39*, 303–308. [CrossRef]
4. Mergerner, K.; Ponchon, T.; Gralnek, I.; Pennazio, M.; Gay, G.; Selby, E.G.; Cellier, C.; Murray, J.; de Franchis, R.; Rosch, T.; et al. Literature review and recommendations for clinical application of small-bowel capsule endoscopy, based on a panel discussion by international experts. Consensus statements for small-bowel capsule endoscopy. *Endoscopy* **2007**, *39*, 303–308.
5. Girelli, C.M.; Porta, P.; Colombo, E.; Lesinigo, E.; Bernasconi, G. Development of a novel index to discriminate bulge from mass on small-bowel capsule endoscopy. *Gastrointest. Endosc.* **2011**, *74*, 1067–1074. [CrossRef]
6. Bilimoria, K.Y.; Bentrem, D.J.; Wayne, J.D.; Ko, C.Y.; Bennett, C.L.; Talamonti, M.S. Small bowel cancer in the United States: Changes in epidemiology, treatment, and survival over the last 20 years. *Ann. Surg.* **2009**, *249*, 63–71. [CrossRef] [PubMed]
7. Bailey, A.A.; Debinski, H.S.; Appleyard, M.N.; Remedios, M.L.; Hooper, J.E.; Walsh, A.J.; Selby, W.S. Diagnosis and outcome of small bowel tumors found by capsule endoscopy: A three-center Australian experience. *Am. J. Gastroenterol.* **2006**, *101*, 2237–2243. [CrossRef] [PubMed]
8. Pasha, S.F.; Sharma, V.K.; Carey, E.J.; Shiff, A.D.; Heigh, R.I.; Gurudu, S.R.; Erickson, P.J.; Post, J.K.; Hara, A.K.; Fleischer, D.E.; et al. Utility of video capsule endoscopy in the detection of small bowel tumors. A single center experience of 1000 consecutive patients. In Proceedings of the 6th International Conference on Capsule Endoscopy, Madrid, Spain, 8–10 June 2007; p. 45.
9. Pennazio, M.; Rondonotti, E.; De franchis, R. Capsule endoscopy in neoplastic diseases. *World J. Gastroenterol.* **2008**, *14*, 5245–5253. [CrossRef] [PubMed]
10. Islam, R.S.; Leighton, J.A.; Pasha, S.F. Evaluation and management of small-bowel tumors in the era of deep enteroscopy. *GIE* **2014**, *79*, 732–740. [CrossRef] [PubMed]
11. Shyung, L.-R.; Lin, S.-C.; Shih, S.-C.; Chang, W.-H.; Chu, C.-H.; Wang, T.-E. Proposed scoring system to determine small bowel mass lesions using capsule endoscopy. *J. Formos Med. Assoc.* **2009**, *108*, 533–538. [CrossRef]

12. Barbosa, D.C.; Roupar, D.B.; Ramos, J.C.; Tavares, A.C.; Lima, C.S. Authomatic small bowel tumor diagnosis by using multi-scale wavelet-based analysis in wireless capsule endoscopy images. *BioMed. Eng. OnLine* **2012**, *11*, 3. [CrossRef] [PubMed]
13. Kodogiannis, V.; Boulougoura, M.; Wadge, E.; Lygouras, J. The usage of soft-computing methodologies in interpreting capsule endoscopy. *Eng. Appl. Artif. Intell.* **2007**, *20*, 539–553. [CrossRef]
14. Rodrigues, J.P.; Pinho, R.; Rodrigues, A.; Silva, J.; Ponte, A.; Sousa, M.; Carvalho, J. Validation of SPICE, a method to differentiate small bowel submucosal lesions from innocent bulges on capsule endoscopy. *Rev. Esp. Enferm. Dig.* **2017**, *109*, 106–113. [CrossRef]

© 2019 by the authors. Licensee MDPI, Basel, Switzerland. This article is an open access article distributed under the terms and conditions of the Creative Commons Attribution (CC BY) license (http://creativecommons.org/licenses/by/4.0/).

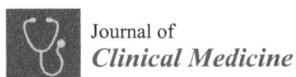

Article

A Systematic Review, Meta-Analysis, and Meta-Regression Evaluating the Efficacy and Mechanisms of Action of Probiotics and Synbiotics in the Prevention of Surgical Site Infections and Surgery-Related Complications

Karolina Skonieczna-Żydecka [1], Mariusz Kaczmarczyk [2], Igor Łoniewski [1], Luis F. Lara [3], Anastasios Koulaouzidis [4], Agata Misera [5], Dominika Maciejewska [1] and Wojciech Marlicz [6,*]

[1] Department of Biochemistry and Human Nutrition, Pomeranian Medical University, Szczecin 71-460, Poland; karzyd@pum.edu.pl (K.S.-Ż.); sanprobi@sanprobi.pl (I.Ł.); dmaciejewska.pum@gmail.com (D.M.)
[2] Department of Clinical and Molecular Biochemistry, Pomeranian Medical University, Szczecin 70-111, Poland; mariush@pum.edu.pl
[3] Division of Gastroenterology, Hepatology, and Nutrition, The Ohio State University Wexner Medical Center, Columbus, OH 43210, USA; Luis.Lara@osumc.edu
[4] Centre for Liver & Digestive Disorders, Royal Infirmary of Edinburgh, Edinburgh EH16 4SA, UK; akoulaouzidis@hotmail.com
[5] Department of Child and Adolescent Psychiatry, Charité Universitätsmedizin, Berlin 13353, Germany; agata.misera@charite.de
[6] Department of Gastroenterology, Pomeranian Medical University, Szczecin 71-252, Poland
* Correspondence: marlicz@hotmail.com; Tel.: +48-91-425-3231

Received: 10 November 2018; Accepted: 13 December 2018; Published: 16 December 2018

Abstract: Intestinal microbiota play an important role in the pathogenesis of surgical site infections (SSIs) and other surgery-related complications (SRCs). Probiotics and synbiotics were found to lower the risk of surgical infections and other surgery-related adverse events. We systematically reviewed the approach based on the administration of probiotics and synbiotics to diminish SSIs/SRCs rates in patients undergoing various surgical treatments and to determine the mechanisms responsible for their effectiveness. A systematic literature search in PubMed/MEDLINE/Cochrane Central Register of Controlled Trials from the inception of databases to June 2018 for trials in patients undergoing surgery supplemented with pre/pro/synbiotics and randomized to the intervention versus placebo/no treatment and reporting on primarily: (i) putative mechanisms of probiotic/symbiotic action, and secondarily (ii) SSIs and SRCs outcomes. Random-effect model meta-analysis and meta-regression analysis of outcomes was done. Thirty-five trials comprising 3028 adult patients were included; interventions were probiotics ($n = 16$) and synbiotics ($n = 19$ trials). We found that C-reactive protein (CRP) and Interleukin-6 (IL-6) were significantly decreased (SMD: -0.40, 95% CI $[-0.79, -0.02]$, $p = 0.041$; SMD: -0.41, 95% CI $[-0.70, -0.02]$, $p = 0.006$, respectively) while concentration of acetic, butyric, and propionic acids were elevated in patients supplemented with probiotics (SMD: 1.78, 95% CI [0.80, 2.76], $p = 0.0004$; SMD: 0.67, 95% CI [0.37, -0.97], $p = 0.00001$; SMD: 0.46, 95% CI [0.18, 0.73], $p = 0.001$, respectively). Meta-analysis confirmed that pro- and synbiotics supplementation was associated with significant reduction in the incidence of SRCs including abdominal distention, diarrhea, pneumonia, sepsis, surgery site infection (including superficial incisional), and urinary tract infection, as well as the duration of antibiotic therapy, duration of postoperative pyrexia, time of fluid introduction, solid diet, and duration of hospital stay ($p < 0.05$). Probiotics and synbiotics administration counteract SSIs/SRCs via modulating gut-immune response and production of short chain fatty acids.

Keywords: surgical site infections (SSIs); probiotics; prebiotics; synbiotics; surgery; adverse events; microbiota; meta-analysis; systematic review

1. Introduction

One of the most challenging health care issues worldwide are surgical site infections (SSIs) [1,2]. Timely administration of effective preoperative antibiotics along with other perioperative quality control interventions recommended by various guidelines [3–5] have resulted in a significant reduction of the rate of SSIs. Despite these efforts, globally SSIs occur in 9–22% of procedures, with a direct correlation with the human developmental index [1]. SSIs result in prolonged hospitalizations, unscheduled re-admissions, extended duration of antibiotic therapy, increase mortality rate, and pose high costs to healthcare systems. Therefore, it is of priority to look for other effective, evidence-based interventions capable of reducing the incidence of life-threatening SSIs [6–8].

There is increasing evidence that human intestinal microbiota play an important role in the pathogenesis of SSIs. Although historically, gut flora has been considered as a pathogen in human infections [9], recent studies show that alteration of the human microbiome (dysbiosis) may play a role in the pathogenesis of SSIs and other surgery-related complications (SRCs) [10–12]. Human gut microbiota composition fluctuates on a daily basis depending predominantly on diet, but also exercise, medications, and exposure to stressful events [13–16]. The general health status of a patient scheduled for surgery is of particular interest, and the make-up of the microbiota could be of particular interest, because it is believed that the majority of hospital infections originate from the patient's own microbiota, in part due to noxious and stressful surgical preparatory procedures [2]. Supporting the role of microbiota, it has been shown that mechanic bowel preparation (MBP) before gut resection, accompanied by oral antibiotic therapy, reduces the number of infectious complications, including anastomotic leakages by almost half [17]. However, multiple studies have reported vast disturbances in microbial counts and diversity following these procedures that may itself create microbiota disturbances with health consequences [18,19].

The surgical procedure itself and other pathology not even related to the gastrointestinal tract may be a major cause of alterations in the intestinal microbiota. There are numerous examples in the literature. Dysbiosis has been described in the excluded colon after small bowel stoma [20]. Major burn injury was described to reduce two major phyla within the human gut and to increase *Gammaproteobacteria* class involved in SSIs [21]. Significant changes of gut flora with increased virulent *Escherichia coli, Pseudomonas aeruginosa,* and *Enterococcus faecalis* counts have been described with surgical procedures [21–23]. Surgical reconstructions of the gastrointestinal (GI) tract may delay the microbiota refaunation [24,25], and result in enhanced virulent phenotype expression [26]. In severe injuries, more virulent pathogens may predominate in the intestinal ecosystem [27], disrupt the intestinal barrier structure and function, which facilitates the bacterial translocation, and may result in SSIs.

It thus appears that manipulating gut microbiota composition to a healthier variety could be promising. Administration of beneficial microbes (probiotics), fiber (prebiotics), or both (synbiotics) could be an attractive strategy to diminish the incidence of SSIs [28]. There are randomized, double-blind, placebo-controlled trials and meta-analyses that support the efficacy of this strategy [28–33]. A recently published meta-analysis aimed to find evidence on prebiotics, probiotics, and synbiotics supplementation on postoperative complications (mostly infective) in surgical patients [28,29,32,34]. Additionally, Wu et al. [29] estimated the efficacy of probiotics and antibiotics combination in the prevention of SSIs and the decrease of antibiotics usage in colorectal surgery, and Kasatpibal et al. [28] conducted a network meta-analysis (NMA) to evaluate the efficacy of probiotics, prebiotics, and synbiotics in reducing SSIs as well as other postoperative complications. Although probiotics have already been used as prophylaxis against SSIs, to the best of our knowledge, none of the guidelines recommend their use. Among the reasons could be lack of data on the precise mechanisms of such interventions in lowering the risk of SSIs and the fact that studies aimed at elucidating the effect of probiotic action on mucosal and stool microbiota lack correlation with clinical outcomes [35].

Therefore, this systematic review was performed to study the role of probiotics and synbiotics in the prevention of SSIs and SRCs. In particular, our study aimed to evaluate:

a. The mechanism of action of probiotics and synbiotics in prevention of SSIs;
b. The influence of probiotics on gut microbiota alterations related to the surgery;
c. A possibility to establish recommendations concerning strain(s), dose, and mode of administration of probiotic in the prevention of SSI and SRCs.

A random-effect model meta-analysis to determine putative mechanisms associated with such intervention was also performed. The meta-analysis (MA) evaluated all available data on the usefulness of probiotics in the prevention of SSIs/SRCs in patients undergoing abdominal surgery. The findings could result in a call to determine the appropriateness of implementation probiotics into clinical practice and consideration for inclusion in guidelines as a potentially cost-effective and life-saving therapy. Finally, a meta-regression was performed in order to try to identify a particular probiotic strain of formula, dose, and duration of the probiotic supplementation, which could be recommended as treatment to prevent SSIs.

2. Materials and Methods

2.1. Search Strategy and Inclusion Criteria

Two independent authors (K.S.-Z., M.K.) searched PubMed/MEDLINE/Cochrane Central Register of Controlled Trials from the inception of databases until 1 June 2018 in English for human trials assessing the efficacy of pre/pro/synbiotic administration in reducing the incidence of SSIs and SRCs. The following search terms with medical subject headings (MeSH–**bold font**) Supplementary Concept Record terms (SCR *italic font*) and free text terms were used: ("**probiotics**" OR probiotic * OR "**prebiotics**" OR symbiotic * OR fiber OR "**dietary fiber**" OR microbiota *) AND (operation OR "surgical procedure" OR "**surgical procedures, operative**" OR "**general surgery**" OR surgery OR **transplantation** OR "surgical operation" OR surgery OR "abdominal surgery" OR "colorectal surgery" OR "colectomy" OR "small bowel surgery" OR **hepatectomy** OR "biliary surgery" OR "pancreas surgery" OR proctology * OR proctocolonic surgery * OR intestine surgery *) AND (readmission OR "readmission rate" OR **mortality** OR **morbidity** OR **sepsis** OR procalcitonin OR **calcitonin** OR leakage OR "surgical infection" OR "surgery site infection" OR leakage OR "anastomotic leakage" OR SSI OR post-operative wound infection * OR postoperative wound infection * OR complication OR **peritonitis** OR **abscess** OR translocation OR **lactulose** OR *zonulin* OR calprotectin OR **ileus** OR "postoperative ileus"). Apart from the electronic search, a manual review of reference lists from existing meta-analyses and relevant reviews was performed.

We used the following inclusion criteria:

1. treatment with pro-/pre-/synbiotics;
2. randomisation to pre/pro/synbiotic versus placebo/monotherapy/standard care; and
3. available meta-analyzable endpoint/change score data on outcomes placed below.
4. if a study contained more than two arms, the data were abstracted separately for each comparator.

2.2. Data Abstraction

Two authors (K.S.-Z., M.K.) independently, in accordance with the Preferred Reporting Items for Systematic Reviews and Meta-Analyses (PRISMA) [36], abstracted information from each study, including details of the study (e.g., study design, treatment protocol, duration, number of subjects, gut barrier and SRCs parameters, and risk of bias), intervention (e.g., pre/pro/symbiotic, agent name, dosage, and duration of treatment), and primary patient characteristics (e.g., age, sex, and reason for the surgery). In case of missing data, a request letter for additional information was sent to authors. Any inconsistencies were referred by the senior author (W.M.).

2.3. Outcomes

The primary outcomes that were extracted from each study were the gut-related parameters associated with the putative mechanism of pre/pro/symbiotic action: bacterial translocation, lactulose/mannitol ratio, short chain fatty acids production, zonulin, calprotectin, gut microbiota composition, diamine oxidase (DAO) activity, as well as non-specific indices of inflammation such as C-reactive protein (CRP), interleukin-6 (IL-6) plasma concentration and white blood cells (WBC) count. To update the data reported by other authors on the effectiveness of pre/pro/synbiotics evaluating such interventions in the prevention of SSIs/SRCs the following secondary outcomes were evaluated: abdominal distention, anastomotic leakage, diarrhea, intraabdominal abscess, mortality, methicilin resistant *staphylococcus aureus* infection, peritonitis, pneumonia, re-operation, sepsis, SSIs, superficial incisional SSIs, deep organ/space SSIs, urinary tract infections, blood loss, duration of antibiotic therapy, duration of postoperative pyrexia, the time of implementation of fluid and solid diet, hospital and intensive care unit stay duration, and operating time.

2.4. Data Synthesis and Statistical Analysis

A random effects meta-analysis [37] of outcomes for which at least three studies contributed data was conducted using software (Comprehensive Meta-Analysis, version 3.3.070; http://www.meta-analysis.com). The between-study variance (τ^2) was estimated using the method of moments (DerSimonian and Laird) and the assumption of homogeneity in effects was tested using the Q statistic with a k-1 degree of freedom (k—the number of studies). Pooled standardized mean difference (SMD) in change score/endpoint scores was used to analyze group differences in case of continuous variables. For nominal outcomes the summary risk ratio (RR) was calculated. A two-tailed Z test was used to test the null hypothesis that the summary effect is zero. In addition to classical meta-analysis, a meta-regression was performed under the random-effects model for both continuous and nominal study level covariates. The regression models with single covariates were fit. Funnel plots were inspected to quantify whether publication bias could have influenced the results. The Egger's regression intercept test for asymmetry of the funnel plots was used. The statistical significance was adopted at two-side p value < 0.05.

2.5. Risk of Bias

Two authors (K.S.-Z. and M.K.) independently assessed the risk of bias using the Cochrane Collaboration's tool for assessing risk of bias [38]. When a discrepancy occurred, a third author (I.Ł.) was involved. The quality of a study was reported as high when there were more than three low risk of bias assessments.

3. Results

3.1. Search Results

The initial search yielded 2872 citations. Of these, 2822 were duplicates and/or removed after title/abstract evaluation. Five manuscripts were identified using a manual search. Forty-seven articles underwent a full-text review, and some were excluded because they were reviews/meta-analysis/systematic review ($N = 8$), in the Chinese language ($N = 2$), mice model ($N = 1$), and contained no meta-analyzable infectious related data/end-points ($N = 1$). Eventually, 35 studies were included in the meta-analysis [39–73] (Figure 1).

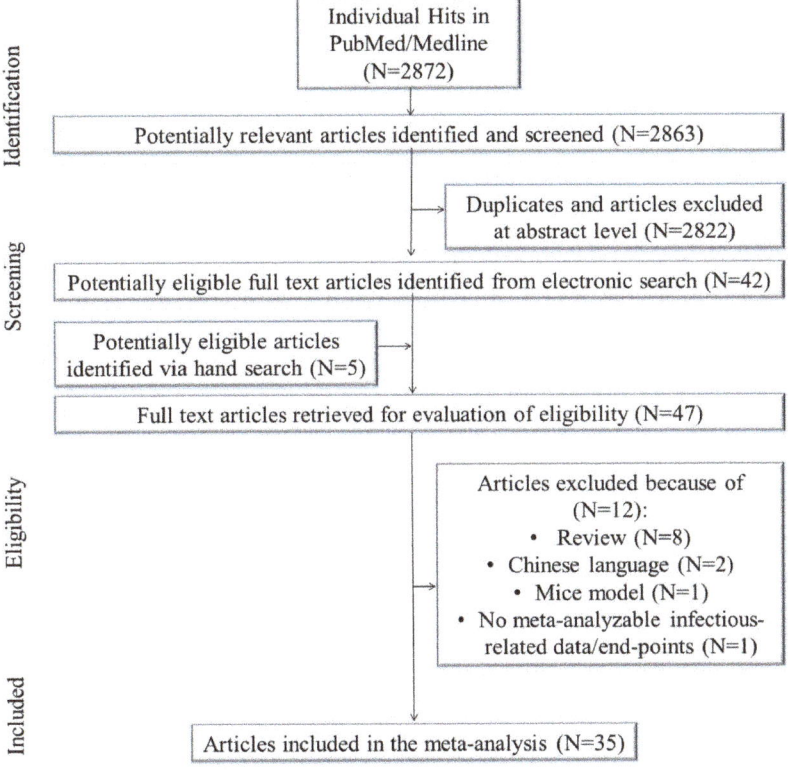

Figure 1. Study flow chart.

3.2. Study, Patient and Treatment Characteristics

Of the 35 studies included, the majority were double-blind trials (N = 17) [39,42,45–47,49–52,56,60,61, 64,71–74]. The mean study duration was 14.5 ± 5.58 (range: 3–28) days. In 16 studies [39,41,42,46,49–54,56, 63–65,69,70], probiotic intervention was used, while synbiotics were administered in 19 trials [40,43–45,47, 48,55,57–62,66–68,71–73]. There were two major groups per surgery performed: hepatopancreatobillary (N = 15) [40,43,46,51,54,58,63,64,66–68,70–73] and colorectal (N = 11) [31,41,47,49–52,56,61,62,65]. In seven studies [42,44,45,48,53,55,60] the procedure was not specified. Two trials involved oesophagectomy [57,59]. The most commonly utilized comparator was placebo (N = 15) [31,42,43,45,47,49–52,56,60,63,64,69,70]. There were 3028 patients included, with a male predominance (n = 1748, 57.73%). Details are given in Table 1.

Table 1. Study characteristics.

Study	Reference	Study (Country)	Study Focus/ Primary Study Outcome	Blinding	Trial Duration (Days)	ROB*	Operation Name	Duration of Probiotic Therapy Pre/Postoperatively (Days)	Probiotic/Synbiotic Content	Probiotic Dose	Comparator	N Total Randomized/ Analysed	Age (Years)	Male (%)	Primary Disease
1	[41]	Aisu 2015 (Japan)	SSIs and the immune response, intestinal microbiota, and surgical outcome	Psr	ND	2	CRC surgery	3–15/NR	*Enterococcus faecalis* T110, *Clostridium butyricum* TO-A, *Bacillus mesentericus* TO-A	2 mg, 10 mg, 10 mg, 6 tablets/day	No intervention	156/156	68.57 ± 12.49	91 (58.33)	CRC
2	[45]	Anderson 2003 (U.K.)	BT, gastric colonisation, systemic inflammation, and septic morbidity	DB	12	5	Elective laparotomy	12/4	*Lactobacillus acidophilus* La5, *Lactobacillus bulgaricus*, *Bifidobacterium lactis* Bb-12, *Streptococcus thermophilus*; Prebiotic: oligofructose	4×10^9 CFU; 16 g; 3 × day	PBO	137/137	71 #	80 (58.39)	GI malignancy
3	[46]	Diepenhorst 2011 (The Netherlands)	BT, intestinal barrier function	DB	14	3	Elective pylorus-preserving pancreaticoduodenectomy	7/7	*Lactobacillus acidophilus* W70, *Lactobacillus salivarius* W24, *Lactococcus lactis* W58, *Bifidobacterium Bifidum* W23, *Bifidobacterium infantis* W52 *Lactobacillus acidophilus* W70, *Lactobacillus salivarius* W24, *Lactococcus lactis* W58, *Bifidobacterium Bifidum* W23, *Bifidobacterium infantis* W52 + SDD	3 g; 2 × day (an equivalent of 10^{10} CFU)	Standard care	20/20	64 # 60 #	10 (50) 9 (45)	Periampullary or ampullary pancreatic malignancy
4	[43]	Eguchi 2011 (Japan)	Infectious complications	OL	16	1	Living donor LT	2/14	*Lactobacillus casei* Strain Shirota, *Bifidobacterium breve* Strain Yakult; Prebiotic: GOS	20 mg + 15 mg + 15 mg; 3 × day	PBO	50/50	56.5 ± NR	29 (58)	Liver cirrhosis due to HCV
5	[47]	Flesch 2017 (Brazil)	Surgical wound infection	DB	19	2	Colorectal resection	5/14	*Lactobacillus acidophilus* NCFM, *Lactobacillus rhamnosus* HN001, *Lactobacillus paracasei Lactobacillus plantarum* c-37, *Bifidobacterium lactis* HN019; Prebiotic: FOS	10^9 each, 6 g/2 sachets 2 × day	PBO	100/91	62.93 ± 12.32	37 (40.66)	Colorectal adenocarcinoma
6	[64]	Grąt 2017 (Poland)	Pre- and post-transplant patient outcomes	DB	Varia, depending on the listing for LT	6	LT	Varia depending on listing for LT, up to 10 weeks	*Lactococcus lactis* PB411, *Lactobacillus casei* PB121, *Lactobacillus acidophilus* PB111, *Bifidobacterium bifidum* PB211	3×10^9 CFU	PBO	55/44	50.95	34 (77.27)	ALD

Table 1. Cont.

Study	Reference	Study (Country)	Study Description					Treatment Description				Subjects Description			
			Study Focus/ Primary Study Outcome	Blinding	Trial Duration (Days)	ROB*	Operation Name	Duration of Probiotic Therapy Pre/Postoperatively (Days)	Probiotic/Synbiotic Content	Probiotic Dose	Comparator	N Total Randomized/ Analysed	Age (Years)	Male (%)	Primary Disease
7	[48]	Horvat 2010 (Slovenia)	Systemic inflammatory response and clinical outcome	DB	NR	3	Abdominal surgery	3/NR	*Pediacoccus pentosaceus* 5-33:3, *Leuconostoc mesenteroides* 32–77:1, *Lactobacillus paracasei* subsp. *Paracasei* 19, *Lactobacillus plantarum* 2362; Prebiotic: 2.5 g betaglucan, 2.5 g inulin, 2.5 g pectin, 2.5 g resistant starch	40 billion, 10 g of fibers, 2 × day	Bowel cleansing	76/40	62 #	20 (50)	Colon adenocarcinoma
8	[40]	Kanazawa 2005 (Japan)	Intestinal integrity, microflora, and surgical outcome	NR	14	1	Combined liver and extrahepatic bile duct resection with hepaticojejunostomy	0/14	*Bifidobacterium breve* Strain Yakult, *Lactobacillus casei* Strain Shirota; Prebiotic: GOS **	10^8/g each; 3 g day; 12 g/day	Prebiotic	76/48	63.25 #	21 (44)	Perihilar cholangiocarcinoma
9	[44]	Komatsu 2016 (Japan)	Surgical outcome	OL	≤17	5	Laparoscopy	7–11/6	*Lactobacillus casei* strain Strain Shirota; Prebiotic: GOS, *Bifidobacterium breve* Strain Yakult.	4×10^{10}, 2.5 g, 1×10^{10}	No intervention	54/44	63.75 ± 9.64	29 (65.91)	Elective laparoscopic colorectal surgery
10	[49]	Kotzampassi 2015 (Greece)	Prophylaxis for complications after colorectal surgery	DB	16	5	Colorectal surgery for cancer.	1/14	*Lactobacillus acidophilus* LA-5, *Lactobacillus plantarum*, *Bifidobacterium lactis* BB-12, *Saccharomyces boulardii*	1.75×10^9 CFU, 0.5×10^9 CFU, 1.75×10^9, 1.5×10^9 CFU per capsule, 2 × day	No intervention	370/362	67.23 ± 11.11	210 (58.01)	CRC
11	[42]	Liu 2010 (China)	Gut barrier function and the surgical outcome	DB	16	4	Laparotomy	6/10	*Lactobacillus plantarum* CGMCC No. 1258, *Lactobacillus acidophilus* LA-11, *Bifidobacterium longum* BL-88	2.6×10^{14} CFU, 2 g/day	PBO	168/164	66.14 ± 11.69	115 (70.12)	CRC
12	[50]	Liu 2013 (China)	Serum zonulin concentrations and postoperative infectious complications	DB	16	5	Colorectal carcinoma surgery	6/10	*Lactobacillus plantarum* CGMCC No. 1258, *Lactobacillus acidophilus* LA-11, *Bifidobacterium longum* BL-88	2.6×10^{14} CFU, 2 g/day	PBO	114/100	65.5 ± 10.45	59 (59)	CRC
13	[51]	Liu 2015 (China)	Serum zonulin levels and postoperative infectious complications	DB	16	5	Colectomy + resection for metastatic tumor/segmental hepatectomy	6/10	*Lactobacillus plantarum* CGMCC No. 1258, *Lactobacillus acidophilus* LA-11, *Bifidobacterium longum* BL-88	2.6×10^{14} CFU, 2 g/day	PBO	161/150	65.06 ± 11.73	78 (52)	CRC
											PBO	134/117	62.84 ± 17.17	70 (59.83)	Colon cancer + Colorectal liver metastases

Table 1. Cont.

Study	Reference	Study (Country)	Study Focus/ Primary Study Outcome	Blinding	Trial Duration (Days)	ROB*	Operation Name	Duration of Probiotic Therapy Pre/Postoperatively (Days)	Probiotic/Synbiotic Content	Probiotic Dose	Comparator	N Total Randomized/ Analysed	Age (Years)	Male (%)	Primary Disease
												Study Description		**Subjects Description**	
									Treatment Description						
14	[52]	Mangell 2012 (Sweden)	Intestinal load of potentially pathogenic bacteria, BT, and cell proliferation	DB	13	4	Colonic resection	8/5	Lactobacillus plantarum 299v	10^{11} CFU	PBO	72/64	72 #	36 (56.25)	Adenocarcinoma
15	[53]	Mcnaught 2002 (U.K.)	BT, gastric colonization, and septic complications	OL	9	1	Major abdominal surgery	7–12/4–9	Lactobacillus plantarum 299v	10^7/mL; preoperatively 4000 mL, postoperatively 800 mL	No intervention	129/129	68.5 #	75 (58.14)	CRC
16	[65]	Mizuta 2016 (Japan)	Immune functions, systemic inflammatory responses, postoperative infectious complications	SB	≤28	2	CRC resection	7–14/7	Bifidobacterium Longum BB536	5×10^{10} CFU, 2 g	No intervention	60/60	70.01 ± 9.96	35 (58.33)	CRC
17	[54]	Nomura 2007 (Japan)	Surgical outcome	NR	≥3	1	Pancreaticoduodenectomy, Whipple	3–15/until discharge	Enterococcus faecalis T-110, Clostridium butyricum TO-A, Bacillus mesentericus TO-A	6×10^7 CFU	No intervention	70/64	66 #	39 (60.94)	Pancreatico-billiary disease
18	[55]	Okazaki 2013 (Japan)	Gut microbiota, infectious complications	OL	17	1	Abdominal surgery	7/10	Lactobacillus casei Strain Shirota and BBG-01, Bifidobacterium breve Strain Yakult; Prebiotic: GOS	Biolactis powder (1 g/day) and BBG-01 (1 g/day), GOS: 5 g, 3 × day	No intervention	53/48	78.5 #	26 (54.17)	Upper digestive illness
19	[63]	Rammohan 2015 (India)	Postoperative infectious complications, clinical outcome	SB (patients)	15	3	Frey procedure for chronic hepatitis	5/10	Streptococcus faecalis T-110, Clostridium butyricum TO-A, Bacillus mesentericus TO-A, Lactobacillus sporogenes; Prebiotic: FOS	60 million, 4 million, 2 million, 100 million,	PBO	79/75	43.29 ± 8.96	48 (64)	Chronic hepatitis
20	[72]	Rayes 2007 (Germany/U.K.)	Postoperative bacterial infection	DB	9	2	Pylorus-preserving, Pancreatoduodenectomy	1/8	Pediacoccus pentosaceus 5-33:3; Leuconostoc mesenteroides 77:1; Lactobacillus paracasei subspecies paracasei F19; Lactobacillus plantarum 2362; Prebiotic: bioactive fibers—2.5 g of each betaglucan, inulin, pectin, and resistant starch.	10^{10}, 10 g	Fiber	89/80	58.5 ± NR	45 (56.3)	Carcinoma (pancreas)

Table 1. Cont.

Study	Reference	Study (Country)	Study Focus/ Primary Study Outcome	Blinding	Trial Duration (Days)	ROB*	Operation Name	Duration of Probiotic Therapy Pre/Postoperatively (Days)	Probiotic/Synbiotic Content	Probiotic Dose	Comparator	N Total Randomized/ Analysed	Age (Years)	Male (%)	Primary Disease
21	[71]	Rayes 2005 (Germany/U.K.)	Infectious complications	DB	14	3	LT	0/14	Pediacoccus pentosaceus 5-33:3; Leuconostoc mesenteroides 77:1; Lactobacillus paracasei subspecies paracasei F19; Lactobacillus plantarum 2362; Prebiotic: bioactive fibers—2.5 g of each betaglucan, inulin, pectin, and resistant starch	10^{10}, 20 g	Fiber	66/66	51.5 ± 2	38 (57.6)	Na
22	[70]	Rayes 2002 a (Multicenter)	Early postoperative infections	OL	12	0	LT	0/12	Lactobacillus plantarum 299v; 2 × day	1×10^9, oat fibers	PBO + fiber	105/69	48.47 ± 2.49	30 (47.6)	Na
23	[69]	Rayes 2002 (Germany)	Postoperative bacterial infection, clinical outcome	OL	4	0	Major abdominal surgery	0/4	Lactobacillus plantarum 299; Prebiotic: oat fiber	1×10^9	PBO + fiber	90/60	60.5 ± 13.59	30 (50)	Liver, pancreatic, gastric resection
24	[73]	Rayes 2012 (Germany)	Liver regeneration after hepatectomy	DB	11	2	Hepatectomy	1/10	Pediacoccus pentosaceus 5-33:3; Leuconostoc mesenteroides 77:1; Lactobacillus paracasei subspecies paracasei F19; Lactobacillus plantarum 2362; Prebiotic: bioactive fibers—2.5 g of each betaglucan, inulin, pectin, and resistant starch	10^{10}, 20 g	Fiber	19/19	60.05 ± 13.89	14 (73.7)	Colorectal metastasis
25	[62]	Reddy 2007 (Denmark/U.K.)	Prevalence of Enterobacteriaceae, inflammatory response including septic morbidity	OL	1	1	Elective CRC surgery	1/0	Lactobacillus acidophilus La5, Lactobacillus bulgaricus, Bifidobacterium lactis, BB-12, Streptococcus thermophilus; Prebiotic: oligofructose	4×10^9 CFU, 15 g, 2 × day	Neomycin + MBP	88/42	70.6 #	22 (52.4)	Anterior resection
26	[61]	Sadahiro 2014 (Japan)	Incisional SSI, organ/space SSI, remote infection, leakage, CD toxin	DB	18	6	Curative resection of CRC	7/11	Bifidobacterium bifidum; Prebiotic: multioligosaccharide	1×10^9/day	Antibiotic, mechanical bowel preparation	294/194	66.7 ± 10.72	107 (55.2)	CRC
27	[60]	Sommacal 2015 (Brazil)	Postoperative morbidity and mortality	DB	14	7	Periampullary cancer: resective and palliative surgery	4/10	Lactobacillus acidophilus 10, Lactobacillus rhamnosus HS 111, Lactobacillus casei 10, Bifidobacterium bifidum; Prebiotic: FOS	1×10^9 CFU, 1×10^9 CFU, 1×10^9 CFU, 1×10^9 CFU, 100 mg	PBO	48/46	59.5 #	NR	Periampullary cancer

Table 1. Cont.

Study	Reference	Study (Country)	Study Focus/ Primary Study Outcome	Blinding	Trial Duration (Days)	ROB*	Operation Name	Duration of Probiotic Therapy Pre/Postoperatively (Days)	Probiotic/Synbiotic Content	Probiotic Dose	Comparator	N Total Randomized/ Analysed	Age (Years)	Male (%)	Primary Disease
28	[67]	Sugawara 2006 (Japan)	Intestinal barrier function, immune responses, systemic inflammatory responses, microflora, and surgical outcome	OL	28	2	Liver and extrahepatic bile duct resection with hepaticojejunostomy	14/14	Lactobacillus casei strain Shirota, Bifidobacterium breve strain Yakult; Prebiotic: GOS	80 mL: 4 × 10^{10}, 100 mL: 1 × 10^{10}, 15 g/day	Synbiotic only post-operatively	101/81	63.15 ± 8.84	46 (56.79)	Perihilar cholangiocarcinoma
29	[59]	Tanaka 2012 (Japan)	Postoperative infections	SB	21	3	Oesophagectomy	1/21	Lactobacillus casei strain Shirota, Bifidobacterium breve strain Yakult; Prebiotic: GOS	1 × 10^{10}/g, 1 × 10^{10}/g; (PRE:3 g/day; POST: 2 g/day) GOS (PRE:15 g, POST:10 g)	Streptococcus faecalis	64/64	62.15 ± 7.74	51 (79.7)	Oesophagal cancer
30	[58]	Usami 2011 (Japan)	Intestinal integrity, systemic inflammatory response, and microflora, surgical outcome	OL	26	4	Hepatic surgery	14/12	Lactobacillus casei strain Shirota, Bifidobacterium breve strain Yakult; Prebiotic: GOS	1 × 10^8/g, 1 × 10^8/g, 10 g	No intervention	67/61	65.42 ± 9.86	55 (90.2)	Primary or metastatic liver cancer
31	[39]	Yang 2016 (China)	Postoperative infections	DB	12	5	Radical CRC resection	5/7	Bifidobacterium longum, Lactobacillus acidophilus Enterococcus faecalis	≥1.0 × 10^7 CFU/g, ≥1.0 × 10^7 CFU/g, ≥1.0 × 10^7 CFU/g	PBO	79/60	63.03 ± 11.70	27 (45)	CRC
32	[57]	Yokoyama 2014 (Japan)	Intestinal microenvironment, BT to mlns, postoperative bacteraemia	OL	21	5	Oesophagectomy	7/14	PRE:Lactobacillus casei strain Shirota, Bifidobacterium breve strain Yakult; Prebiotic: 15 g GOS; POST:Lactobacillus casei strain Shirota Bifidobacterium breve strain Shirota Yakult; Prebiotic: 15 g GOS	PRE: 4 × 10^{10}, 1 × 10^{10}, 15 g; POST: 1 × 10^8/g, 1 × 10^8/g, 15 g	No intervention	42/42	65.5 #	37 (88.1)	Oesophagal cancer
33	[66]	Yokoyama 2016 (Japan)	BT to mlns and blood, postoperative infectious complications	OL	7	2	Pancreatoduodenectomy	7/0	Lactobacillus casei Strain Shirota, Bifidobacterium breve strain Strain Yakult; Prebiotic: GOS	80 mL: 4 × 10^{10}, 100 mL: 1 × 10^{10}, 15 g/day	No intervention	45/44	65 #	12 (27.27)	Pancreatic cancer

Table 1. Cont.

Study	Reference	Study Description				Treatment Description					Subjects Description		
		Study (Country)	Study Focus/ Primary Study Outcome	Blinding	Trial Duration (Days)	ROB*	Operation Name	Probiotic/Synbiotic Content	Probiotic Dose	Duration of Probiotic Therapy Pre/ Postoperatively (Days)	Comparator	N Total Randomized/ Analysed	Age (Years)	Male (%)	Primary Disease
34	[56]	Zhang 2012 (China)	Postoperative infections and related complications	DB	3	5	Radical CRC resection with laparotomy	Bifidobacterium longum, Lactobacillus acidophilus, Enterococcus faecalis	0.21 g (10^8 CFU/g)	3/0	PBO	60/60	64.5 #	24 (60)	CRC
35	[68]	Zhang 2013 (Australia)	Assessing the impact on bacterial sepsis and wound complications	OL	?	2	LT	Lactobacillus Acidophilus LA-14, Lactobacillus Plantarum 115, Bifidobacterium Lactis BL-04, Lactobacillus Casei LC-11, Lactobacillus Rhamnosus LR-32, Lactobacillus Brevis Bv-35; Prebiotic: fiber	15.5 × 10^9, 5.0 × 10^9, 2.0 × 10^9, 1.5 × 10^9, 1.5 × 10^9, 1.5 × 10^9 CFU	0/?	Fiber	67/67	56.01 ± 10.98	36 (53.73)	NR

*—number of low risk judgements; **—enetral feeding, #—median, CFU—colony forming units, DB—double blind, SB—single blind, CRC—colorectal cancer, GI—gastrointestinal, LT—liver transplantation, GOS—galactoologosaccharides, FOS—fructooligosaccharides, OL—open label, PsR—pseudorandomisation, SDD—standard decontamination of the digestive tract, BT—bacterial transolcation, MLN—mesenteric lymph node, ALD—alcoholic liver disease, CRC—colorectal cancer, SDD—selective decontamination of the digestive tract.

3.3. Microbiota and Putative Mechanism of Probiotic/Synbiotics' Action in SSIs/SRCs Prevention—Primary Outcomes

Gut microbiota analyses were present in 14 studies [40–44,52,55–59,64,65,67]. The results confirmed postoperative microbiome alterations in study groups compared to controls. Most studies identified *Lactobacillus* (phylum *Firmicutes*) and *Bifidobacterium* (phylum *Actinobacteria*) as beneficial for the outcomes. Nine studies [40–42,55–57,59,67] reported elevations in *Bifidobacterium* genus (or its particular species) including patients supplemented with microbial agents, but did not reach statistical significance for a benefit. *Lactobacillus* concentrations were elevated post-surgery in six studies [40,57,59,64,67,75]. In contrast, decreased numbers of beneficial microbes and increased abundance of harmful species (*Enterobacteriaceae, Pseudomonas, Staphylococcus,* and *Candida*) were reported in a few no-intervention groups [40,42,44,57]. One study [56] reported a *Bifidobacterium/E. coli* ratio. In two studies [43,58], there were no significant differences in bacterial species abundance between the groups. For example, Usami et al. [58] concluded that two weeks after the surgery microbiota composition resembled that of before the surgery regardless of the intervention. However, changes of fecal microbiota composition observed by Usami et al. [58] were not consistent with results reported by other authors [67]. Reasons for this discrepancy might be associated with the difference in intestinal microbiota between liver cirrhosis and biliary surgery patients and/or no administration of enteral nutrition in their study [40,67]. Details are given in Table 2.

Putatively factors associated with the mechanism of pro/synbiotic action were searched with a focus on gut barrier integrity. These included: (i) bacterial translocation, (ii) lactulose/mannitol permeability test, and (iii) short chain fatty acids (butyrate, acetate, propionate) concentration, as well as non-specific markers of inflammation: (iv) C-reactive protein, (v) IL-6, and (vi) WBC counts. Diamine oxidase (DAO) activity was analyzed in two studies only [40,58], therefore excluded from metanalysis. CRP and IL-6 were significantly decreased (SMD: -0.40, 95% CI $[-0.79, -0.02]$, $p = 0.041$; SMD: -0.41, 95% CI $[-0.70, -0.12]$, $p = 0.006$, respectively) and short chain fatty acids (SCFAs)–acetic, butyric and propionic acids–were elevated (SMD: 1.78, 95% CI [0.80, 2.76], $p = 0.0004$; SMD: 0.67, 95% CI [0.37, 0.97], $p = 0.00001$; SMD: 0.46, 95% CI [0.18, 0.73], $p = 0.001$, respectively) in patients supplemented with probiotics. No other statistically significant results were found. Results are presented in Table 3 and Figures 2–9.

Table 2. Gut microbiota alterations following probiotic treatment.

Reference	Country	Gut Microbiota Changes after the Surgery/Intervention
Aisu 2015	Japan	Probiotic group: the mean proportion of *Bifidobacterium* increased between 4.6 ± 1.97 and 9.1 ± 1.89%. No-probiotic group: the mean proportion of *Bifidobacterium* decreased between 7.06(1.95)% And 5.53(±1.93)
Eguchi 2011	Japan	No significant changes in bacterial species abundance between the groups. In 25% of patients under immunosuppression *Enterococcus* spp evident in both groups
Grat 2017	Poland	Probiotic group: *Bacteroides* spp. count increased in comparison to pre-trial values ($p = 0.008$). *Enterococcus* spp. abundance significantly increased ($p = 0.04$) and a tendency towards increased number of *Lactobacillus* spp. ($p = 0.07$) as compared to no-probiotic group
Kanazawa 2005	Japan	Synbiotic group: beneficial bacteria (including *Lactobacillus* and *Bifidobacterium*) count increased after surgery, in comparison to controls ($p < 0.05$). No-synbiotic group: harmful microorganisms (including *Enterobacteriaceae*, *Pseudomonas*, and *Candida*) increased in comparison to synbiotic group ($p < 0.05$). *Enterococci* abundance increased after surgery in both groups, with no significant intergroup differences.
Komatsu 2016	Japan	Synbiotic group: Total bacteria, dominant obligate anaerobes (such as *Clostridium leptum* subgroup or *Bifidobacterium*), and facultative anaerobes (*Lactobacillus* species) significantly increased. The abundance of *Enterobacteriaceae*, *Staphylococcus* (MSCNS), and *Pseudomonas* decreased compared to the control group ($p < 0.05$). *Bifidobacterium* and *L. casei* subgroup numbers and *C. perfringens*, *L. gasseri* subgroup, *L. reuteri* subgroup, and *L. sakei* subgroup increased and decreased respectively regarding preoperative concentrations ($p < 0.05$). No synbiotic group: total bacteria, dominant obligate anaerobes (*C. coccoides* group, *C. leptum* subgroup, *Bacteroides fragilis* group, *Bifidobacterium*, *Prevotella*, and *Lactobacillus* species) counts decreased while the numbers of *Enterobacteriaceae*, *Staphylococcus* (MSCNS), *Pseudomonas*, and *C. difficile* increased in comparison to the preoperative values ($p < 0.05$).
Liu 2010	China	Probiotic group: *Bifidobacterium* count increased in comparison to controls and preoperative values. *Enterobacteriaceae*, *Pseudomonas*, and *Candida* numbers were decreased compared to placebo group ($p < 0.05$). Probiotic bacterial richness was enhanced when compared to healthy volunteers and the control group ($p < 0.05$). A higher similarity to the healthy volunteers compared with the control group ($p < 0.05$). No probiotic group: *Enterobacteriaceae*, *Pseudomonas* and *Candida* numbers increased compared to probiotic group ($p < 0.05$) *Enterococci* abundance increased in both groups.
Mangell 2012	Sweden	Probiotic group: *Enterobacteriaceae* count increased significantly in comparison to placebo ($p < 0.001$) but not regarding preoperatively values.
Mizuta 2016	Japan	Probiotic group: Firmicutes decreased (62.31% vs. 56.51%) and Actinobacteria increased (0.7% vs. 1.71%) in comparison to control group ($p < 0.05$). No-probiotic group: Bacteroidetes (24.52% vs. 32.8%) and Proteobacteria (1.74% vs. 3.54%) numbers increased and Firmicutes (66.57% vs. 56.82%) and unclassified bacterial groups (0.5% vs. 0.37%) abundance decreased compared to before the surgery period.
Okazaki 2013	Japan	Synbiotic group: Before surgery *Bifidobacteria* count and numbers of *Enterobacteriaceae* and *Pseudomonas* were significantly increased and decreased, respectively, in comparison to the pre-trial values and the control group ($p < 0.05$). *Bifidobacterium* abundance was significantly increased while *Enterobacteriaceae* and *Staphylococcus* bacteria counts decreased postoperatively in comparison to controls. No-synbiotic group: *Bifidobacterium* number gradually decreased
Sugawara 2006	Japan	Pre-and post-operative probiotic group: *Bifidobacterium* number increased significantly after preoperative treatment ($p < 0.05$), as well as *Lactobacillus* but with no statistical difference ($p > 0.05$). *Bifidobacterium* abundance 1 day before hepatectomy was higher and lower for *Candida* in comparison to the only pre-surgery probiotic group. Anaerobic bacteria numbers were unchanged before and after surgery between the two groups, without intergroup differences.
Tanaka 2012	Japan	Synbiotic group: *Bifidobacterium* and total *Lactobacillus* numbers were significantly higher ($p < 0.01$) when compared to controls. Postoperatively (day 7) the abundance of *Clostridium coccoides* group ($p < 0.01$); *C. leptum* subgroup ($p < 0.01$); *Bacteroides fragilis* subgroup ($p < 0.05$); *Bifidobacterium* ($p < 0.01$), *Atopobium* cluster ($p < 0.05$), *Prevotella* ($p < 0.01$), and *Lactobacillus* ($p < 0.01$) significantly decreased when compared to the pre-operative time point. *Bifidobacterium* and *Lactobacillus* species count were not decreased, but were higher when compared to controls. *Enterobacteriaceae*, *Staphylococcus*, and *Pseudomonas* species numbers were significantly lower in comparison to the second group patients. Collectively (3 weeks post-surgery) *Bifidobacterium* abundance was significantly higher and *Enterobacteriaceae* count was lower in the synbiotic group ($p < 0.05$).

Table 2. Cont.

Reference	Country	Gut Microbiota Changes after the Surgery/Intervention
Usami 2011	Japan	Synbiotic group: Fecal anaerobic bacteria, including *Bacteroidaceae*, as well as *Bifidobacterium* genus were decreased compared to before the trial (post-operative days 6–8). The numbers of *Candida* were increased in this time point. In contrast, two weeks after the surgery, these numbers started to resemble values before hepatectomy (*Bacteroidaceae*: 10.0 ± 0.4 vs. 10.1 ± 0.3, *Bifidobacterium*: 10.0 ± 0.7 vs. 10.0 ± 0.6, *Candida*: 3.4 ± 1.4 vs. 3.1 ± 1.0 log10 CFU/g of feces. No-synbiotic group: Two weeks after the surgery, particular bacteria numbers started to resemble values before hepatectomy (*Bacteroidaceae*: 10.0 ± 0.5 vs. 9.9 ± 0.4, *Bifidobacterium*: 9.8 ± 0.8 vs. 9.5 ± 0.7, *Candida*: 4.1 ± 1.6 vs. 4.1 ± 1.9 log10 CFU/g of feces. Subgroup comparison between normal liver and chronic liver damage, including chronic hepatitis, liver fibrosis, and cirrhosis in either group found no significant differences
Yokoyama 2014	Japan	Synbiotic group: A week post-surgery, *Bifidobacterium* and *Lactobacillus* counts increased and *Enterobacteriaceae* and *Pseudomonas* decreased in comparison to pre-operative values and the control group ($p < 0.05$). The numbers of *Staphylococcus*, *Pseudomonas*, and *Enterobacteriaceae* were significantly decreased 21 days post-surgery when compared to the no-synbiotic group and pre-surgery time (except for *Pseudomonas*). No-synbiotic group: *Pseudomonas*, *Staphylococcus*, and *Enterobacteriaceae* levels were increased post-operatively in comparison to the intervention group ($p < 0.05$).
Zhang 2012	China	Probiotic group: During preoperative treatment (3 days before surgery), the reversal of the *Bifidobacterium*/*E. coli* ratio inversion in comparison to day−6 (0.26 ± 0.32 and 1.26 ± 0.28 log10/g, respectively, $p < 0.001$) and controls (1.26 ± 0.28 and 0.27 ± 0.34 log10/g, respectively, $p < 0.001$). Postoperatively decreased *E coli* count compared to controls (8.29 ± 0.27 log10/g and 9.67 ± 0.17 log10/g, respectively, $p < 0.001$), and *B. longum* increased (8.43 ± 0.17 log10/g and 7.94 ± 0.11 log10/g, respectively; $p < 0.001$). No-probiotic group: Postoperative *Bifidobacterium*/*E. coli* ratio inversion in comparison to 6 days before surgery (0.14 ± 0.20 and 0.26 ± 0.32, respectively, $p < 0.001$) and probiotic group (0.14 ± 0.20 and 1.73 ± 0.22, $p < 0.001$).

Table 3. Primary outcomes associated with gut barrier implicated in potential mechanisms of probiotic/synbiotic action.

Outcome	SMD (95% CI)	Z-Value	References	Heterogeneity	Tau	Intercept (95% CI) [†]	Meta-Regression Coefficients
CRP	−0.40 (−0.79, −0.02)	−2.04 $p = 0.041$	Kanazawa, 2005 Yokoyama, 2014 Usami, 2011 Tanaka, 2012 Rayes, 2002 Sugawara, 2006	Q = 16.1 $p = 0.007$ (df = 5) $I^2 = 69$	$\tau^2 = 0.159$ $\tau = 0.399$	8.59 (−13.42, 30.59) $p = 0.339$	Dose: −0.32 ($p = 0.158$) Intervention: NOT ESTIMABLE Operation (Hepatobiliary vs. Gut): −0.69 ($p = 0.075$), (Mixed vs. Gut): −0.34, $p = 0.515$ ROB (Low vs. High): −0.28 ($p = 0.539$) Duration: −0.02 ($p = 0.477$) Timing (Post vs. Peri): 0.08 ($p = 0.871$)
IL-6	−0.41 (−0.70, −0.12)	−2.77 $p = 0.006$	Zhang, 2012 Usami, 2011 Sugawara, 2006 Mizuta, 2016	Q = 4.03 $p = 0.258$ (df = 3) $I^2 = 25.6$	$\tau^2 = 0.022$ $\tau = 0.150$	−2.18 (−39.73, 35.38) $p = 0.826$	Dose: −0.09 ($p = 0.538$) Intervention (Synbiotic vs. Probiotic): 0.36 ($p = 0.159$) Operation (Hepatobiliary vs. Gut): 0.36 ($p = 0.159$) ROB (Low vs. High): −0.27 ($p = 0.383$) Duration: 0.01 ($p = 0.231$) Timing (Pre vs. Peri): −0.22 ($p = 0.580$)
WBC	−0.60 (−1.45, 0.24)	−1.40 $p = 0.162$	Kanazawa, 2005 Yokoyama, 2014 Usami, 2011 Tanaka, 2012 Rayes, 2002a Sugawara, 2006	Q = 70 $p < 0.0001$ (df = 5) $I^2 = 93$	$\tau^2 = 1.033$ $\tau = 1.016$	0.09 (−38.14, 38.32) $p = 0.995$	Dose: −0.03 ($p = 0.965$) Intervention: NOT ESTIMABLE Operation (Mixed vs. Gut): −1.45 ($p = 0.078$) ROB (Low vs. High): −1.42 ($p = 0.089$) Duration: 0.05 ($p = 0.515$) Timing (Post vs. Peri): −1.13 ($p = 0.223$)
L/M	−0.28 (−0.82, 0.27)	−1.00 $p = 0.316$	Kanazawa, 2005 Liu, 2010 Liu, 2013 Sugawara, 2006	Q = 19.5 $p = 0.0002$ (df = 3) $I^2 = 85$	$\tau^2 = 0.257$ $\tau = 0.507$	8.66 (−14.75, 32.07) $p = 0.252$	Dose: −0.28 ($p = 0.323$) Intervention (Synbiotic vs. Probiotic): 0.46 ($p = 0.435$) Operation (Mixed vs. Gut): 0.46 ($p = 0.435$) ROB (Low vs. High): 0.46 ($p = 0.435$) Duration: −0.002 ($p = 0.968$) Timing (Post vs. Peri): 0.59 ($p = 0.376$)
Butyrate	0.67 (0.37, 0.97)	4.40 $p = 0.00001$	Kanazawa, 2005 Komatsu, 2016 Okazaki, 2013 Sugawara, 2006	Q = 5.04 $p = 0.169$ (df = 3) $I^2 = 40.4$	$\tau^2 = 0.037$ $\tau = 0.193$	1.37 (−8.79, 11.53) $p = 0.622$	Dose: NOT ESTIMABLE Intervention: NOT ESTIMABLE Operation: NOT ESTIMABLE ROB (Low vs. High): 0.22 ($p = 0.572$) Duration: 0.02 ($p = 0.510$) Timing (Post vs. Peri): 0.45 ($p = 251$)
Acetate	1.78 (0.80, 2.76)	3.55 $p = 0.0004$	Kanazawa, 2005 Komatsu, 2016 Okazaki, 2013 Sugawara, 2006	Q = 41.4 $p < 0.00001$ (df = 3) $I^2 = 93$	$\tau^2 = 0.912$ $\tau = 0.955$	2.65 (−26.40, 31.71) $p = 0.732$	Dose: NOT ESTIMABLE Intervention: NOT ESTIMABLE Operation: NOT ESTIMABLE ROB (Low vs. High): −0.27 ($p = 0.851$) Duration: −0.10 ($p = 0.118$) Timing (Post vs. Peri): −0.25 ($p = 0.850$)
Propionate	0.46 (0.18, 0.73)	3.23 $p = 0.001$	Kanazawa, 2005 Komatsu, 2016 Okazaki, 2013 Sugawara, 2006	Q = 4.58 $p = 0.206$ (df = 3) $I^2 = 34.4$	$\tau^2 = 0.028$ $\tau = 0.166$	−1.99 (−11.22, 7.24) $p = 0.451$	Dose: NOT ESTIMABLE Intervention: NOT ESTIMABLE Operation: NOT ESTIMABLE ROB (Low vs. High): −0.38 ($p = 0.074$) Duration: −0.04 ($p = 0.049$) Timing (Post vs. Peri): 0.18 ($p = 0.675$)

[†] Egger's regression intercept test for asymmetry of the funnel plots; Dose – dose of probiotic (log), ROB – risk of bias, Post – post operation, Pre – pre operation, Peri – peri operation, SSI-surgical site infection.

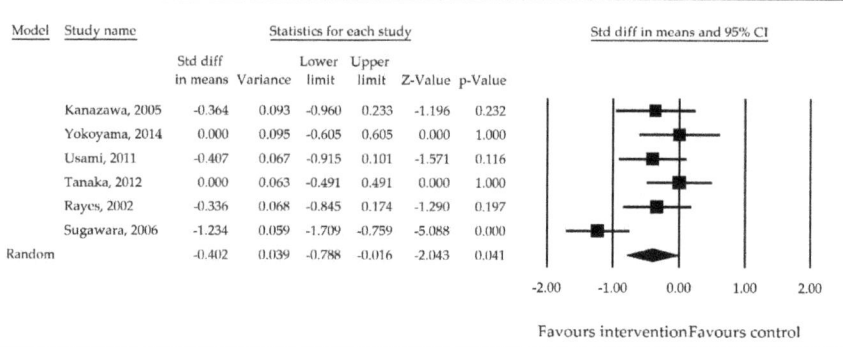

Figure 2. The effect size (standardized mean difference) for the concentration of CRP in patients taking probiotics (intervention) vs. no probiotics (control).

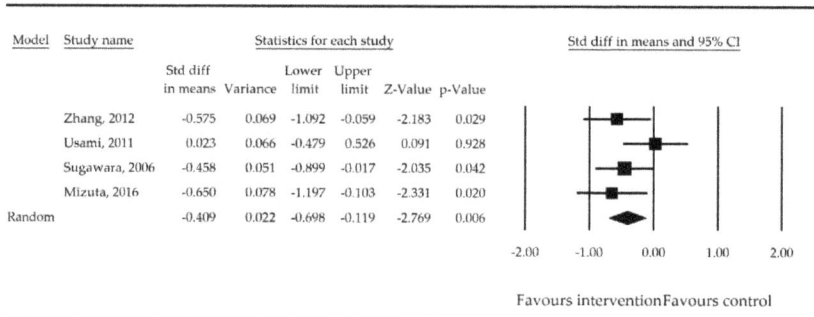

Figure 3. The effect size (standardized mean difference) for the concentration of IL-6 in patients taking probiotics (intervention) vs. no probiotics (control).

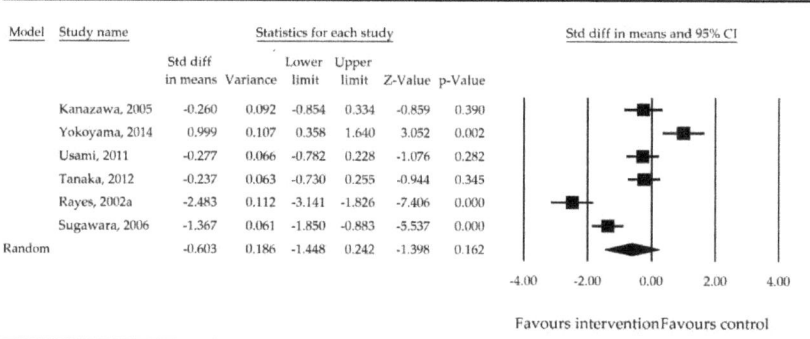

Figure 4. The effect size (standardized mean difference) for the concentration of WBC in patients taking probiotics (intervention) vs. No probiotics (control).

L/M

Model	Study name	Std diff in means	Variance	Lower limit	Upper limit	Z-Value	p-Value
	Kanazawa, 2005	0.185	0.091	-0.408	0.778	0.612	0.540
	Liu, 2010	0.000	0.040	-0.392	0.392	0.000	1.000
	Liu, 2013	-0.977	0.030	-1.315	-0.638	-5.653	0.000
	Sugawara, 2006	-0.226	0.050	-0.663	0.211	-1.013	0.311
Random		-0.278	0.077	-0.822	0.266	-1.002	0.316

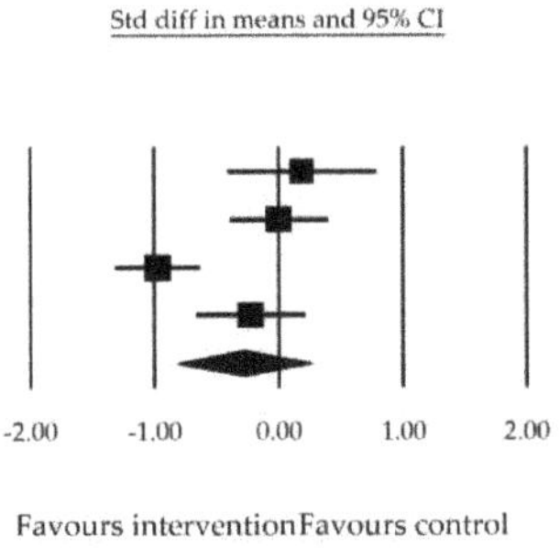

Favours intervention Favours control

Figure 5. The effect size (standardized mean difference) for the lactulose/mannitol (L/M) ratio in patients taking probiotics (intervention) vs. no probiotics (control).

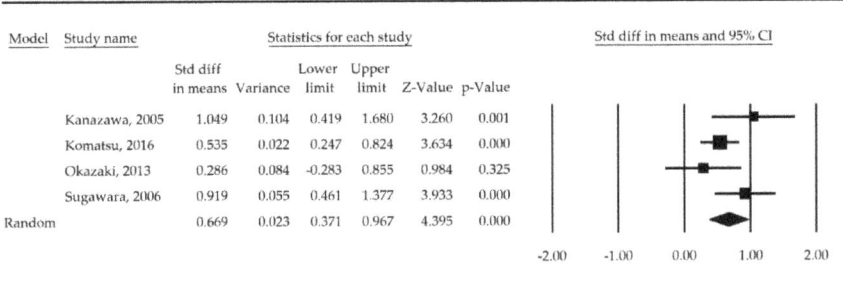

Figure 6. The effect size (standardized mean difference) for the concentration of butyrate ratio in patients taking probiotics (intervention) vs. no probiotics (control).

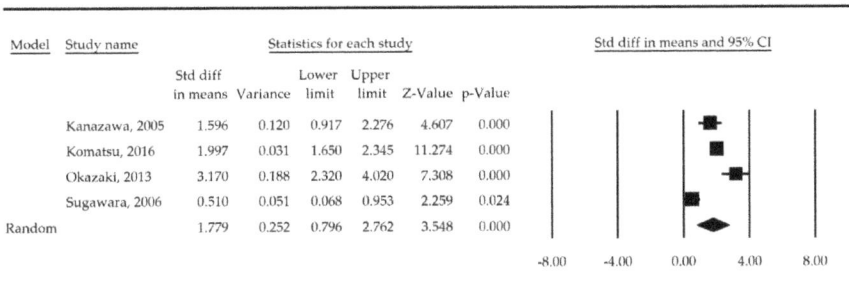

Figure 7. The effect size (standardized mean difference) for the concentration of acetic ratio in patients taking probiotics (intervention) vs. no probiotics (control).

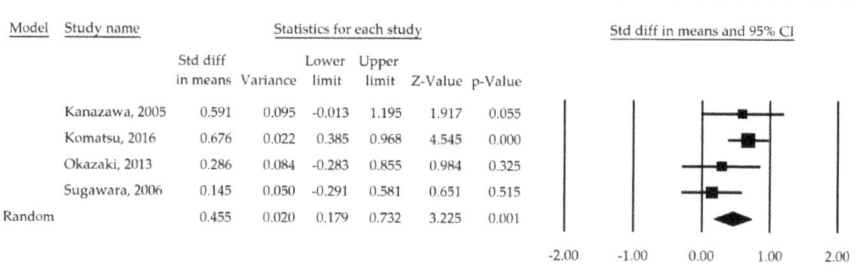

Figure 8. The effect size (standardized mean difference) for the concentration of propionic ratio in patients taking probiotics (intervention) vs. no probiotics (control).

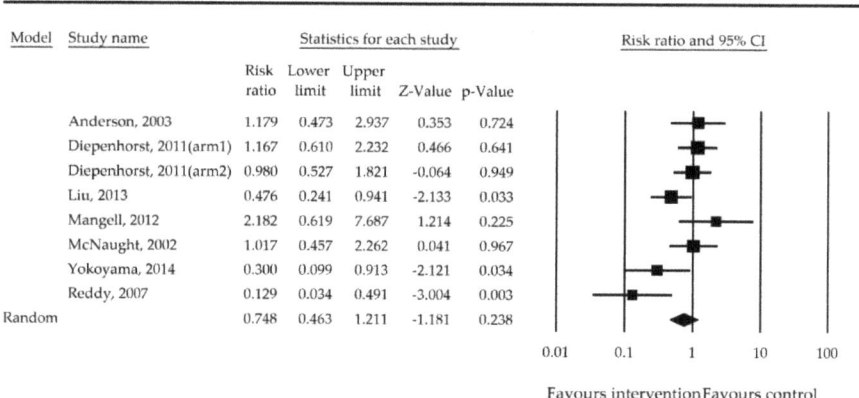

Figure 9. The effect size (risk ratio) for the overall effects of probiotics in the prevention of bacterial translocation.

3.4. Surgery Related Complications (SRCs) and Secondary Outcomes

To evaluate the effectiveness of pro/synbiotic interventions in reducing the incidence of SSIs/SRCs, data was extracted from common surgery-related clinical outcomes. Consequently, meta-analyses were conducted on parameters reported in at least three studies and the data confirmed that microbial supplementation was associated with a significant reduction in the incidence of SSIs and SRCs including: (i) abdominal distention, (ii) diarrhea, (iii) pneumonia, (iv) sepsis, (v) superficial incisional infection, (vi) urinary tract infection, (vii) duration of antibiotic therapy, (viii) duration of postoperative pyrexia, (ix) time of fluid introduction and (x) solid diet, and (xi) duration of hospital stay. Data are given in Supplementary Table S1. Representative forest plots of secondary outcomes are presented in Supplementary Figures S1 and S2. Other forest plots are available upon request.

To obtain data useful for drawing clinical recommendations and new guidelines a meta-regression was conducted (Table 3). Based on the analysis of the selected studies, it was not possible to find a particular probiotic formula or strain, its dose or duration of the probiotic supplementation that could be recommended to manage either primary or secondary outcomes analyzed in this study ($p > 0.05$).

An inverse correlation was only found for propionic acid concentration. For every increase of one unit (day) in treatment duration, the SDM for propionate decreased by 0.0355 ($p = 0.049$). Also effect sizes were found to be independent of the timing of the intervention (pre + post vs. only post-surgery). It was not possible to show whether the quality of the trial could have influenced its results ($p > 0.05$).

3.5. Risk of Bias

An analysis of the overall risk of bias from the studies included in the meta-analysis was limited by restricted information being provided. For example, random sequence generation bias could not be determined in 15 studies and allocation concealment bias could not be studied in 13 papers. The unclear risk of bias in performance, detection, short-term outcomes, and reporting sections were reported in 9, 11, 3, and 12 studies, respectively. It was not possible to determine other risks of bias in 24 papers. Overall, 14 studies were of high quality and 21 of low quality. One study achieved maximum points of low risk assessments (i.e., 7 points) and only two studies achieved no low risk of bias assessments points (i.e., 0 points). The results are in Table S2 (Supplementary Material).

4. Discussion

To the best of our knowledge this meta-analysis of 35 trials and 3028 patients is the first one to exclusively investigate the effect and possible mechanism of action of pro-/synbiotics to lower the risk of SSIs and SRCs. The study shows that microbial agents administered perioperatively have the potential to increase the abundance of beneficial bacteria within the gut, elevate the synthesis of short chain fatty acids and thus reduce the immune response. Consequently, it appears to indicate that pro-/synbiotics may serve as preventive strategy toward SSIs and SRCs.

The data are mounting that the host complex of bacteria, fungi, viruses, and *Archaea* contribute to human biology [76]. In patients scheduled for elective abdominal surgery, the gut microbiota might undergo alterations that have an impact on surgery outcomes. In this study in patients not treated with any microbial agents perioperatively, the predominance of beneficial microbes was decreased, but the counts of potentially harmful ones were elevated. Eubiosis and a proper abundance of protective bacteria in the gut may protect the host against pathogens [75]. In this meta-analysis, the majority of the studies showed that pro-/synbiotic treatment reduced the number of *Enterobacteriaceae*. However, Mangel et al. [52] showed opposing results and observed increased abundance of *Enterobacteriaceae* in patients undergoing colon resection who received a probiotic. The explanation of this phenomenon is not clear. One reason might be too short of a probiotic administration to reduce potential pathogen counts, while another could be associated with oatmeal used as a prebiotic, which could act as a substrate for intestinal bacteria, and the third one is that lactobacilli given orally did not survive the passage through the gastrointestinal tract. Another explanation is a different response of *Enterobacteriaceae* genera to probiotic administration (reduction in the numbers of one genera by the probiotic may result in an expansion of another). This is also of interest as lipopolysaccharide (LPS) attached to the membrane surface of Gram-negative microbes [77,78] may result in enhanced virulence phenotype expression [26]. In severe injuries, more virulent pathogens may predominate in the intestinal ecosystem [27], disrupt the intestinal barrier structure, and function and facilitate bacterial translocation resulting in SSIs and SRCs.

The steady state composition of gut microbiota is crucial in maintaining gut homeostasis [79]. The mechanisms that are implicated in the pathogenesis of complications in patients in the perioperative period are complex. Initially, a healthy microbiota produces lactic acid, which is metabolized to short chain fatty acids (SCFAs), the latter ones are directly related to fecal *Bifidobacterium* count [66]. SCFAs, predominantly butyrate, are crucial for proper gut barrier structure and function [80,81]. After abdominal surgeries and in the course of multiple nonsurgical diseases, beneficial butyrate, acetate, and propionate concentration diminish as a consequence of the deterioration of lactic acid metabolism, as well as fasting [82]. Butyrate, apart from being an energy source for colonocytes, stimulates mucus production and tight junction proteins synthesis [75].

It has been found to inhibit the expression of virulence genes [83] and restrict the growth of *Pseudomonas aueroginosa*, a collagenase producer, implicated in the pathogenesis of anastomotic leakage [84,85]. Butyrate controls the function of regulatory T cells in a microbe-associated context [86] and suppresses inflammation via nuclear factor kappa-light-chain-enhancer of activated B cells (NF-kB) signaling [87]. It also stabilizes the hypoxia inducible factor involved in the augmentation of the barrier function [88]. This meta-analysis shows that the concentrations of acetic, butyric, and propionic acids were elevated in patients supplemented with probiotics. Surprisingly, a meta-regression indicated that the longer duration of probiotic intervention, the smaller the effect size for propionic acid. This seems to be in contrast with mechanistic studies in which propionic acid was discovered to act as an immunosuppressant [89]. This metabolite possesses anti-fungal and anti-bacterial effects [90] responsible for the inhibition of invasion genes in *Salmonella typhimurium*. Propionic acid is able to diminish the synthesis of eicosanoids via lowering the activity of cyclooxygenase [91,92]. Although the acid may inhibit mitogen-activating lymphocytes proliferation, different studies found that the inhibitory effects may be positively correlated with its concentration [93–95]. The discrepancies between concentrations inside and outside the visceral compartment may at least partly explain the observed results. It should be pointed out that this data was extracted from four studies, so the results need to be interpreted with caution [40,44,55,67]. More studies evaluating SCFAs concentration in surgical patients are needed to confirm this finding.

It was also found that in patients supplemented with pro-/synbiotics, the concentration of CRP and IL-6 were significantly decreased in comparison to non-treated patients. As antigens flow through the disrupted intestinal barrier, the activation of the immune response in *lamina propria* and the production of inflammatory mediators take place. IL-6 and CRP were found to be at higher serum concentrations in patients with low DAO activity following the surgery [58]. This is crucial as DAO being produced at the tip of the villi reflects the integrity of the small intestine barrier. The enzyme serum concentration is of small bowel origin [96–98] and its activity was found to be diminished following major hepatectomy [40,58,67]. This study shows that pro-/synbiotic intervention significantly lowered the concentration of IL-6 and CRP. The body of evidence states that IL-6 signaling plays a pivotal role in epithelial stem cells and intraepithelial lymphocytes proliferation and may be involved in wound healing [99]. Recently, Kuhn et al. [100] discovered that intraepithelial lymphocyte-derived IL-6 served positively toward barrier function via claudin-1 protein expression and increased mucus thickness [100]. Although CRP production in hepatocytes was found not to be influenced by medical therapies [101], the most recent meta-analysis by Mazidi et al. proved that probiotic administration may significantly reduce serum CRP with a weighted mean difference (WMD) of -1.35 mg/L; however, that study was not limited to surgical patients only [102].

Gut-derived bacteremia is a result of elevated intestinal permeability which further makes antigens flow through the epithelium, elevate serum inflammatory mediators [58], and enhance bacterial translocation to mesenteric lymph nodes after interventions such as a hepatectomy [103] and an esophagectomy [104]. In this study, it was not possible to demonstrate that microbial intervention diminished the risk of bacterial translocation. However, studies evaluating the bacterial translocation were based on culture-based methods and such methodology was valid to evaluate the presence of well-cultured bacteria only [66]. Culture-independent molecular techniques and sophisticated bioinformatic analyses should therefore be implemented in future trials to evaluate bacterial translocation and assess the functionality of translocated microorganisms in patients in perioperative periods.

This updated systematic review found that patients treated perioperatively with pro-/synbiotics had lower relative risk toward (i) abdominal distention, (ii) diarrhea, (iii) pneumonia, (iv) sepsis, (v) superficial incisional infection, (vi) urinary tract infection, (vii) duration of antibiotic therapy, (viii) duration of postoperative pyrexia, (ix) time of fluid introduction and (x) solid diet, and (xi) duration of hospital stay, and supports other observations [28,29,32].

This study also shows that biochemical parameters associated with the gut barrier were improved in patients treated with pro-/synbiotics, supporting the hypothesis that SSIs and SRCs are actually in large part sourced from the patient's own gut flora. This is in line with a recent SR by Lederer et al. [105] who reported that the gut microbiome was responsible for postoperative complications including anastomotic leakage and wound infection. The data was not robust enough to establish recommendations for the use of beneficial bacteria in SSIs/SRCs prevention. The limitations of the available data did not allow us to determine which probiotics strain is the optimal choice, particular clinical situations where they could prove beneficial, how long the intervention should last, and the optimal dose of the supplement. The study was unable to establish that synbiotics should be used first-line to reduce specific SSIs and SRCs, which contrasts with the network meta-analysis by Kasatpibal et al. [28]. Apart from different methodological approach, this study included more patients (2952 vs. 3028) but excluded studies in a non-English language that may partly explain the discrepancies. Therefore, on the basis of the results of this study, microbial supplements in general, without strain recommendation in perioperative period, could be advocated. Taking into account the documented stability and safety of probiotics available on the market, the findings could explain the lack of current implementation of probiotics/synbiotics into SSIs/SRCs prevention clinical guidelines. More high-quality studies are needed to draw detailed protocols to evaluate particular probiotic strains, optimal duration of their supplementation, objective outcomes measurements, and maybe even stratify by surgery types to understand the roles. Nevertheless, the evidence is strong to already support dietary supplementation with probiotics in patients undergoing major abdominal surgeries. This topic seems to be of high priority as Berrios-Torres et al. [4] in their recent Centers for Disease Control and Prevention Guideline for the Prevention of Surgical Site Infection stated that antimicrobial prophylaxis should be administered only when indicated based on published clinical practice guidelines. The evidence is mounting that the longer post-surgical antibiotic administration, the greater the frequency of SSIs [1]. Antibiotic administration was found to elevate the risk toward inflammatory disorders, predominantly due to commensal bacteria translocation through the gut barrier, thus disturbing the microecological niche within the gut [106]. Also, antibiotic gut decontamination may activate dormant spores, which consequently results in severe infectious complications [107]. Recently, the 6th National Audit Project of the Royal College of Anaesthetists reported antibiotic-induced life-threatening anaphylaxis as well [108]. However, one of the current widely agreed and recommended intervention to decrease the incidence of SSIs/SRCs is perioperative antibiotic administration.

Postsurgical complications (PSCs) are currently one of the most challenging health care issues worldwide [1,2]. Moreover, these unpredictable post-surgical events result in unscheduled readmissions, extended antibiotic therapy, and elevated mortality rate, but importantly generate additional costs of treatment. For example, Tanner et al., evaluated that in the U.K., SSIs secondary to colorectal surgery generated an extra cost of more than £10.000 with only 15% met in primary care [109]. More recently, Straatman et al. [110] pointed that in Netherlands, complications following major abdominal surgery may generate as much as 240% higher costs of treatment, depending on the clinical course of PSC. In the USA, the mean cost for a hospital stay was found to be approximately twice as high in patients with complications compared with those suffering from no PSCs. Consequently, total profit margin was estimated to be about 5.7% lower in patients with complications [111]. On the other hand, as reported by Keenan et al. [112], introducing a preventive strategy, e.g., SSI bundle in colorectal surgery, may significantly diminish the incidence of SSIs, and consequently, health care costs. As our paper provides evidence linking PSCs to host intestinal microenvironment, maintaining healthy microbiota—at least during the hospital stay—to reducing the incidence of these life-threatening events seems to be one of these cost-effective regimens [6–8]. Indeed, our study has shown that probiotic intervention significantly decreased the duration of antibiotic therapy (SMD: -0.597, 95% CI: -1.093, -0.10, $p = 0.018$) and overall length of hospital stay (SMD: -0.479, 95% CI: (-0.660, -0.297, $p = 0.0000002$). The reduction of these variables, together with the lowest incidence of PSCs reported in our study, extrapolate to a reduction in the cost of a patient's stay in a hospital. This is in line with the assumptions made recently by Wu et al. [34] who analyzed two studies of Liu et al. [50,51] and reported a lower hospital charge concerning patients receiving probiotics in comparison to the placebo groups. Finally, it was concluded [34] that probiotic prophylaxis in surgery wards may decrease the hospital costs.

Several limitations of this MA require underlining. These include (i) a small number of double-blind clinical trials; (ii) heterogeneous study aims, patient groups, intervention characteristics, and study targets; (iii) a limited number of reported outcomes; and (iv) meta-regression analyses were conducted only for exploratory reasons due to different subsets of patients and treatments. The overall moderate quality of the studies may have significantly influenced the study outcomes. Nevertheless, despite these limitations, this is the first, comprehensive SR/MA that shows a beneficial effect of pro-/synbiotics in reducing the incidence of SSIs/SRCs likely via modulating gut related immune response and production of SCFA.

In conclusion, our MA supports that pro-/synbiotics as a class can have an effect on the outcome, but more granular data on particular types and concentrations cannot be recommended. The effect on SSIs/SRCs is complex, including the modulation of CRP and WBC counts, as well as alteration of SCFAs synthesis and others that need further clarification. More high-quality studies are needed to draw detailed protocols to evaluate particular probiotic strains and optimal duration of their supplementation in patients undergoing surgical procedures. However, the evidence presented in this systematic review strongly supports that dietary supplementation with probiotics in patients undergoing major abdominal surgeries has a beneficial effect.

Supplementary Materials: The following are available online at http://www.mdpi.com/2077-0383/7/12/556/s1. Figure S1: The effect size (risk ratio) for the overall effects of probiotics in the prevention of pneumonia. Figure S2: The effect size (risk ratio) for the overall effects of probiotics in the prevention of surgical site infection. Table S1: The efficacy of probiotics to counteract surgery related complications (SRCs). Table S2: Risk of bias assessment.

Author Contributions: Conceptualization, K.S.-Ż., M.K., I.Ł., and W.M.; Data curation, K.S.-Ż., M.K., L.F.L., A.K., and W.M.; Formal analysis, K.S.-Ż., M.K., I.Ł., A.M., D.M., and W.M.; Investigation, K.S.-Ż., M.K., I.Ł., L.F.L., A.K., A.M., D.M., and W.M.; Methodology, K.S.-Ż.; Project administration, K.S.-Ż.; Software, M.K.; Supervision, I.Ł., L.F.L., A.K., and W.M.; Visualization, M.K.; Writing original draft, K.S.-Ż.; Writing review and editing, K.S.-Ż., M.K., I.Ł., L.F.L., A.K., A.M., D.M., and W.M.

Funding: This research received no external funding.

Conflicts of Interest: Igor Loniewski and Wojciech Marlicz are cofounders and shareholders at Sanprobi company, a producer and distributor of probiotics. Karolina Skonieczna-Żydecka received honoraria from a probiotic company. Other authors have nothing to disclose.

Data Source: Data presented in this manuscript were discussed in the presidential choice session of the WGO-GAT International Conference, Bangkok, 5–8 Dec 2018.

References

1. GlobalSurg Collaborative. Surgical site infection after gastrointestinal surgery in high-income, middle-income, and low-income countries: A prospective, international, multicentre cohort study. *Lancet Infect. Dis.* **2018**, *18*, 516–525. [CrossRef]
2. Guyton, K.; Alverdy, J.C. The gut microbiota and gastrointestinal surgery. *Nat. Rev. Gastroenterol. Hepatol.* **2017**, *14*, 43–54. [CrossRef] [PubMed]
3. WHO. Global Guidelines on the Prevention of Surgical Site Infection. Available online: http://www.who.in t/gpsc/ssi-guidelines/en/ (accessed on 7 September 2018).
4. Berríos-Torres, S.I.; Umscheid, C.A.; Bratzler, D.W.; Leas, B.; Stone, E.C.; Kelz, R.R.; Reinke, C.E.; Morgan, S.; Solomkin, J.S.; Mazuski, J.E.; et al. Centers for Disease Control and Prevention Guideline for the Prevention of Surgical Site Infection, 2017. *JAMA Surg.* **2017**, *152*, 784–791. [CrossRef]
5. Ban, K.A.; Minei, J.P.; Laronga, C.; Harbrecht, B.G.; Jensen, E.H.; Fry, D.E.; Itani, K.M.F.; Dellinger, E.P.; Ko, C.Y.; Duane, T.M. American College of Surgeons and Surgical Infection Society: Surgical Site Infection Guidelines, 2016 Update. *J. Am. Coll. Surg.* **2017**, *224*, 59–74. [CrossRef] [PubMed]
6. Stone, P.W.; Braccia, D.; Larson, E. Systematic review of economic analyses of health care-associated infections. *Am. J. Infect. Control* **2005**, *33*, 501–509. [CrossRef] [PubMed]

7. *WHO Guidelines for Safe Surgery 2009: Safe Surgery Saves Lives*; WHO Guidelines Approved by the Guidelines Review Committee; World Health Organization: Geneva, Switzerland, 2009; ISBN 978-92-4-159855-2.
8. Nguyen, N.; Yegiyants, S.; Kaloostian, C.; Abbas, M.A.; Difronzo, L.A. The Surgical Care Improvement project (SCIP) initiative to reduce infection in elective colorectal surgery: Which performance measures affect outcome? *Am. Surg.* **2008**, *74*, 1012–1016.
9. Altemeier, W.A.; Culbertson, W.R.; Hummel, R.P. Surgical considerations of endogenous infections—Sources, types, and methods of control. *Surg. Clin. N. Am.* **1968**, *48*, 227–240. [CrossRef]
10. Brial, F.; Le Lay, A.; Dumas, M.-E.; Gauguier, D. Implication of gut microbiota metabolites in cardiovascular and metabolic diseases. *Cell. Mol. Life Sci.* **2018**, *75*, 3977–3990. [CrossRef]
11. Marlicz, W.; Yung, D.E.; Skonieczna-Żydecka, K.; Loniewski, I.; van Hemert, S.; Loniewska, B.; Koulaouzidis, A. From clinical uncertainties to precision medicine: The emerging role of the gut barrier and microbiome in small bowel functional diseases. *Expert Rev. Gastroenterol. Hepatol.* **2017**, *11*, 961–978. [CrossRef]
12. Clemente, J.C.; Manasson, J.; Scher, J.U. The role of the gut microbiome in systemic inflammatory disease. *BMJ* **2018**, *360*, j5145. [CrossRef]
13. Spadoni, I.; Zagato, E.; Bertocchi, A.; Paolinelli, R.; Hot, E.; Sabatino, A.D.; Caprioli, F.; Bottiglieri, L.; Oldani, A.; Viale, G.; et al. A gut-vascular barrier controls the systemic dissemination of bacteria. *Science* **2015**, *350*, 830–834. [CrossRef] [PubMed]
14. Foster, J.A.; Rinaman, L.; Cryan, J.F. Stress & the gut-brain axis: Regulation by the microbiome. *Neurobiol. Stress* **2017**, *7*, 124–136. [PubMed]
15. Sonnenburg, J.L.; Bäckhed, F. Diet-microbiota interactions as moderators of human metabolism. *Nature* **2016**, *535*, 56–64. [CrossRef] [PubMed]
16. David, L.A.; Materna, A.C.; Friedman, J.; Campos-Baptista, M.I.; Blackburn, M.C.; Perrotta, A.; Erdman, S.E.; Alm, E.J. Host lifestyle affects human microbiota on daily timescales. *Genome Biol.* **2014**, *15*, R89. [CrossRef] [PubMed]
17. Scarborough, J.E.; Mantyh, C.R.; Sun, Z.; Migaly, J. Combined Mechanical and Oral Antibiotic Bowel Preparation Reduces Incisional Surgical Site Infection and Anastomotic Leak Rates after Elective Colorectal Resection: An Analysis of Colectomy-Targeted ACS NSQIP. *Ann. Surg.* **2015**, *262*, 331–337. [CrossRef] [PubMed]
18. Bretagnol, F.; Panis, Y.; Rullier, E.; Rouanet, P.; Berdah, S.; Dousset, B.; Portier, G.; Benoist, S.; Chipponi, J.; Vicaut, E.; et al. Rectal cancer surgery with or without bowel preparation: The French GRECCAR III multicenter single-blinded randomized trial. *Ann. Surg.* **2010**, *252*, 863–868. [CrossRef] [PubMed]
19. Bachmann, R.; Leonard, D.; Delzenne, N.; Kartheuser, A.; Cani, P.D. Novel insight into the role of microbiota in colorectal surgery. *Gut* **2017**, *66*, 738–749. [CrossRef]
20. Hartman, A.L.; Lough, D.M.; Barupal, D.K.; Fiehn, O.; Fishbein, T.; Zasloff, M.; Eisen, J.A. Human gut microbiome adopts an alternative state following small bowel transplantation. *Proc. Natl. Acad. Sci. USA* **2009**, *106*, 17187–17192. [CrossRef]
21. Shimizu, K.; Ogura, H.; Asahara, T.; Nomoto, K.; Matsushima, A.; Hayakawa, K.; Ikegawa, H.; Tasaki, O.; Kuwagata, Y.; Shimazu, T. Gut microbiota and environment in patients with major burns—A preliminary report. *Burns* **2015**, *41*, e28–e33. [CrossRef]
22. Earley, Z.M.; Akhtar, S.; Green, S.J.; Naqib, A.; Khan, O.; Cannon, A.R.; Hammer, A.M.; Morris, N.L.; Li, X.; Eberhardt, J.M.; et al. Burn Injury Alters the Intestinal Microbiome and Increases Gut Permeability and Bacterial Translocation. *PLoS ONE* **2015**, *10*, e0129996. [CrossRef]
23. Wang, F.; Li, Q.; He, Q.; Geng, Y.; Tang, C.; Wang, C.; Li, J. Temporal variations of the ileal microbiota in intestinal ischemia and reperfusion. *Shock* **2013**, *39*, 96–103. [CrossRef] [PubMed]
24. Gralka, E.; Luchinat, C.; Tenori, L.; Ernst, B.; Thurnheer, M.; Schultes, B. Metabolomic fingerprint of severe obesity is dynamically affected by bariatric surgery in a procedure-dependent manner. *Am. J. Clin. Nutr.* **2015**, *102*, 1313–1322. [CrossRef] [PubMed]
25. Fan, P.; Li, L.; Rezaei, A.; Eslamfam, S.; Che, D.; Ma, X. Metabolites of Dietary Protein and Peptides by Intestinal Microbes and their Impacts on Gut. *Curr. Protein Pept. Sci.* **2015**, *16*, 646–654. [CrossRef] [PubMed]
26. Ojima, M.; Motooka, D.; Shimizu, K.; Gotoh, K.; Shintani, A.; Yoshiya, K.; Nakamura, S.; Ogura, H.; Iida, T.; Shimazu, T. Metagenomic Analysis Reveals Dynamic Changes of Whole Gut Microbiota in the Acute Phase of Intensive Care Unit Patients. *Dig. Dis. Sci.* **2016**, *61*, 1628–1634. [CrossRef] [PubMed]

27. Zaborin, A.; Smith, D.; Garfield, K.; Quensen, J.; Shakhsheer, B.; Kade, M.; Tirrell, M.; Tiedje, J.; Gilbert, J.A.; Zaborina, O.; et al. Membership and Behavior of Ultra-Low-Diversity Pathogen Communities Present in the Gut of Humans during Prolonged Critical Illness. *mBio* **2014**, *5*, e01361-14. [CrossRef] [PubMed]
28. Kasatpibal, N.; Whitney, J.D.; Saokaew, S.; Kengkla, K.; Heitkemper, M.M.; Apisarnthanarak, A. Effectiveness of Probiotic, Prebiotic, and Synbiotic Therapies in Reducing Postoperative Complications: A Systematic Review and Network Meta-analysis. *Clin. Infect. Dis.* **2017**, *64*, S153–S160. [CrossRef] [PubMed]
29. Wu, X.-D.; Xu, W.; Liu, M.-M.; Hu, K.-J.; Sun, Y.-Y.; Yang, X.-F.; Zhu, G.-Q.; Wang, Z.-W.; Huang, W. Efficacy of prophylactic probiotics in combination with antibiotics versus antibiotics alone for colorectal surgery: A meta-analysis of randomized controlled trials. *J. Surg. Oncol.* **2018**, *117*, 1394–1404. [CrossRef]
30. Arumugam, S.; Lau, C.S.M.; Chamberlain, R.S. Probiotics and Synbiotics Decrease Postoperative Sepsis in Elective Gastrointestinal Surgical Patients: A Meta-Analysis. *J. Gastrointest. Surg.* **2016**, *20*, 1123–1131. [CrossRef]
31. Yang, Z.; Wu, Q.; Liu, Y.; Fan, D. Effect of Perioperative Probiotics and Synbiotics on Postoperative Infections after Gastrointestinal Surgery: A Systematic Review with Meta-Analysis. *JPEN J. Parenter. Enter. Nutr.* **2017**, *41*, 1051–1062. [CrossRef]
32. Lytvyn, L.; Quach, K.; Banfield, L.; Johnston, B.C.; Mertz, D. Probiotics and synbiotics for the prevention of postoperative infections following abdominal surgery: A systematic review and meta-analysis of randomized controlled trials. *J. Hosp. Infect.* **2016**, *92*, 130–139. [CrossRef]
33. Sawas, T.; Al Halabi, S.; Hernaez, R.; Carey, W.D.; Cho, W.K. Patients Receiving Prebiotics and Probiotics Before Liver Transplantation Develop Fewer Infections Than Controls: A Systematic Review and Meta-Analysis. *Clin. Gastroenterol. Hepatol.* **2015**, *13*, 1567–1574. [CrossRef] [PubMed]
34. Wu, X.-D.; Liu, M.-M.; Liang, X.; Hu, N.; Huang, W. Effects of perioperative supplementation with pro-/synbiotics on clinical outcomes in surgical patients: A meta-analysis with trial sequential analysis of randomized controlled trials. *Clin. Nutr.* **2018**, *37*, 505–515. [CrossRef] [PubMed]
35. Suez, J.; Zmora, N.; Zilberman-Schapira, G.; Mor, U.; Dori-Bachash, M.; Bashiardes, S.; Zur, M.; Regev-Lehavi, D.; Ben-Zeev Brik, R.; Federici, S.; et al. Post-Antibiotic Gut Mucosal Microbiome Reconstitution Is Impaired by Probiotics and Improved by Autologous FMT. *Cell* **2018**, *174*, 1406–1423.e16. [CrossRef] [PubMed]
36. Shamseer, L.; Moher, D.; Clarke, M.; Ghersi, D.; Liberati, A.; Petticrew, M.; Shekelle, P.; Stewart, L.A.; PRISMA-P Group. Preferred reporting items for systematic review and meta-analysis protocols (PRISMA-P) 2015: Elaboration and explanation. *BMJ* **2015**, *350*, g7647. [CrossRef] [PubMed]
37. DerSimonian, R.; Laird, N. Meta-analysis in clinical trials. *Control. Clin. Trials* **1986**, *7*, 177–188. [CrossRef]
38. Higgins, J.P.T.; Altman, D.G.; Gøtzsche, P.C.; Jüni, P.; Moher, D.; Oxman, A.D.; Savović, J.; Schulz, K.F.; Weeks, L.; Sterne, J.A.C. The Cochrane Collaboration's tool for assessing risk of bias in randomised trials. *BMJ* **2011**, *343*, d5928. [CrossRef]
39. Yang, Y.; Xia, Y.; Chen, H.; Hong, L.; Feng, J.; Yang, J.; Yang, Z.; Shi, C.; Wu, W.; Gao, R.; et al. The effect of perioperative probiotics treatment for colorectal cancer: Short-term outcomes of a randomized controlled trial. *Oncotarget* **2016**, *7*, 8432–8440. [CrossRef]
40. Kanazawa, H.; Nagino, M.; Kamiya, S.; Komatsu, S.; Mayumi, T.; Takagi, K.; Asahara, T.; Nomoto, K.; Tanaka, R.; Nimura, Y. Synbiotics reduce postoperative infectious complications: A randomized controlled trial in biliary cancer patients undergoing hepatectomy. *Langenbeck's Arch. Surg.* **2005**, *390*, 104–113. [CrossRef]
41. Aisu, N.; Tanimura, S.; Yamashita, Y.; Yamashita, K.; Maki, K.; Yoshida, Y.; Sasaki, T.; Takeno, S.; Hoshino, S. Impact of perioperative probiotic treatment for surgical site infections in patients with colorectal cancer. *Exp. Ther. Med.* **2015**, *10*, 966–972. [CrossRef]
42. Liu, Z.; Qin, H.; Yang, Z.; Xia, Y.; Liu, W.; Yang, J.; Jiang, Y.; Zhang, H.; Yang, Z.; Wang, Y.; et al. Randomised clinical trial: The effects of perioperative probiotic treatment on barrier function and post-operative infectious complications in colorectal cancer surgery—A double-blind study: Randomised clinical trial: Perioperative probiotics on colon cancer. *Aliment. Pharmacol. Ther.* **2011**, *33*, 50–63.
43. Eguchi, S.; Takatsuki, M.; Hidaka, M.; Soyama, A.; Ichikawa, T.; Kanematsu, T. Perioperative synbiotic treatment to prevent infectious complications in patients after elective living donor liver transplantation: A prospective randomized study. *Am. J. Surg.* **2011**, *201*, 498–502. [CrossRef] [PubMed]

44. Komatsu, S.; Sakamoto, E.; Norimizu, S.; Shingu, Y.; Asahara, T.; Nomoto, K.; Nagino, M. Efficacy of perioperative synbiotics treatment for the prevention of surgical site infection after laparoscopic colorectal surgery: A randomized controlled trial. *Surg. Today* **2016**, *46*, 479–490. [CrossRef] [PubMed]
45. Anderson, A.D.G. Randomised clinical trial of synbiotic therapy in elective surgical patients. *Gut* **2004**, *53*, 241–245. [CrossRef] [PubMed]
46. Diepenhorst, G.M.P.; van Ruler, O.; Besselink, M.G.H.; van Santvoort, H.C.; Wijnandts, P.R.; Renooij, W.; Gouma, D.J.; Gooszen, H.G.; Boermeester, M.A. Influence of prophylactic probiotics and selective decontamination on bacterial translocation in patients undergoing pancreatic surgery: A randomized controlled trial. *Shock* **2011**, *35*, 9–16. [CrossRef] [PubMed]
47. Flesch, A.T.; Tonial, S.T.; Contu, P.D.C.; Damin, D.C. Perioperative synbiotics administration decreases postoperative infections in patients with colorectal cancer: A randomized, double-blind clinical trial. *Rev. Col. Bras. Cir.* **2017**, *44*, 567–573. [CrossRef] [PubMed]
48. Horvat, M.; Krebs, B.; Potrč, S.; Ivanecz, A.; Kompan, L. Preoperative synbiotic bowel conditioning for elective colorectal surgery. *Wien. Klin. Wochenschr.* **2010**, *122*, 26–30. [CrossRef]
49. Kotzampassi, K.; Stavrou, G.; Damoraki, G.; Georgitsi, M.; Basdanis, G.; Tsaousi, G.; Giamarellos-Bourboulis, E.J. A Four-Probiotics Regimen Reduces Postoperative Complications after Colorectal Surgery: A Randomized, Double-Blind, Placebo-Controlled Study. *World J. Surg.* **2015**, *39*, 2776–2783. [CrossRef] [PubMed]
50. Liu, Z.-H.; Huang, M.-J.; Zhang, X.-W.; Wang, L.; Huang, N.-Q.; Peng, H.; Lan, P.; Peng, J.-S.; Yang, Z.; Xia, Y.; et al. The effects of perioperative probiotic treatment on serum zonulin concentration and subsequent postoperative infectious complications after colorectal cancer surgery: A double-center and double-blind randomized clinical trial. *Am. J. Clin. Nutr.* **2013**, *97*, 117–126. [CrossRef]
51. Liu, Z.; Li, C.; Huang, M.; Tong, C.; Zhang, X.; Wang, L.; Peng, H.; Lan, P.; Zhang, P.; Huang, N.; et al. Positive regulatory effects of perioperative probiotic treatment on postoperative liver complications after colorectal liver metastases surgery: A double-center and double-blind randomized clinical trial. *BMC Gastroenterol.* **2015**, *15*, 34. [CrossRef]
52. Mangell, P.; Thorlacius, H.; Syk, I.; Ahrné, S.; Molin, G.; Olsson, C.; Jeppsson, B. Lactobacillus plantarum 299v Does Not Reduce Enteric Bacteria or Bacterial Translocation in Patients Undergoing Colon Resection. *Dig. Dis. Sci.* **2012**, *57*, 1915–1924. [CrossRef]
53. McNaught, C.E. A prospective randomised study of the probiotic Lactobacillus plantarum 299V on indices of gut barrier function in elective surgical patients. *Gut* **2002**, *51*, 827–831. [CrossRef] [PubMed]
54. Nomura, T.; Tsuchiya, Y.; Nashimoto, A.; Yabusaki, H.; Takii, Y.; Nakagawa, S.; Sato, N.; Kanbayashi, C.; Tanaka, O. Probiotics reduce infectious complications after pancreaticoduodenectomy. *Hepatogastroenterology* **2007**, *54*, 661–663. [PubMed]
55. Okazaki, M.; Matsukuma, S.; Suto, R.; Miyazaki, K.; Hidaka, M.; Matsuo, M.; Noshima, S.; Zempo, N.; Asahara, T.; Nomoto, K. Perioperative synbiotic therapy in elderly patients undergoing gastroenterological surgery: A prospective, randomized control trial. *Nutrition* **2013**, *29*, 1224–1230. [CrossRef] [PubMed]
56. Zhang, J.-W.; Du, P.; Yang, B.-R.; Gao, J.; Fang, W.-J.; Ying, C.-M. Preoperative Probiotics Decrease Postoperative Infectious Complications of Colorectal Cancer. *Am. J. Med. Sci.* **2012**, *343*, 199–205. [CrossRef] [PubMed]
57. Yokoyama, Y.; Nishigaki, E.; Abe, T.; Fukaya, M.; Asahara, T.; Nomoto, K.; Nagino, M. Randomized clinical trial of the effect of perioperative synbiotics *versus* no synbiotics on bacterial translocation after oesophagectomy: Synbiotic treatment for patients who undergo oesophagectomy. *Br. J. Surg.* **2014**, *101*, 189–199. [CrossRef] [PubMed]
58. Usami, M.; Miyoshi, M.; Kanbara, Y.; Aoyama, M.; Sakaki, H.; Shuno, K.; Hirata, K.; Takahashi, M.; Ueno, K.; Tabata, S.; et al. Effects of Perioperative Synbiotic Treatment on Infectious Complications, Intestinal Integrity, and Fecal Flora and Organic Acids in Hepatic Surgery with or without Cirrhosis. *J. Parenter. Enter. Nutr.* **2011**, *35*, 317–328. [CrossRef] [PubMed]
59. Tanaka, K.; Yano, M.; Motoori, M.; Kishi, K.; Miyashiro, I.; Ohue, M.; Ohigashi, H.; Asahara, T.; Nomoto, K.; Ishikawa, O. Impact of perioperative administration of synbiotics in patients with esophageal cancer undergoing esophagectomy: A prospective randomized controlled trial. *Surgery* **2012**, *152*, 832–842. [CrossRef] [PubMed]

60. Sommacal, H.M.; Bersch, V.P.; Vitola, S.P.; Osvaldt, A.B. Perioperative synbiotics decrease postoperative complications in periampullary neoplasms: A randomized, double-blind clinical trial. *Nutr. Cancer* **2015**, *67*, 457–462. [CrossRef]
61. Sadahiro, S.; Suzuki, T.; Tanaka, A.; Okada, K.; Kamata, H.; Ozaki, T.; Koga, Y. Comparison between oral antibiotics and probiotics as bowel preparation for elective colon cancer surgery to prevent infection: Prospective randomized trial. *Surgery* **2014**, *155*, 493–503. [CrossRef]
62. Reddy, B.S.; MacFie, J.; Gatt, M.; Larsen, C.N.; Jensen, S.S.; Leser, T.D. Randomized clinical trial of effect of synbiotics, neomycin and mechanical bowel preparation on intestinal barrier function in patients undergoing colectomy. *Br. J. Surgery* **2007**, *94*, 546–554. [CrossRef]
63. Rammohan, A.; Sathyanesan, J.; Rajendran, K.; Pitchaimuthu, A.; Perumal, S.K.; Balaraman, K.; Ramasamy, R.; Palaniappan, R.; Govindan, M. Synbiotics in Surgery for Chronic Pancreatitis: Are They Truly Effective? A Single-blind Prospective Randomized Control Trial. *Ann. Surg.* **2015**, *262*, 31–37. [CrossRef] [PubMed]
64. Grąt, M.; Wronka, K.M.; Lewandowski, Z.; Grąt, K.; Krasnodębski, M.; Stypułkowski, J.; Hołówko, W.; Masior, Ł.; Kosińska, I.; Wasilewicz, M.; et al. Effects of continuous use of probiotics before liver transplantation: A randomized, double-blind, placebo-controlled trial. *Clin. Nutr.* **2017**, *36*, 1530–1539. [CrossRef] [PubMed]
65. Mizuta, M.; Endo, I.; Yamamoto, S.; Inokawa, H.; Kubo, M.; Udaka, T.; Sogabe, O.; Maeda, H.; Shirakawa, K.; Okazaki, E.; et al. Perioperative supplementation with bifidobacteria improves postoperative nutritional recovery, inflammatory response, and fecal microbiota in patients undergoing colorectal surgery: A prospective, randomized clinical trial. *Biosci. Microbiota Food Health* **2016**, *35*, 77–87. [CrossRef] [PubMed]
66. Yokoyama, Y.; Asahara, T.; Nomoto, K.; Nagino, M. Effects of Synbiotics to Prevent Postoperative Infectious Complications in Highly Invasive Abdominal Surgery. *Ann. Nutr. Metab.* **2017**, *71*, 23–30. [CrossRef]
67. Sugawara, G.; Nagino, M.; Nishio, H.; Ebata, T.; Takagi, K.; Asahara, T.; Nomoto, K.; Nimura, Y. Perioperative Synbiotic Treatment to Prevent Postoperative Infectious Complications in Biliary Cancer Surgery: A Randomized Controlled Trial. *Ann. Surg.* **2006**, *244*, 706–714. [CrossRef] [PubMed]
68. Zhang, Y.; Chen, J.; Wu, J.; Chalson, H.; Merigan, L.; Mitchell, A. Probiotic use in preventing postoperative infection in liver transplant patients. *Hepatobiliary Surg. Nutr.* **2013**, *2*, 6.
69. Rayes, N.; Hansen, S.; Seehofer, D.; Müller, A.R.; Serke, S.; Bengmark, S.; Neuhaus, P. Early enteral supply of fiber and Lactobacilli versus conventional nutrition: A controlled trial in patients with major abdominal surgery. *Nutrition* **2002**, *18*, 609–615. [CrossRef]
70. Rayes, N.; Seehofer, D.; Hansen, S.; Boucsein, K.; Müller, A.R.; Serke, S.; Bengmark, S.; Neuhaus, P. Early enteral supply of lactobacillus and fiber versus selective bowel decontamination: A controlled trial in liver transplant recipients. *Transplantation* **2002**, *74*, 123–128. [CrossRef]
71. Rayes, N.; Seehofer, D.; Theruvath, T.; Schiller, R.A.; Langrehr, J.M.; Jonas, S.; Bengmark, S.; Neuhaus, P. Supply of Pre- and Probiotics Reduces Bacterial Infection Rates After Liver Transplantation-A Randomized, Double-Blind Trial. *Am. J. Transplant.* **2005**, *5*, 125–130. [CrossRef]
72. Rayes, N.; Seehofer, D.; Theruvath, T.; Mogl, M.; Langrehr, J.M.; Nüssler, N.C.; Bengmark, S.; Neuhaus, P. Effect of Enteral Nutrition and Synbiotics on Bacterial Infection Rates After Pylorus-preserving Pancreatoduodenectomy: A Randomized, Double-blind Trial. *Ann. Surg.* **2007**, *246*, 36–41. [CrossRef]
73. Rayes, N.; Pilarski, T.; Stockmann, M.; Bengmark, S.; Neuhaus, P.; Seehofer, D. Effect of pre- and probiotics on liver regeneration after resection: A randomised, double-blind pilot study. *Benef. Microbes* **2012**, *3*, 237–244. [CrossRef] [PubMed]
74. Horvath, A.; Leber, B.; Schmerboeck, B.; Tawdrous, M.; Zettel, G.; Hartl, A.; Madl, T.; Stryeck, S.; Fuchs, D.; Lemesch, S.; et al. Randomised clinical trial: The effects of a multispecies probiotic vs. placebo on innate immune function, bacterial translocation and gut permeability in patients with cirrhosis. *Aliment. Pharmacol. Ther.* **2016**, *44*, 926–935. [CrossRef] [PubMed]
75. Komatsu, S.; Yokoyama, Y.; Nagino, M. Gut microbiota and bacterial translocation in digestive surgery: The impact of probiotics. *Langenbeck's Arch. Surg.* **2017**, *402*, 401–416. [CrossRef] [PubMed]
76. Lynch, S.V.; Pedersen, O. The Human Intestinal Microbiome in Health and Disease. *N. Engl. J. Med.* **2016**, *375*, 2369–2379. [CrossRef] [PubMed]
77. Rizzatti, G.; Lopetuso, L.R.; Gibiino, G.; Binda, C.; Gasbarrini, A. Proteobacteria: A Common Factor in Human Diseases. Available online: https://www.hindawi.com/journals/bmri/2017/9351507/ (accessed on 8 September 2018).

78. Lupp, C.; Robertson, M.L.; Wickham, M.E.; Sekirov, I.; Champion, O.L.; Gaynor, E.C.; Finlay, B.B. Host-mediated inflammation disrupts the intestinal microbiota and promotes the overgrowth of Enterobacteriaceae. *Cell Host Microbe* **2007**, *2*, 119–129. [CrossRef] [PubMed]
79. Hiippala, K.; Jouhten, H.; Ronkainen, A.; Hartikainen, A.; Kainulainen, V.; Jalanka, J.; Satokari, R. The Potential of Gut Commensals in Reinforcing Intestinal Barrier Function and Alleviating Inflammation. *Nutrients* **2018**, *10*, 988. [CrossRef]
80. Fukuda, S.; Toh, H.; Hase, K.; Oshima, K.; Nakanishi, Y.; Yoshimura, K.; Tobe, T.; Clarke, J.M.; Topping, D.L.; Suzuki, T.; et al. Bifidobacteria can protect from enteropathogenic infection through production of acetate. *Nature* **2011**, *469*, 543–547. [CrossRef]
81. Canani, R.B.; Costanzo, M.D.; Leone, L.; Pedata, M.; Meli, R.; Calignano, A. Potential beneficial effects of butyrate in intestinal and extraintestinal diseases. *World J. Gastroenterol.* **2011**, *17*, 1519–1528. [CrossRef]
82. Hayakawa, M.; Asahara, T.; Henzan, N.; Murakami, H.; Yamamoto, H.; Mukai, N.; Minami, Y.; Sugano, M.; Kubota, N.; Uegaki, S.; et al. Dramatic changes of the gut flora immediately after severe and sudden insults. *Dig. Dis. Sci.* **2011**, *56*, 2361–2365. [CrossRef]
83. Gantois, I.; Ducatelle, R.; Pasmans, F.; Haesebrouck, F.; Hautefort, I.; Thompson, A.; Hinton, J.C.; Van Immerseel, F. Butyrate specifically down-regulates salmonella pathogenicity island 1 gene expression. *Appl. Environ. Microbiol.* **2006**, *72*, 946–949. [CrossRef]
84. Seal, J.B.; Morowitz, M.; Zaborina, O.; An, G.; Alverdy, J.C. The molecular Koch's postulates and surgical infection: A view forward. *Surgery* **2010**, *147*, 757–765. [CrossRef] [PubMed]
85. Olivas, A.D.; Shogan, B.D.; Valuckaite, V.; Zaborin, A.; Belogortseva, N.; Musch, M.; Meyer, F.; Trimble, W.L.; An, G.; Gilbert, J.; et al. Intestinal tissues induce an SNP mutation in Pseudomonas aeruginosa that enhances its virulence: Possible role in anastomotic leak. *PLoS ONE* **2012**, *7*, e44326. [CrossRef] [PubMed]
86. Furusawa, Y.; Obata, Y.; Fukuda, S.; Endo, T.A.; Nakato, G.; Takahashi, D.; Nakanishi, Y.; Uetake, C.; Kato, K.; Kato, T.; et al. Commensal microbe-derived butyrate induces the differentiation of colonic regulatory T cells. *Nature* **2013**, *504*, 446–450. [CrossRef] [PubMed]
87. Inan, M.S.; Rasoulpour, R.J.; Yin, L.; Hubbard, A.K.; Rosenberg, D.W.; Giardina, C. The luminal short-chain fatty acid butyrate modulates NF-kappaB activity in a human colonic epithelial cell line. *Gastroenterology* **2000**, *118*, 724–734. [CrossRef]
88. Kelly, C.J.; Zheng, L.; Campbell, E.L.; Saeedi, B.; Scholz, C.C.; Bayless, A.J.; Wilson, K.E.; Glover, L.E.; Kominsky, D.J.; Magnuson, A.; et al. Crosstalk between Microbiota-Derived Short-Chain Fatty Acids and Intestinal Epithelial HIF Augments Tissue Barrier Function. *Cell Host Microbe* **2015**, *17*, 662–671. [CrossRef] [PubMed]
89. Al-Lahham, S.H.; Peppelenbosch, M.P.; Roelofsen, H.; Vonk, R.J.; Venema, K. Biological effects of propionic acid in humans; metabolism, potential applications and underlying mechanisms. *Biochim. Biophys. Acta (BBA)-Mol. Cell Biol. Lipids* **2010**, *1801*, 1175–1183. [CrossRef] [PubMed]
90. Lawhon, S.D.; Maurer, R.; Suyemoto, M.; Altier, C. Intestinal short-chain fatty acids alter Salmonella typhimurium invasion gene expression and virulence through BarA/SirA. *Mol. Microbiol.* **2002**, *46*, 1451–1464. [CrossRef]
91. Dannhardt, G.; Lehr, M. Nonsteriodal Antiinflammatory Agents, XVII: Inhibition of Bovine Cyclooxygenase and 5-Lipoxygenase by N-Alkyldiphenyl-pyrrolyl Acetic and Propionic Acid Derivatives. *Arch. Pharm.* **1993**, *326*, 157–162. [CrossRef]
92. Bos, C.L.; Richel, D.J.; Ritsema, T.; Peppelenbosch, M.P.; Versteeg, H.H. Prostanoids and prostanoid receptors in signal transduction. *Int. J. Biochem. Cell Biol.* **2004**, *36*, 1187–1205. [CrossRef]
93. Curi, R.; Bond, J.A.; Calder, P.C.; Newsholme, E.A. Propionate regulates lymphocyte proliferation and metabolism. *Gen. Pharmacol. Vasc. Syst.* **1993**, *24*, 591–597. [CrossRef]
94. Wajner, M.; Santos, K.D.; Schlottfeldt, J.L.; Rocha, M.P.; Wannmacher, C.M. Inhibition of mitogen-activated proliferation of human peripheral lymphocytes in vitro by propionic acid. *Clin. Sci.* **1999**, *96*, 99–103. [CrossRef] [PubMed]
95. Cavaglieri, C.R.; Nishiyama, A.; Fernandes, L.C.; Curi, R.; Miles, E.A.; Calder, P.C. Differential effects of short-chain fatty acids on proliferation and production of pro- and anti-inflammatory cytokines by cultured lymphocytes. *Life Sci.* **2003**, *73*, 1683–1690. [CrossRef]
96. Luk, G.D.; Bayless, T.M.; Baylin, S.B. Diamine oxidase (histaminase). A circulating marker for rat intestinal mucosal maturation and integrity. *J. Clin. Investig.* **1980**, *66*, 66–70. [CrossRef] [PubMed]

97. Buffoni, F. Histaminase and Related Amine Oxidases. *Pharmacol. Rev.* **1966**, *18*, 1163–1199. [PubMed]
98. Honzawa, Y.; Nakase, H.; Matsuura, M.; Chiba, T. Clinical significance of serum diamine oxidase activity in inflammatory bowel disease: Importance of evaluation of small intestinal permeability. *Inflamm. Bowel Dis.* **2011**, *17*, E23–25. [CrossRef] [PubMed]
99. Kuhn, K.A.; Manieri, N.A.; Liu, T.-C.; Stappenbeck, T.S. IL-6 Stimulates Intestinal Epithelial Proliferation and Repair after Injury. *PLoS ONE* **2014**, *9*, e114195. [CrossRef] [PubMed]
100. Kuhn, K.A.; Schulz, H.M.; Regner, E.H.; Severs, E.L.; Hendrickson, J.D.; Mehta, G.; Whitney, A.K.; Ir, D.; Ohri, N.; Robertson, C.E.; et al. Bacteroidales recruit IL-6-producing intraepithelial lymphocytes in the colon to promote barrier integrity. *Mucosal Immunol.* **2018**, *11*, 357–368. [CrossRef]
101. Henriksen, M.; Jahnsen, J.; Lygren, I.; Stray, N.; Sauar, J.; Vatn, M.H.; Moum, B.; IBSEN Study Group. C-reactive protein: A predictive factor and marker of inflammation in inflammatory bowel disease. Results from a prospective population-based study. *Gut* **2008**, *57*, 1518–1523. [CrossRef]
102. Mazidi, M.; Rezaie, P.; Ferns, G.A.; Vatanparast, H. Impact of Probiotic Administration on Serum C-Reactive Protein Concentrations: Systematic Review and Meta-Analysis of Randomized Control Trials. *Nutrients* **2017**, *9*, 20. [CrossRef]
103. Mizuno, T.; Yokoyama, Y.; Nishio, H.; Ebata, T.; Sugawara, G.; Asahara, T.; Nomoto, K.; Nagino, M. Intraoperative bacterial translocation detected by bacterium-specific ribosomal rna-targeted reverse-transcriptase polymerase chain reaction for the mesenteric lymph node strongly predicts postoperative infectious complications after major hepatectomy for biliary malignancies. *Ann. Surg.* **2010**, *252*, 1013–1019. [PubMed]
104. Nishigaki, E.; Abe, T.; Yokoyama, Y.; Fukaya, M.; Asahara, T.; Nomoto, K.; Nagino, M. The detection of intraoperative bacterial translocation in the mesenteric lymph nodes is useful in predicting patients at high risk for postoperative infectious complications after esophagectomy. *Ann. Surg.* **2014**, *259*, 477–484. [CrossRef] [PubMed]
105. Lederer, A.-K.; Pisarski, P.; Kousoulas, L.; Fichtner-Feigl, S.; Hess, C.; Huber, R. Postoperative changes of the microbiome: Are surgical complications related to the gut flora? A systematic review. *BMC Surg.* **2017**, *17*, 125. [CrossRef] [PubMed]
106. Knoop, K.A.; McDonald, K.G.; Kulkarni, D.H.; Newberry, R.D. Antibiotics promote inflammation through the translocation of native commensal colonic bacteria. *Gut* **2016**, *65*, 1100–1109. [CrossRef] [PubMed]
107. Britton, R.A.; Young, V.B. Role of the Intestinal Microbiota in Resistance to Colonization by Clostridium difficile. *Gastroenterology* **2014**, *146*, 1547–1553. [CrossRef] [PubMed]
108. NAP6 Report—The National Institute of Academic Anaesthesia. Available online: http://www.nationalauditprojects.org.uk/NAP6Report (accessed on 26 May 2018).
109. Tanner, J.; Khan, D.; Aplin, C.; Ball, J.; Thomas, M.; Bankart, J. Post-discharge surveillance to identify colorectal surgical site infection rates and related costs. *J. Hosp. Infect.* **2009**, *72*, 243–250. [CrossRef]
110. Straatman, J.; Cuesta, M.A.; De Lange-de Klerk, E.S.; Van Der Peet, D.L. Hospital Cost-Analysis of Complications after Major Abdominal Surgery. *DSU* **2015**, *32*, 150–156. [CrossRef]
111. Healy, M.A.; Mullard, A.J.; Campbell, D.A.; Dimick, J.B. Hospital and Payer Costs Associated with Surgical Complications. *JAMA Surg.* **2016**, *151*, 823–830. [CrossRef]
112. Keenan, J.E.; Speicher, P.J.; Thacker, J.K.M.; Walter, M.; Kuchibhatla, M.; Mantyh, C.R. The preventive surgical site infection bundle in colorectal surgery: An effective approach to surgical site infection reduction and health care cost savings. *JAMA Surg.* **2014**, *149*, 1045–1052. [CrossRef]

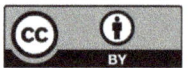

© 2018 by the authors. Licensee MDPI, Basel, Switzerland. This article is an open access article distributed under the terms and conditions of the Creative Commons Attribution (CC BY) license (http://creativecommons.org/licenses/by/4.0/).

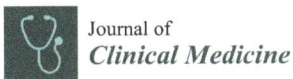
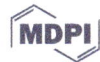

Article

Validity of Capsule Endoscopy in Monitoring Therapeutic Interventions in Patients with Crohn's Disease

Masanao Nakamura [1,*], Takeshi Yamamura [2], Keiko Maeda [2], Tsunaki Sawada [2], Yasuyuki Mizutani [1], Takuya Ishikawa [1], Kazuhiro Furukawa [1], Eizaburo Ohno [1], Hiroki Kawashima [1], Ryoji Miyahara [1], Anastasios Koulaouzidis [3], Yoshiki Hirooka [2] and the Nagoya University Crohn's Disease Study Group [1]

1. Department of Gastroenterology & Hepatology, Nagoya University Graduate School of Medicine, 65 Tsuruma-cho, Showa-ku, Nagoya 466-8550, Japan; y-mizu@med.nagoya-u.ac.jp (Y.M.); ishitaku@med.nagoya-u.ac.jp (T.I.); kazufuru@med.nagoya-u.ac.jp (K.F.); eono@med.nagoya-u.ac.jp (E.O.); h-kawa@med.nagoya-u.ac.jp (H.K.); myhr@med.nagoya-u.ac.jp (R.M.)
2. Department of Endoscopy, Nagoya University Hospital, Nagoya 466-8550, Japan; tyamamu@med.nagoya-u.ac.jp (T.Y.); kmaeda@med.nagoya-u.ac.jp (K.M.); t.sawada@med.nagoya-u.ac.jp (T.S.); hirooka@med.nagoya-u.ac.jp (Y.H.)
3. Endoscopy Unit, The Royal Infirmary of Edinburgh, Edinburgh EH16 4SA, UK; akoulaouzidis@hotmail.com
* Correspondence: makamura@med.nagoya-u.ac.jp; Tel.: +81-52-744-2172; Fax: 81-52-744-2180

Received: 8 September 2018; Accepted: 25 September 2018; Published: 29 September 2018

Abstract: Mucosal healing in Crohn's disease (CD) can be evaluated by capsule endoscopy (CE). However, only a few studies have utilized CE to demonstrate the therapeutic effect of medical treatment. We sought to evaluate the validity of using CE to monitor the effect of medical treatment in patients with CD. One hundred ($n = 100$) patients with CD were enrolled. All patients had a gastrointestinal (GI) tract patency check prior to CE. Patients with baseline CE Lewis score (LS) ≤ 135 were included in the non-active CD group and ended the study. In those with LS > 135 (active CD group), additional treatment was administered, regardless of symptoms, as per the treating clinician's advice. Patients of the active CD group underwent follow-up CE assessment 6 months later. Out of 92 patients with confirmed GI patency who underwent CE, 40 (43.4%) had CE findings of active inflammation. Of 29 patients with LS > 135 who received additional medications and underwent follow-up CE, improvement of the LS was noted in 23 (79.3%) patients. Eleven patients were asymptomatic but received additional medications; 8 (72.7%) had improvement of the LS. This study demonstrated that additional treatment even for patients with CD in clinical remission and active small-bowel inflammation on CE can reduce mucosal damage.

Keywords: capsule endoscopy; Crohn's disease; mucosal healing; small bowel

1. Introduction

The main goal in the treatment for Crohn's disease (CD) is mucosal healing (MH). MH is predictive of reduced subsequent disease activity and clinical upset, and decreased need for further active treatment [1–3]. Several modalities are used in assessing overall disease activity and MH in CD. For instance, faecal calprotectin (FC) is a simple, non-invasive, and readily available tool; however, its accuracy in evaluating active small-bowel (SB) mucosal lesions in CD has often been debated [4]. Although cross-sectional imaging has been traditionally used in the evaluation of SB CD [5,6], endoscopy remains the 'gold standard' for assessing SB MH because it provides direct and clear observation of the SB mucosa.

Capsule endoscopy (CE) enables physicians to visualize the SB in a non-invasive manner. Hence, CE allows detection of SB mucosal lesions, as well as linear ulceration and luminal stenosis [7]. Recently, Esaki et al. [8] reported that CE enables the identification of SB damage in 88% of patients with established SB CD. Capsule retention is a potentially serious complication of CE; however, the rate of this complication decreases substantially if gastrointestinal (GI) patency is assessed prior to performing regular CE [9,10]. Consequently, CE is recommended as the initial diagnostic modality for SB assessment in patients with suspected CD and negative ileocolonoscopy [11].

To quantify/categorize SB inflammation, Gralnek et al. [12] developed a CE index, the Lewis score (LS), comprising 3 parameters: villous oedema, mucosal ulcer(s), and luminal stenosis. A LS < 135 indicates normal or insignificant mucosal inflammation, LS 135–790 indicates mild mucosal inflammation, and LS ≥ 790 indicates moderate-to-severe inflammation. LS has been validated in the diagnosis and follow-up of established CD [13]. Stratifying SB inflammatory activity at the time of diagnosis has relevant prognostic value in patients with isolated SB CD [14]. A CE-based assessment of SB MH is reported to be useful for predicting long-term clinical remission in CD [15]. Moreover, several retrospective studies have highlighted the potential effect of CE on the therapeutic management of patients with established CD [16–18].

However, a high percentage of patients in clinical remission have findings suggestive of on-going inflammatory activity, as evidenced by C-reactive protein (CRP) and FC levels, CE, and cross-sectional imaging [19]. Kopylov et al. [20] demonstrated that a positive CRP level was found in 30.8% of patients with CD in clinical remission, while a high LS on CE was found in 84.6%. Nevertheless, patients with CD who are clinically asymptomatic may not wish to receive additional treatment, and/or physicians may be reluctant to recommend additional treatment in such situations.

Therefore, the aim of this prospective study was to evaluate using CE additional treatment in patients with inflammatory activity, regardless of the presence of clinical symptoms.

2. Patients & Methods

2.1. Patients

This prospective, multicenter study was conducted in hospitals affiliated with the Department of Gastroenterology & Hepatology at Nagoya University Graduate School of Medicine. Key inclusion criteria were patients with established CD who were >10-years-old and scheduled to receive a PillCam patency capsule (PPC), and thereafter CE. For patients to be eligible for inclusion, the colon had to be clear of any inflammation, as confirmed using a conventional colonoscopy. Key exclusion criteria were the presence of any contraindications to anti-tumor necrosis factor (anti-TNF) agents and/or those who were considered non-appropriate candidates by their physician.

2.2. Study Protocol

The study protocol involved two rounds of CE. Patients with CD referred for CE evaluation were informed of the study, aims, and its protocol. Once consent was obtained, patients who accepted to participate underwent the baseline CE at their local hospital. For every patient who was considered for study inclusion, the absence of colonic inflammation, confirmed by a conventional colonoscopy, was necessary. PPC was used before CE, including follow-ups, in all patients who agreed to participate. The PPC consists of lactose and 10% barium, which dissolves when intestinal fluids come into contact with them through a window at the edges of the PPC. PPC is similar to the second-generation Agile patency capsule, with the only difference being that the radiofrequency identification tag has been removed [10] (Figure 1). GI patency was evaluated either by confirming excretion of an intact PPC or by obtaining a plain abdominal X-ray and/or computed tomography (CT), generally between 30 and 33 h after PPC ingestion. The capsules used for CE were PillCam®SB2 or SB3 (manufactured by Medtronic, Minneapolis, MN, USA), which measure 26 × 11 mm and are propelled by peristalsis. All subjects whose GI patency was confirmed underwent CE, at their earliest convenience, following an overnight fast without prokinetics or prior laxative bowel preparation. Patients whose GI patency was not confirmed were excluded from further participation in this study. Following anonymization, the CE videos were sent to Nagoya University Hospital via the Nagoya network system, as described in References [21,22]. Two expert CE readers (MN, TY) independently reviewed each CE and calculated the LS. They also read the second CE videos and remained blinded to the treatment provided following the baseline CE reports. SB cleansing was evaluated in four grades according to previous literature [23,24]. In cases of any discordance in LS results, the experts discussed all relevant CE images and provided final LS by consensus agreement. The report of each CE was then sent back to the local hospital and further clinical management was left with the treating physician/team. Clinical data related to PPC and CE, including adverse events, were collected.

Figure 1. PillCam patency capsule.

Clinical remission was defined as a CD activity index (CDAI) score < 150. Since a LS < 135 can occasionally be associated with the presence of aphtha(e) or villous/fold oedema on CE, only a LS =0 was defined as complete MH. If LS $\leq$ 135 on baseline CE, suggestive of normal or clinically insignificant mucosal inflammatory change [25], the patient finished the study (non-active CD group). In the case of LS > 135, the treating teams could proceed with additional treatment, regardless of the presence of any clinical symptoms (active CD group). For patients of the active group, the follow-up CE was scheduled 6 months later, and it was performed with the same protocol as the baseline one.

2.3. Evaluations

Comparison was made between the clinical background and the baseline CE findings between the active and non-active groups. Additional therapeutic effects were evaluated in the active group, especially in asymptomatic patients, who underwent follow-up CEs. Primary outcome was any reported change in CE findings between the two CE procedures. Key secondary outcomes were changes in the CDAI and CRP level at the time of follow-up CE (for the active group), as well as any adverse events of PPC and CE procedures.

2.4. Statistical Analysis

The statistical software package SPSS for Windows (SPSS Inc., Chicago, IL, USA) was used for data analysis. The Wilcoxon signed-rank test was used to compare the LS based on CE and changes in each marker before and after any additional treatment. Patients' demographic data at the baseline examination was compared between the active and non-active groups using the Mann-Whitney U test or χ^2 test. In all analyses, a p value < 0.05 was considered statistically significant.

2.5. Ethical Considerations

This study was approved by the ethics Committee of Nagoya University Hospital. This study was registered in the University Hospital Medical Information Network, a clinical trials registry (UMIN000008486). Written informed consent was obtained from all participants.

3. Results

Between September 2012 and April 2016, 100 patients were referred for CE and approached for inclusion in this study at the Nagoya University Hospital and its 5 affiliated hospitals, as shown in

Figure 2. Of these patients, 92 had confirmed GI patency and were eventually included in this study. Absence of colonic inflammation was confirmed, prior to study entry, with a conventional colonoscopy which was performed at a median of 14 (range 1–29) months prior to inclusion in the study.

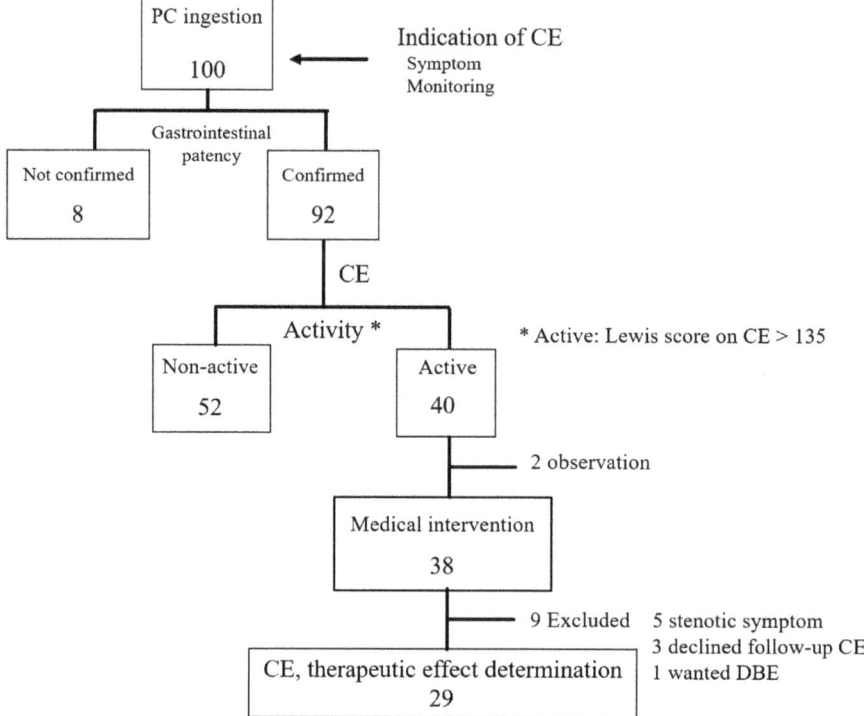

Figure 2. Flow chart of present study. Abbreviations PC, patency capsule; CE, capsule endoscopy; DBE, double balloon enteroscopy.

In the 92 baseline CEs, the grades of SB cleansing (for the whole SB) were excellent, good, fair, and poor in 19, 59, 12, and 2 patients, respectively. Of 92 patients, 40 (43.4%) had findings of active CD (*active CD group*); clinically, 28/40 patients were symptomatic. Their symptoms were diarrhea ($n = 20$), abdominal pain ($n = 4$), bloody stool (n = 3), and abdominal fullness ($n = 1$). The remainder ($n = 52$), with LS < 135 on baseline CE, comprised the *non-active CD group*. CDAI scores were not significantly different between the two groups; however, LS was significantly higher in the active group than in the non-active CD group. Hemoglobin and serum albumin levels were significantly lower in the active group than in the non-active CD group (Table 1).

Table 1. Demographic data of the patients at the point of study inclusion.

	Total	Active Group	Non Active Group	p Value
N	92	40	52	
Age, mean ± SD, years old	37.2 ± 12.3	37.5 ± 12.3	37.1 ± 12.9	0.8624
Gender, M/F	68/24	29/11	39/13	0.9751
BMI	21.3 ± 3.2	21.5 ± 3.6	21.1 ± 2.9	0.603
Duration of disease, mean ± SD, months	117.1 ± 96.7	93.9 ± 73.3	135 ± 108.8	0.093
Montreal classification				
Age at diagnosis				
<17 years	7	3	4	
17–40 years	70	30	40	
>40 years	15	7	8	
Location				
L1—ileal	38	17	21	
L2—colonic	0			
L3—ileocolonic	54	23	31	
Behavior				
B1—Non-stricturing, non-penetrating	72	28	44	
B2—Stricturing	15	9	6	
B3—Penetrating	5	3	2	
p-perianal disease	9	6	3	
History of GI surgery	53/92	25/40	28/52	0.5353
Ileo-colonic resection	26	12	14	
Ileal resection	21	9	12	
Ileo-colonic resection plus Ileal resection	4	3	1	
Colonic resection	2	1	1	
Any symptom	28/92	19/40	9/52	0.0038
CDAI	104 ± 56	116 ± 72	95 ± 39	0.277
Laboratory data				
CRP (mg/dL), mean ± SD	0.36 ± 0.62	0.53 ± 0.75	0.24 ± 0.47	0.0761
Hb (g/dL), mean ± SD	13.3 ± 2.1	12.7 ± 2.5	13.8 ± 1.6	0.0201
Albumin (g/dL), mean ± SD	4.0 ± 0.5	3.9 ± 0.5	4.2 ± 0.4	0.0014
Indication of CE				
Symptom(s)	28	19	9	
diarrhea	20	15	5	
abdominal pain	4	2	2	
bloody stools	3	2	1	
abdominal fullness	1	0	1	
Monitoring	64	21	43	
PPC and CE				
PPC intact body excretion	62/92	26/40	36/52	0.8377
Gastric transit time (min.)	45.5 ± 42.4	45.6 ± 40.3	47.2 ± 44.3	0.9904
SBTT (min.)	248.8 ± 128.8	270.7 ± 149.5	231.7 ± 108.5	0.3042
Lewis score, mean ± SD	396 ± 706	844 ± 892	52.1 ± 66.1	<0.0001
Treatment				
Anti TNF-α agent	54/92	23/40	31/52	
5-ASA	78/92	35/40	43/52	
Immunomodulator	14/92	5/40	9/52	
Elemental diet	57/92	23/40	34/52	

We defined as regular use of non-steroidal anti-inflammatory drugs (NSAIDs), the use of this class of medications for more than 6 months irrespective of type and dose. This was clarified by review of the medical charts and patient interview. None of the patients regularly had used NSAIDs before and/or after CEs. Of 38/40 patients of the active CD group who received additional anti-inflammatory treatment(s) (infliximab, $n = 8$; 5-aminosalicylic acid, $n = 7$; azathioprine, $n = 6$; adalimumab, $n = 4$; elemental diet, $n = 2$; prednisolone, $n = 1$; and mercaptopurine, $n = 1$), 29/40 (72%) underwent follow-up CEs to assess the therapeutic effect on MH.

Following additional treatment for 6 months, the mean LS improved from 691 ± 126 to 394 ± 99. Villous oedema before and after treatment was detected in 20 and 11 patients, respectively. Of all the 29 patients who had ulcers at baseline CE, 19 improved and 4 no longer had an ulcer. The LS of 4 patients who had a baseline LS > 1000 decreased; however, only 2/29 patients achieved MH (Table 2).

The mean CDAI score and LS significantly improved 6 months after the start of additional treatment (Table 3), although the mean CRP level did not improve dramatically.

Table 2. 29 cases where intervention.

Case	Medicine	Intervention	Lewis Score							
			Total Score		Villous Edema		Ulcer		Stenosis	
			Pre	Post	Pre	Post	Pre	Post	Pre	Post
1	Infliximab	dose up 5 ⇒ 10 mg/kg	2914	2824	112	112	450	360	2352	2352
2	Infliximab	introduction 5 mg/kg	2585	280	8	0	225	0	2352	280
3	Adalimumab	introduction 160 mg	2140	600	340	0	1800	600	0	0
4	Azathiopurin	introduction 50 mg	1012	337	112	112	900	225	0	0
5	mercaptopurine	introduction 20 mg	900	1368	0	168	900	1200	0	0
6	5-ASA	dose up 3000 ⇒ 4000 mg	712	712	112	112	600	600	0	0
7	Infliximab	introduction 5 mg/kg	712	421	112	0	600	225	0	196
8	Adalimumab	introduction 160 mg	654	0	204	0	450	0	0	0
9	Adalimumab	introduction 160 mg	600	0	0	0	600	0	0	0
10	Infliximab	dose up 5 ⇒ 10 mg/kg	562	196	112	0	450	0	0	196
11	5-ASA	dose up 1500 ⇒ 2000 mg	562	225	112	0	450	225	0	0
12	5-ASA	introduction 3000 mg	562	337	112	112	450	225	0	0
13	Infliximab	introduction 5 mg/kg	562	233	112	8	450	225	0	0
14	Azathiopurin	introduction 50 mg	504	180	204	0	300	180	0	0
15	Prednisolone	introduction 20 mg	458	450	8	0	450	450	0	0
16	5-ASA	dose up 2000 ⇒ 3000 mg	458	147	8	12	450	135	0	0
17	Azathiopurin	introduction 50 mg	450	458	0	8	450	450	0	0
18	Adalimumab	introduction 160 mg	436	225	136	0	300	225	0	0
19	Elemental diet	dose up	429	225	204	0	225	225	0	0
20	Elemental diet	dose up	412	225	112	0	300	225	0	0
21	Infliximab	dose up 5 ⇒ 10 mg/kg	412	225	112	0	300	225	0	0
22	Infliximab	introduction 5 mg/kg	337	135	112	0	225	135	0	0
23	Azathiopurin	introduction 50 mg	300	278	0	8	300	270	0	0
24	Azathiopurin	dose up 50 ⇒ 75 mg	300	180	0	0	300	180	0	0
25	Azathiopurin	introduction 50 mg	233	143	8	8	225	135	0	0
26	Infliximab	dose up 5 ⇒ 10 mg/kg	225	233	0	8	225	225	0	0
27	5-ASA	dose up 2000 ⇒ 3000 mg	225	225	0	0	225	225	0	0
28	5-ASA	dose up 1500 ⇒ 3000 mg	225	450	0	0	225	450	0	0
29	5-ASA	dose up 2000 ⇒ 3000 mg	180	135	0	0	180	135	0	0

Table 3. Biomarker levels at baselines and 6 months later.

	Pre-Treatment	Post-Treatment	p Value
CDAI	102 (5–253)	68 (0–231)	0.0057
Lewis score	458 (180–2914)	233 (0–2824)	0.0004
CRP level (mg/dL)	0.55 ± 0.80	0.30 ± 0.51	0.0652
WBC count (/μL)	6822 ± 2602	5920 ± 1807	0.1663
Hb level (g/dL)	12.7 ± 2.5	13.2 ± 1.9	0.7843
Plt count($\times 1000/mm^3$)	26.6 ± 6.1	26.7 ± 7.0	0.5014
Albumin level (g/dL)	3.9 ± 0.6	4.1 ± 0.5	0.1297

Data are presented as a mean ± standard deviation. CDAI, Crohn's disease activity index; CRP, C-reactive protein; WBC, white blood cell; Hb, hemoglobin; Plt, platelet.

All 7 patients who received additional treatment with biologics had improvement of LS on repeat CE (Figure 3). Of the 11 patients who were asymptomatic, 4 received 5-ASA, 3 received biologics, 2 received immunomodulators, 1 received prednisolone, and 1 received elemental diet as additional treatment (Figure 4). LS improvement was noted in 8/11 (72.7%) patients; however, none of them achieved MH. No adverse events occurred throughout the study, as no retention of PPC or capsule was noted. Of 29 patients who received additional treatment and underwent follow-up CE, 23 patients' clinical course could be confirmed post-study in November 2017. During the median follow-up 36 months, 12 patients did not undergo change in treatment, although 10 patients were given additional treatment and 1 underwent surgery.

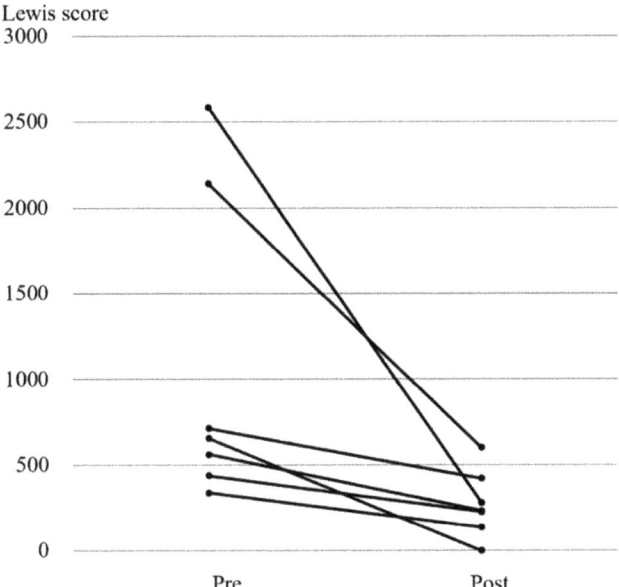

Figure 3. Changes in the Lewis scores in patients who received biologics as additional treatment. Abbreviations Pre, pre-treatment; post, post-treatment.

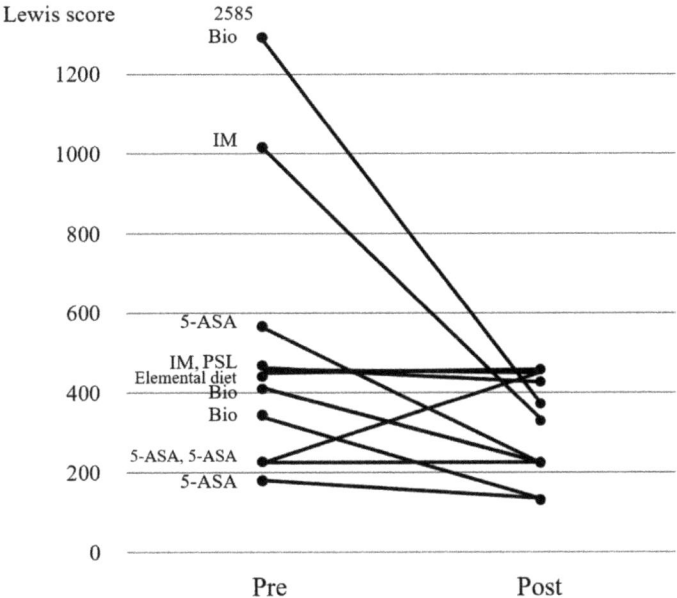

Figure 4. Changes in the Lewis scores in asymptomatic patients before and after treatment. Bio, biologic; IM, infliximab; 5-ASA, 5-aminosalicylic acid; PSL, prednisolone; pre, pre-treatment; post, post-treatment.

4. Discussion

Our study confirms LS improvement in 23/29 patients (79.3%), irrespective of symptoms status, who received additional treatment for active CD based on the findings of baseline CE. Interestingly, 8/11 asymptomatic CD patients (72.7%) had improvement in their LS, regardless of the type of additional treatment provided. These results underline a couple of key points. First, asymptomatic CD patients may require additional treatment or simply increasing the dose of their existing therapeutic regimen to achieve MH. Additional medication had a positive effect in both asymptomatic and symptomatic CD patients, as shown in Figures 2–4. Second, CE is a valid tool in evaluating both therapeutic effect, as well as confirming MH in patients with asymptomatic (active) CD.

In CD, it remains controversial whether the physician should set the therapeutic target at MH or clinical remission. If the therapeutic goal is MH rather than clinical (symptoms) remission, this can only be evaluated by endoscopy. The POCER study suggested that monitoring using early colonoscopy and treatment step-up was better in preventing postoperative CD recurrence, than conventional drug therapy alone [26]. On the other hand, Kim et al. reported that endoscopic monitoring did not significantly contribute to the non-hospitalization rate associated with CD, compared with ulcerative colitis [27]. However, the definition of MH remains unclear. Total disappearance of mucosal ulcerations has the advantage of providing irrefutable evidence of MH, but this strict 'black-and-white' goal may be difficult to achieve [28]. For instance, a patient with numerous deep mucosal ulcerations in whom treatment leads to healing of all but a superficial mucosal ulceration will be classified as a 'non-responder'.

To date, only few studies have shown the necessity and effectiveness of additional treatment for CD patients in clinical remission and endoscopically-confirmed active lesions, although the significance of monitoring has been widely recognized. Once the therapeutic effects for such patients have been clarified, physicians may recommend a change of the medication regimen. Under the notion of treat-to-target, Ungar et al. suggested a significant association between serum levels of anti-TNF agents and the level of mucosal healing as the therapeutic goal [29]. Physicians may modify the dose of biologic treatment with reference to the serum levels even if patients have no symptoms. The CALM study demonstrated the significance of tight control, including timely escalation with anti-TNF therapy. Combining clinical symptoms with biomarkers in patients with early CD results in better clinical and endoscopic outcomes than symptom-driven decisions alone [30]. This study also supported the importance of tight control in CD by evaluating treatment outcomes in asymptomatic patients.

The development and introduction of a new, more effective drug will provide better CD monitoring. Endoscopic findings may become the best way to evaluate MH in CD because endoscopy provides direct visualization of the intestinal mucosa and enables physicians to detect even subtle mucosal lesions. However, it is unclear whether small lesions affect the long-term clinical outcome in CD. Moreover, it is questionable whether physicians can determine MH in patients with small lesions. LS calculation does not include the evaluation of such lesions. Therefore, MH according to LS means that there is no mucosal ulcer, but this does not preclude the presence of erosions or mucosal aphtha(e). Niv score or CECDAI, on the other hand, classifies erosion and small ulcers <5 mm under the same category [31,32]. It may be necessary to evaluate the outcome of patients with and without erosions.

If physicians can ignore small lesions to consider the long-term outcome of CD, abdominal ultrasonography and magnetic resonance enterography (MRE) will also be excellent modalities to evaluate MH. Koulaouzidis et al. reported that the LS appears to have only a fair correlation with the FC level, as well as other serological markers of inflammation [33]. FC level does not seem to be a reliable biomarker for significant SB inflammation. Nevertheless, an FC level ≥ 76 μg/g may be associated with appreciable visual inflammation on SB CE in patients with a prior negative diagnostic workup, and it may become the surrogate marker of CD.

This study has few limitations. The overall sample size of this study was small. This study focused on the Lewis score for next treatment, and laboratory data or calprotectin was not collected on follow-up. Of the patients with active CD based on CE, the percentage of patients who received an intervention was low because five patients had developed small-bowel stenosis, as demonstrated on a CT scan. The others did not wish to receive additional treatment. The kind of intervention depended on the physician and patients according to the protocol. Therefore, the balance between the degree of CD activity and kind of medication may not always be suitable. In conclusion, this prospective, multi-center study demonstrated that additional treatment regardless of clinical remission reduces mucosal inflammation in CD.

Author Contributions: Conceptualization, M.N., T.S. and Y.M.; Data curation, T.Y., K.M., T.S., K.F. and Nagoya University Crohn's Disease Study Group; Formal analysis, M.N., T.I., E.O. and H.K.; Investigation, M.N.; Methodology, M.N. and T.Y.; Critical review of the manuscript versions, A.K.; Validation, R.M.; Visualization, Y.M.; Writing—original draft, M.N.; Writing—review & editing, A.K.; Approval of this study, Y.H.

Funding: This research received no external funding.

Acknowledgments: For Data Availability, The data used to support the findings of this study are available from the corresponding author upon request.

Conflicts of Interest: The authors declare that there is no conflict of interest regarding the publication of this article.

Abbreviations

5-aminosalicylic acid (5-ASA), C-reactive protein (CRP), Crohn disease (CD), Crohn's disease activity index (CDAI), capsule endoscopy (CE), double-balloon endoscopy (DBE), faecal calprotectin (FC), gastrointestinal (GI), Lewis score (LS), mucosal healing (MH), non-steroidal anti-inflammatory drugs (NSAIDs), PillCam patency capsule (PPC).

References

1. Baert, F.; Moortgat, L.; Van Assche, G.; Caenepeel, P.; Vergauwe, P.; De Vos, M.; Stokkers, P.; Hommes, D.; Rutgeerts, P.; Vermeire, S.; et al. Belgian Inflammatory Bowel Disease Research Group; North-Holland Gut Club. Mucosal healing predicts sustained clinical remission in patients with early-stage Crohn's disease. *Gastroenterology* **2010**, *138*, 463–468. [CrossRef] [PubMed]
2. Peyrin-Biroulet, L.; Ferrante, M.; Magro, F.; Campbell, S.; Franchimont, D.; Fidder, H.; Strid, H.; Ardizzone, S.; Veereman-Wauters, G.; Chevaux, J.B.; et al. Results from the 2nd Scientific Workshop of the ECCO. I: Impact of mucosal healing on the course of inflammatory bowel disease. *J. Crohns Colitis* **2011**, *5*, 477–483. [CrossRef] [PubMed]
3. Frøslie, K.F.; Jahnsen, J.; Moum, B.A.; Vatn, M.H.; IBSEN Group. Mucosal healing in inflammatory bowel disease: Results from a Norwegian population-based cohort. *Gastroenterology* **2007**, *133*, 412–422.
4. Sipponen, T.; Savilahti, E.; Kolho, K.L.; Nuutinen, H.; Turunen, U.; Farkkila, M. Crohn's disease activity assessed by fecal calprotectin and lactoferrin: Correlation with Crohn's disease activity index and endoscopic findings. *Inflamm. Bowel Dis.* **2008**, *14*, 40–46. [CrossRef] [PubMed]
5. Kopylov, U.; Klang, E.; Yablecovitch, D.; Lahat, A.; Avidan, B.; Neuman, S.; Levhar, N.; Greener, T.; Rozendorn, N.; Beytelman, A.; et al. Magnetic resonance enterography versus capsule endoscopy activity indices for quantification of small bowel inflammation in Crohn's disease. *Ther. Adv. Gastroenterol.* **2016**, *9*, 655–663. [CrossRef] [PubMed]
6. Moy, M.P.; Kaplan, J.L.; Moran, C.J.; Winter, H.S.; Gee, M.S. MR enterographic findings as biomarkers of mucosal healing in young patients with Crohn disease. *Am. J. Roentgenol.* **2016**, *207*, 896–902. [CrossRef] [PubMed]
7. Kopylov, U.; Koulaouzidis, A.; Klang, E.; Carter, D.; Ben-Horin, S.; Eliakim, R. Monitoring of small bowel Crohn's disease. *Expert Rev. Gastroenterol. Hepatol.* **2017**, *11*, 1014–1058. [CrossRef] [PubMed]
8. Esaki, M.; Matsumoto, T.; Watanabe, K.; Arakawa, T.; Naito, Y.; Matsuura, M.; Nakase, H.; Hibi, T.; Matsumoto, T.; Nouda, S.; et al. Use of capsule endoscopy in patients with Crohn's disease in Japan: A multicenter survey. *J. Gastroenterol. Hepatol.* **2014**, *29*, 96–101. [CrossRef] [PubMed]
9. Nemeth, A.; Kopylov, U.; Koulaouzidis, A.; Wurm Johansson, G.; Thorlacius, H.; Amre, D.; Eliakim, R.; Seidman, E.G.; Toth, E. Use of patency capsule in patients with established Crohn's disease. *Endoscopy* **2016**, *48*, 373–379. [CrossRef] [PubMed]

10. Nakamura, M.; Hirooka, Y.; Yamamura, T.; Miyahara, R.; Watanabe, O.; Ando, T.; Ohmiya, N.; Goto, H. Clinical usefulness of novel tag-less Agile patency capsule prior to capsule endoscopy for patients with suspected small bowel stenosis. *Dig. Endosc.* **2015**, *27*, 61–66. [CrossRef] [PubMed]
11. Pennazio, M.; Spada, C.; Eliakim, R.; Keuchel, M.; May, A.; Mulder, C.J.; Rondonotti, E.; Adler, S.N.; Albert, J.; Baltes, P.; et al. Small-bowel capsule endoscopy and device-assisted enteroscopy for diagnosis and treatment of small-bowel disorders: European Society of Gastrointestinal Endoscopy (ESGE) Clinical Guideline. *Endoscopy* **2015**, *47*, 352–376. [CrossRef] [PubMed]
12. Gralnek, I.M.; Defranchis, R.; Seidman, E.; Leighton, J.A.; Legnani, P.; Lewis, B.S. Development of a capsule endoscopy scoring index for small bowel mucosal inflammatory change. *Aliment. Pharmacol. Ther.* **2008**, *27*, 146–154. [CrossRef] [PubMed]
13. Koulaouzidis, A.; Douglas, S.; Plevris, J.N. Lewis score correlates more closely with fecal calprotectin than Capsule Endoscopy Crohn's Disease Activity Index. *Dig. Dis. Sci.* **2012**, *57*, 987–993. [CrossRef] [PubMed]
14. Dias de Castro, F.; Boal Carvalho, P.; Monteiro, S.; Rosa, B.; Firmino-Machado, J.; Moreira, M.J.; Cotter, J. Lewis score—Prognostic value in patients with isolated small bowel Crohn's disease. *J. Crohns Colitis* **2015**, *9*, 1146–1151. [CrossRef] [PubMed]
15. Niv, Y. Small-bowel mucosal healing assessment by capsule endoscopy as a predictor of long-term clinical remission in patients with Crohn's disease: A systematic review and meta-analysis. *Eur. J. Gastroenterol. Hepatol.* **2017**, *29*, 844–848. [CrossRef] [PubMed]
16. Long, M.D.; Barnes, E.; Isaacs, K.; Morgan, D.; Herfarth, H.H. Impact of capsule endoscopy on management of inflammatory bowel disease: A single tertiary care center experience. *Inflamm. Bowel Dis.* **2011**, *17*, 1855–1862. [CrossRef] [PubMed]
17. Lorenzo-Zúñiga, V.; de Vega, V.M.; Domènech, E.; Cabré, E.; Mañosa, M.; Boix, J. Impact of capsule endoscopy findings in the management of Crohn's Disease. *Dig. Dis. Sci.* **2010**, *55*, 411–414. [CrossRef] [PubMed]
18. Sidhu, R.; McAlindon, M.E.; Drew, K.; Hardcastle, S.; Cameron, I.C.; Sanders, D.S. Evaluating the role of small-bowel endoscopy in clinical practice: The largest single-centre experience. *Eur. J. Gastroenterol. Hepatol.* **2012**, *24*, 513–519. [CrossRef] [PubMed]
19. Annese, V.; Daperno, M.; Rutter, M.D.; Amiot, A.; Bossuyt, P.; East, J.; Ferrante, M.; Götz, M.; Katsanos, K.H.; Kießlich, R.; et al. European evidence based consensus for endoscopy in inflammatory bowel disease. *J. Crohns Colitis* **2013**, *7*, 982–1018. [CrossRef] [PubMed]
20. Kopylov, U.; Yablecovitch, D.; Lahat, A.; Neuman, S.; Levhar, N.; Greener, T.; Klang, E.; Rozendorn, N.; Amitai, M.M.; Ben-Horin, S.; et al. Detection of small bowel mucosal healing and deep remission in patients with known small bowel Crohn's disease using biomarkers, capsule endoscopy, and imaging. *Am. J. Gastroenterol.* **2015**, *110*, 1316–1323. [CrossRef] [PubMed]
21. Goto, H.; Nakamura, M.; Ohmiya, N.; Hirooka, Y.; Itoh, A. Establishment of an interpretation system for video capsule endoscopy for obscure gastrointestinal bleeding. *J. Gastroenterol.* **2010**, *45*, 468–469. [CrossRef] [PubMed]
22. Goto, H.; Nakamura, M.; Ohmiya, N. Advanced network system for reading capsule endoscopy images. *Dig. Endosc.* **2013**, *25*, 91. [CrossRef] [PubMed]
23. Brotz, C.; Nandi, N.; Conn, M.; Daskalakis, C.; DiMarino, M.; Infantolino, A.; Katz, L.C.; Schroeder, T.; Kastenberg, D. A validation study of 3 grading systems to evaluate small-bowel cleansing for wireless capsule endoscopy: A quantitative index, a qualitative evaluation, and an overall adequacy assessment. *Gastrointest. Endosc.* **2009**, *69*, 262–270. [CrossRef] [PubMed]
24. Yung, D.E.; Rondonotti, E.; Sykes, C.; Pennazio, M.; Plevris, J.N.; Koulaouzidis, A. Systematic review and meta-analysis: Is bowel preparation still necessary in small bowel capsule endoscopy? *Expert Rev. Gastroenterol. Hepatol.* **2017**, *11*, 979–993. [CrossRef] [PubMed]
25. Cotter, J.; Dias de Castro, F.; Magalhães, J.; Moreira, M.J.; Rosa, B. Validation of the Lewis score for the evaluation of small-bowel Crohn's disease activity. *Endoscopy* **2015**, *47*, 330–335. [CrossRef] [PubMed]
26. De Cruz, P.; Kamm, M.A.; Hamilton, A.L.; Ritchie, K.J.; Krejany, E.O.; Gorelik, A.; Liew, D.; Prideaux, L.; Lawrance, I.C.; Andrews, J.M.; et al. Crohn's disease management after intestinal resection: A randomised trial. *Lancet* **2015**, *385*, 1406–1417. [CrossRef]
27. Kim, D.H.; Park, S.J.; Park, J.J.; Yun, Y.H.; Hong, S.P.; Kim, T.I.; Kim, W.H.; Cheon, J.H. Effect of follow-up endoscopy on the outcomes of patients with inflammatory bowel disease. *Dig. Dis. Sci.* **2014**, *59*, 2514–2522. [CrossRef] [PubMed]

28. Pineton de Chambrun, G.; Peyrin-Biroulet, L.; Lémann, M.; Colombel, J.F. Clinical implications of mucosal healing for the management of IBD. *Nat. Rev. Gastroenterol. Hepatol.* **2010**, *7*, 15–29. [CrossRef] [PubMed]
29. Ungar, B.; Levy, I.; Yavne, Y.; Yavzori, M.; Picard, O.; Fudim, E.; Loebstein, R.; Chowers, Y.; Eliakim, R.; Kopylov, U.; et al. Optimizing anti-TNF-α therapy: Serum levels of infliximab and adalimumab are associated with mucosal healing in patients with inflammatory bowel diseases. *Clin. Gastroenterol. Hepatol.* **2016**, *14*, 550–557. [CrossRef] [PubMed]
30. Colombel, J.F.; Panaccione, R.; Bossuyt, P.; Lukas, M.; Baert, F.; Vaňásek, T.; Danalioglu, A.; Novacek, G.; Armuzzi, A.; Hébuterne, X.; et al. Effect of tight control management on Crohn's disease (CALM): A multicentre, randomised, controlled phase 3 trial. *Lancet* **2017**, *17*, 32641–32647. [CrossRef]
31. Gal, E.; Geller, A.; Fraser, G.; Levi, Z.; Niv, Y. Assessment and validation of the new capsule endoscopy Crohn's disease activity index (CECDAI). *Dig. Dis. Sci.* **2008**, *53*, 1933–1937. [CrossRef] [PubMed]
32. Niv, Y.; Ilani, S.; Levi, Z.; Hershkowitz, M.; Niv, E.; Fireman, Z.; O'Donnel, S.; O'Morain, C.; Eliakim, R.; Scapa, E.; et al. Validation of the Capsule Endoscopy Crohn's Disease Activity Index (CECDAI or Niv score): A multicenter prospective study. *Endoscopy* **2012**, *44*, 21–26. [CrossRef] [PubMed]
33. Koulaouzidis, A.; Sipponen, T.; Nemeth, A.; Makins, R.; Kopylov, U.; Nadler, M.; Giannakou, A.; Yung, D.E.; Johansson, G.W.; Bartzis, L.; et al. Association between fecal calprotectin levels and small-bowel inflammation score in capsule endoscopy: A multicenter retrospective study. *Dig. Dis. Sci.* **2016**, *61*, 2033–2040. [CrossRef] [PubMed]

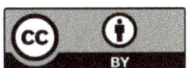

© 2018 by the authors. Licensee MDPI, Basel, Switzerland. This article is an open access article distributed under the terms and conditions of the Creative Commons Attribution (CC BY) license (http://creativecommons.org/licenses/by/4.0/).

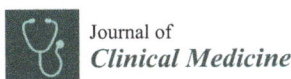

Review
Non-Invasive Biomarkers for Celiac Disease

Alka Singh [1], Atreyi Pramanik [2], Pragyan Acharya [2] and Govind K. Makharia [1,*]

[1] Department of Gastroenterology and Human Nutrition; All India Institute of Medical Sciences, New Delhi-110029, India; singhalka34@gmail.com
[2] Department of Biochemistry, All India Institute of Medical Sciences, New Delhi-110029, India; atreyipram91@gmail.com (A.P.); dr.pragyan.acharya@gmail.com (P.A.)
* Correspondence: govindmakharia@gmail.com or govindmakharia@aiims.edu

Received: 12 May 2019; Accepted: 2 June 2019; Published: 21 June 2019

Abstract: Once thought to be uncommon, celiac disease has now become a common disease globally. While avoidance of the gluten-containing diet is the only effective treatment so far, many new targets are being explored for the development of new drugs for its treatment. The endpoints of therapy include not only reversal of symptoms, normalization of immunological abnormalities and healing of mucosa, but also maintenance of remission of the disease by strict adherence of the gluten-free diet (GFD). There is no single gold standard test for the diagnosis of celiac disease and the diagnosis is based on the presence of a combination of characteristics including the presence of a celiac-specific antibody (anti-tissue transglutaminase antibody, anti-endomysial antibody or anti-deamidated gliadin peptide antibody) and demonstration of villous abnormalities. While the demonstration of enteropathy is an important criterion for a definite diagnosis of celiac disease, it requires endoscopic examination which is perceived as an invasive procedure. The capability of prediction of enteropathy by the presence of the high titer of anti-tissue transglutaminase antibody led to an option of making a diagnosis even without obtaining mucosal biopsies. While present day diagnostic tests are great, they, however, have certain limitations. Therefore, there is a need for biomarkers for screening of patients, prediction of enteropathy, and monitoring of patients for adherence of the gluten-free diet. Efforts are now being made to explore various biomarkers which reflect different changes that occur in the intestinal mucosa using modern day tools including transcriptomics, proteomics, and metabolomics. In the present review, we have discussed comprehensively the pros and cons of available biomarkers and also summarized the current status of emerging biomarkers for the screening, diagnosis, and monitoring of celiac disease.

Keywords: celiac disease; biomarker; serology; enteropathy

1. Introduction

Celiac disease (CeD) is a systemic autoimmune disorder that is induced by the ingestion of gluten protein present in wheat, barley, and rye in genetically predisposed individuals [1]. Once considered to be limited to Western Europe, CeD has now emerged as a major public health problem globally. A recent systematic review suggests that 0.7% (95% Confidence Interval (CI), 0.5–0.9%) of the global population suffers from CeD [2]. With the global population of 6.4 billion, approximately 37–59 million people are estimated to have CeD globally. While the global pool of patients is so large, the majority of patients (83–95%) in developed countries, and possibly even a higher number in developing countries, still remain undiagnosed [3]. This large pool remains unrecognized partly because of the lack of classical gastrointestinal symptoms in approximately half of patients. The spectrum of clinical manifestation of CeD is wide and includes both gastrointestinal symptoms such as chronic diarrhea, dyspepsia, anemia, and failure to thrive and extra-gastrointestinal manifestations such as short stature, dermatitis herpetiformis, infertility, and liver diseases. Recognition of wide spectrum of CeD, simplification of the diagnostic criteria and widespread use of celiac-specific serological tests (anti-tissue transglutaminase antibody, anti-endomysial antibody or anti-deamidated gliadin peptide antibody) have led to an increase in the recognition of CeD globally [4]. There is no single gold standard test for the diagnosis of CeD, and the diagnosis of CeD is based on a combination of clinical manifestations, presence of the celiac-specific serological test and demonstration of villous abnormality on intestinal mucosal biopsies [5]. While the treatment of CeD at present time is life-long gluten-free diet (GFD); a number of drugs including intraluminal gluten degrading enzyme therapies such as latiglutenases, peptide vaccines such as NexVax 2, and zonulin antagonist such as larazotide are being explored as an alternative or additive treatment for patients with CeD.

A biomarker is a defining characteristic that is measured as an indicator of normal biological processes, pathogenic processes, or responses to an exposure or intervention, including therapeutic interventions [6]. Since an ideal biomarker should provide a "signature" for a condition, the development of biomarkers requires several rounds of controlled experimentations, and validation before it can be used in clinical practice. In the present review, we have discussed comprehensively the pros and cons of available biomarkers and we have also summarized the current status of emerging biomarkers for the screening, diagnosis, and monitoring of the disease. For CeD, biomarkers are required for multiple purposes including a) screening of the disease, b) detection/prediction of enteropathy, c) markers of complications, d) monitoring of the disease, and e) assessment of adherence to gluten free diet (GFD). Indeed, enormous efforts have been made in this direction; some of the established and potential biomarkers are summarized in Table 1.

Table 1. Established and potential biomarkers for celiac disease

Types of Biomarkers	Name of the Biomarker
Serological biomarker	Anti-gliadin antibody (AGA) Anti-endomysial antibody (AEA) Anti-tissue transglutaminase (tTG)- TG2, TG6, TG3 Deamidated gliadin peptide (DGP) Synthetic neo-epitopes tTG-DGP complex
Genetic marker	HLA-DQ haplotyping
Biomarkers for the prediction of enteropathy	Cytochrome P450 3A4 (CYP3A4) Plasma citrulline Intestinal-fatty acid binding proteins Regenerating gene1α (Reg 1α)
Biomarkers to predict dietary adherence	Gluten immunogenic peptide (GIP) Mean platelet volume (MPV)
Miscellaneous Biomarkers	miRNA Intestinal permeability

2. Serological Biomarkers

Serological tests are the first line investigation for the screening of patients suspected to have CeD. Until the late 1950s, there was no biomarker for the diagnosis of CeD, and the diagnosis made was on the basis of the presence of suggestive clinical symptoms and resolution of symptoms with a GFD [7]. The advent of methods for obtaining intestinal biopsies such as Crosby capsules and endoscopic techniques, added villous atrophy as one of the most specific requirements for the diagnosis of CeD. The discovery of anti-gliadin antibodies (AGA) in the 1960s was a landmark step in the evolution of the modern-day diagnostic strategy for CeD. AGA remained the first line celiac-specific serological test until the 1990s [8]. In the 1990s, anti-endomysial antibody (AEA) was discovered and a combination of AGA with AEA testing became the standard diagnostic strategy for CeD [9]. With recognition of the high false positive rate for AGA, the use of AGA fell both for the screening and diagnosis of CeD. Further discovery of anti-tissue transglutaminase (tTG) as the substrate for AEA, tTG based enzyme-linked immunoassays (ELISA) became the standard diagnostic test for CeD [10].

2.1. Anti-Gliadin Antibodies

Anti-Gliadin Antibodies (AGA) is produced against gliadin, a prolamin found in wheat and related cereals. Anti-Gliadin Antibodies are of two types IgA-AGA and IgG-AGA. Anti-Gliadin Antibodies is no more used for the diagnosis of CeD because of the advent of more reliable serological tests. However, there has been renewed interest in the utility of AGA. Immunoglobulin G (IgG) AGA and IgA-AGA are now used to recognize other gluten-related disorders such as non-celiac gluten sensitivity, gluten ataxia, and autism [11]. Anti-Gliadin Antibodies (more precisely, IgG dependent AGA) is positive in approximately 50% of patients with non-celiac gluten sensitivity [12,13].

2.2. Anti-Endomysial Antibody

Chorzelski et al. discovered the AEA test, which revolutionized the diagnostic strategy for CeD [14]. Anti-Endomysial Antibody (AEA) is an antibody against the smooth muscle's inter-myofibrillar substance [9]. Earlier, a monkey esophagus was used as a substrate for AEA testing and the use of human umbilical cord as a substrate has enhanced the sensitivity and specificity of AEA [15]. While both sensitivity and specificity of AEA was reported to be >95%, a recent systematic review has reported a lower pooled sensitivity, 73.0% (95% CI, 61.0% to 83.0%), based on the data of newer studies, the specificity however still remains to be 99.0% (95% CI, 98.0% to 99.0%) [16]. While AEA is very specific, detection of AEA requires indirect immunofluorescence, which is labor intensive and time-consuming as compared to the estimation of tTG Ab by ELISA [17].

2.3. Anti-Tissues Transglutaminase Antibody

Transglutaminase (TG) is a calcium-dependent enzyme, which catalyzes the covalent bond and cross-linking of proteins irreversibly [18]. Nine different types of the TG gene have been discovered in mammals, eight codes for catalytically active enzymes and one for an inactive enzyme. These TGs play different roles in different tissues in physiological and pathological conditions. Transglutaminase 1 (TG1) (keratinocyte), TG3 (epidermal), and TG5 are involved in the formation of the cornified envelope during keratinocyte differentiation, thus contribute to the cutaneous barrier function [19]. Transglutaminase 6 (TG6) and TG7 are expressed in testis, lung and brain, but their function is still uncertain [20]. Transglutaminase 2 (TG2) is ubiquitously present in cells and tissues—and hence TG2 is known as "tissue" TG.

Autoantigen against TG2 was identified by Dieterich et al., who also suggested the role of TG2 in the deamidation of the bond between glutamine and lysine, present in gluten [18]. Of all the serological tests, IgA anti-TG2 Ab is the most widely used test both for the diagnosis and initial screening for CeD because of its very high sensitivity and specificity, ease of use, and its quantitative capability. In a recent systematic review, Chou R et al. reported a pooled sensitivity of anti-tTG Ab to be 92.8% (95% CI, 90.3–94.8%); specificity 97.9% (95% CI, 96.4–98.8%); a positive likelihood ratio (LR) of 45.1 (95% CI, 25.1–75.5%) and negative LR of 0.07 (95% CI, 0.05–0.10%) [16]. Immunoglobulin A (IgA) tTG levels also correlate with the degree of severity of mucosal damage, and a titer of 10 folds or higher over the upper limit of normal (ULN) predicts presence of villous abnormality with very high specificity [21].

Antibodies against other TGs have been reported in extra-intestinal forms of gluten-related disorders [22]. Anti-TG3 Ab has been reported in patients having dermatitis herpetiformis [23]. As discussed above, TG6 is found in the brain and anti-TG6 Ab has been reported in gluten-induced neurological diseases such as gluten ataxia [24,25]. The concentration of anti-TG6 Ab has been observed to correlate with longer gluten exposure in them and the level of TG6 decreases after GFD [26]. In a study, 73% of patients with idiopathic sporadic ataxia positive for AGA, were also positive for TG6 antibodies [27].

2.4. Anti-Deamidated Gliadin Peptides

Anti-deamidated gliadin peptides Ab (DGP) is directed against deamidated gliadin peptides and is another serologic marker for the diagnosis of CeD [28]. Initially, IgA DGP was reported to be equally sensitive and specific as IgA tTG Ab, however recent studies have shown that tTG Ab is the most trusted serological test for CeD [29,30]. A recent systematic review and meta-analysis reported the pooled sensitivity of anti-DGP Ab to be 87.8% (95% CI, 85.6–89.9%), and of specificity 94.1% (95% CI, 92.5–95.5%) [16].

2.5. Point-of-Care Test

Point-of-care tests (POCTs) for the diagnosis and monitoring of CeD have been in use for the past one decade, especially in Europe [31,32]. They are easy to perform, do not require a laboratory or experienced laboratory staff, and have a quick turn-around time [33,34]. Therefore, POCTs have the potential to increase CeD diagnosis rates worldwide, facilitate early diagnosis, and reduce cost. POCTs have been shown to be successfully used in various settings including primary care, specialty clinics, and endoscopy suites [35]. The majority of these POCTs are immunochromatographic tests and they are performed in a similar way with whole blood/serum and buffer placed on a test field that diffuses down a test strip [34]. If antibodies (tTG and/or DGP) are present, antigen-antibody complexes are detected by labeled anti-human IgA and/or IgG antibodies. The test is visually read on site after a few minutes as recommended by the manufacturer. A positive test is reflected by the presence of a solid line in the test window and a negative test by the absence of a line in the test window [31–35].

In a recent systematic review and meta-analysis, we observed the pooled sensitivity and specificity of all POCTs (based on tTG or DGP or tTG + anti-gliadin antibodies) for diagnosing CeD to be 94.0% (95% CI, 89.9–96.5%) and 94.4% (95% CI, 90.9–96.5%), respectively. The pooled positive and negative LR for POCTs were 16.7 and 0.06, respectively [36].

2.6. Limitations of Serological Tests

False positive results can occur due to a cross-reaction of antibodies in conditions such as enteric infection, chronic liver disease, congestive heart failure, or hypergammaglobulinemia [37]. The serological tests should ideally be conducted when the patient is on a gluten-containing diet, as being on a low-gluten diet or gluten-free diet can lead to a false negative result [38]. False negative results may also be due to IgA deficiency, which affects 2–3% of the general population [39]. In IgA deficient patients, an IgG -based test such as IgG DGP or IgG anti-tTG antibodies should be performed [12].

A few studies have raised question about the sensitivity of these assays in clinical practice [40,41]. tTG antigens used in these commercial kits are variable, ranging from recombinant human tTG to human tTG cross-linked to gliadin specific peptides [42,43]. In addition, commercial kits typically provide sensitivity and specificity values that are calculated using small, poorly-defined populations, which can be misleading. Several studies comparing different anti-tTG-ab based assays from different manufacturers have revealed variable sensitivities and specificities for detecting CeD; however, most of these studies were small in size and did not have the necessary sample size to accurately comment on the diagnostic accuracies of the testing [22,43–46]. In addition to the possibility of inter-assay variation in the diagnostic performance of commercially available IgA anti-tTG-ab assays, there might be intra-assay variation in the diagnostic performance of these assays for different ethnic populations. Studies from India suggest that the sensitivity of several tTG-ab ELISA assays might be lower in the Indian population than that reported in the Caucasian population [33,36].

3. Genetic Markers

Human Leukocyte Antigen (HLA) DQ Haplotyping

Celiac disease is strongly associated with Human Leukocyte Antigen (HLA) and approximately 95% of CeD patients express HLA-DQ2 encoded by DQA1*05 and DQB1*02 and the rest 5% carry DQ8 alleles encoded by DQA1*03 and DQB1*0302 alleles [47]. The HUGO Gene Nomenclature Committee (http://www.genenames.org/) has shown HLA-DQA1 and HLA-DQB1 class II genes as CELIAC1 [48]. HLA alone accounts for about 40% of genetic heritability for CeD, while 60% genetic susceptibility of CeD by non-HLA genes [49,50]. Other that HLA -DQ2/ DQ8, more than 40 candidate genes have been discovered to be associated with CeD [51,52]. Interestingly, approximately 30% of the general population have HLA-DQ2/DQ8 haplotype, only 3% of them ever develop gluten-related disorders [53].

Human leukocyte antigen typing is not sufficient for the diagnosis of CeD because of its modest sensitivity (HLA-DQ2, 70–99.8%; HLA-DQ8, 1.6–38%) and specificity (HLA-DQ2, 69–77%; HLA-DQ8, 77–85%) [54]. Nevertheless, HLA-DQ typing test has a high negative predictive value that suggests if an individual is negative for HLA-DQ typing, he or she is less likely to have CeD [49]. Human leukocyte antigen (HLA)-DQ typing is mainly used for the exclusion of CeD and it is considered to be an additional test especially in patients where no agreement exists between the serological and histological results.

4. Biomarkers to Predict Presence of Enteropathy

Villous atrophy is the hallmark of CeD, which gets reverted after the institution of GFD. While the clinical response to GFD is evident in weeks and months; reversal of mucosal changes takes months and even years [2,54]. Furthermore, despite GFD, complete villous recovery may not be achieved. The small intestinal mucosal biopsy is the cornerstone for the diagnosis of CeD. In addition to being the gold standard for the initial diagnosis of CeD, periodic biopsies are also recommended for the monitoring of the disease. However, obtaining biopsies is an invasive and expensive procedure (endoscopic examination). Moreover, a correct assessment of biopsies requires an experienced pathologist and well-oriented high-quality biopsy specimens. In fact, an active debate is going on amongst the celiac disease scientific community, whether to do biopsies or skip biopsies in the making of a CeD diagnosis. A relevant question is "can we demonstrate/predict villous atrophy by non-invasive means?"

Enterocytes are very specialized cells and they perform specific functions including absorption of nutrients and secretion of enzymes. Because of the constant exposure of the gastrointestinal (GI) tract to harsh mechanical and chemical conditions, the GI tract has evolved mechanisms to cope with these assaults via a highly regulated process of self-renewal [55]. Most of the epithelial cells are replaced every 3 to 5 days. According to the so-called "Unitarian hypothesis", first proposed by Cheng and Leblond, epithelial cell renewal is driven by a common intestinal stem cell residing within the crypt base [56,57]. From their niche, intestinal stem cells (ISCs) give rise to transit-amplifying cells that migrate upwards and progressively lose their proliferative capability and mature to become fully-differentiated villous epithelial cells (absorptive enterocytes or secretory cells which include goblet cells, enteroendocrine cells, paneth cells, and tuft cells). Each adult crypt harbors approximately 5 to 15 ISCs that are responsible for the daily production of about 300 cells; up to 10 crypts are necessary to replenish the epithelium of a single villus [58]. According to mathematical modeling, approximately 1400 mature enterocytes are shed from a single villus tip in 24 h (2×10^8 cells shed from small intestine every day) [58].

All the changes that occur in the intestinal mucosa include intraepithelial lymphocytosis, heightened apoptosis of enterocytes, heightened regeneration of enterocytes, imbalance in the rate of apoptosis and regeneration leading to decrease in the villous height, enterocyte mass, and increase in the inflammatory cells in the mucosa [59,60].

There are certain molecules which can serve as a biomarker of the enterocyte mass and enterocyte function (citrulline, cytochrome P450 3A4), enterocyte injury (intestinal fatty acid binding protein), and enterocyte regeneration (regenerating gene 1α).

4.1. Cytochrome P450 3A4

Like the liver, intestinal mucosa also has a drug metabolizing enzyme system along with the crypt- villous axis. Cytochrome P450 3A4 is a drug-metabolizing enzyme system expressed abundantly at the tips of the villi, and less abundantly at the crypts [61]. Loss of intestinal villi because of any cause including CeD can lead to a reduction in the activity of CYP3A4. Both the expression and function of CYP3A4 can be assessed to estimate the function of enterocytes. Simvastatin is a lipid-lowering agent that is metabolized by CYP3A4. Therefore, the function of CYP3A4 can be assessed by pharmacokinetics and maximum concentration (C_{max}) of orally administered simvastatin (SV) in blood. While healthy people having normal enterocyte function should have a low level of SV and higher levels of its metabolites in the blood; the levels of SV should be high and its metabolites level should be low in those having enteropathy. Therefore, the assessment of the functional activity of CYP3A4 may serve as a biomarker for enteropathy [62,63].

As a preclinical test of this hypothesis, we measured the plasma concentrations of SV and its major metabolites in mice expressing the human CYP3A4 transgene in the small intestine, in whom acute enteropathy had been induced using polyinosinic-polycytidylic acid (poly I:C). In CYP3A4-humanized mice, a marked decrease in simvastatin metabolism was observed in response to enteropathy. Encouraging results from these experiments motivated us to do a clinical study involving untreated as well as treated patients with CeD along with healthy controls, in order to determine the potential utility of using serum concentrations of SV and/or its metabolites as a tool predicting enteropathy. We included 11 healthy volunteers, 18 newly diagnosed patients with CeD, and 25 patients with CeD who had followed a GFD for more than one year. The C_{max} of orally administered SV, plus its major non-CYP3A4 derived metabolite SV acid (SV_{eq} C_{max}) was measured, and compared to clinical, histological, and serological parameters. Untreated patients with CeD displayed a significantly higher SV_{eq} C_{max} (46 ± 24 nM) compared to treated patients (21 ± 16 nM, $p < 0.001$) or healthy subjects (19 ± 11 nM, $p < 0.005$). SV_{eq} C_{max} correctly predicted the diagnosis in 16/18 untreated celiac patients as well as the recovery status of all follow-up patients. Therefore, SV_{eq} C_{max} is a promising non-invasive marker for the assessment of small intestinal health. Further studies are warranted to establish its clinical utility for assessing the status of villous abnormality in patients with CeD.

4.2. Plasma Citrulline

Citrulline is a non-protein amino acid that is mainly synthesized by the enterocyte and hence the level of citrulline in plasma can represent the synthetic function of the enterocytes [64]. The concept of using citrulline as a marker of enterocyte mass was first provided by Crenn et al. [65]. They reported lower citrulline levels in the plasma of patients with short bowel syndrome compared to controls (20 ± 13 vs. 40 ± 10 µmol L^{-1}, $p < 0.001$). Furthermore, the level of plasma citrulline also correlated with the length of the residual intestine [66]. A lower level of plasma citrulline in comparison to healthy controls has been observed in many small intestinal diseases including CeD, giardiasis, tropical sprue, and small bowel lymphoma. Interestingly, a declining trend in the levels of plasma citrulline was observed with increasing severity of villous atrophy i.e., concentration of citrulline <10 µmol L^{-1} in patients with diffuse total villous atrophy, 10–20 µmol L^{-1} in patients with proximal-only total villous atrophy, and 20–30 µmol L^{-1} for patients with partial villous atrophy. At an optimum cut-off value of plasma citrulline of 20 µmol L^{-1}, the diagnostic accuracy of predicting villous abnormality was 92% with sensitivity and specificity of 95% and 90%, respectively [67].

In a recent study, we have shown that plasma citrulline of <30 µmol L^{-1} indicates the presence of villous abnormality of modified Marsh grade more than 2 with a diagnostic accuracy of 89% with sensitivity and specificity of 78.6% and 95.5%, respectively. Above mentioned statistics suggest that it is possible to predict significant villous abnormality based on the citrulline level even without obtaining duodenal mucosal biopsies in 78.6% patients with 95.5% specificity in patients suspected to have CeD. Therefore, in a clinical context of a positive anti-tTG Ab, if the plasma citrulline is less than 30 µmol L^{-1}, one can predict that there is significant villous atrophy and one can choose to avoid duodenal biopsy for demonstration of villous atrophy. (Under publication) A recent meta-analysis by Fragkos et al. has shown that citrulline levels correlate with small bowel length in patients with short bowel syndrome (r = 0.76) while negatively correlate with the severity of intestinal disease such as CeD, tropical enteropathy, Crohn's disease, mucositis, acute rejection in intestinal transplantation [67].

4.3. Intestinal-Fatty Acid Binding Proteins

Fatty acid-binding proteins (FABPs) are small (14–15 KDa) cytoplasmic proteins involved in the cholesterol and phospholipid metabolism, transport of long-chain fatty acids and maintenance of lipid homeostasis [68]. Fatty acid-binding proteins was first discovered in 1972 and by now nine types of FABP have been identified from the different organs where they are involved in active lipid metabolism. Intestinal type (I-FABP) is specifically expressed in intestine and encoded by the FABP2 gene present on chromosome 4 [69]. Intestinal fatty acid-binding proteins is expressed throughout the intestine, most abundantly in the jejunum, and in greater abundance in enterocytes at the villous tip than in the enterocytes at the crypts.

As I-FABP is expressed in enterocytes, the injury to enterocytes leads to the release of I-FABP at the local sites, which are then absorbed and passes into the circulation. As the levels of I-FABP get elevated in the serum in patients with enterocyte damage, I-FABPs has been considered to be a potential biomarker for the detection of enteropathy [70]. Elevated levels of I-FABP are detected in patients with necrotizing enterocolitis in preterm infants, mesenteric infarction, and intestinal allograft rejection [71–75].

In a study including 96 biopsy-proven adult CeD patients, I-FABP levels were higher in untreated CeD compared with controls (median 691 pg mL^{-1} vs. 178 pg mL^{-1}, $p < 0.001$) and the level declined with GFD [76]. Interestingly, in those patients with CeD, where the FABP levels remained elevated, the biopsy showed persistent histological abnormalities. In another multicenter study, high FABP levels have been shown to predict the diagnosis of CeD in 61/90 (67.8%) children [77].

In a study of treatment naïve patients with CeD, we observed that the optimal cut-off value of plasma I-FABP is ≥1100 pg ml^{-1} in predicting villous abnormalities of modified Marsh grade 2 or more. Using the ROC curve analysis, we observed a diagnostic accuracy of 78% with sensitivity, specificity and odds ratio, LR+ and LR- of 39.7%, 95.5%, 13.9 (95% CI 5.8–33.1%), 8.7 and 0.63, respectively in predicting villous abnormality of modified Marsh grade 2 or more (under publication). We believe that I-FABP may be a good biomarker of enterocyte damage but it requires more studies around the world to understand its consistent performance. There are inconsistencies in the performance of I-FABP as a diagnostic marker as reported in earlier studies [74,76,78].

4.4. Regenerating Gene1α

Human *Reg1α* is a member of the multigene family and it plays a role in the regeneration of cells [79]. There are four types of the Reg gene, Reg1α is one of them which is also known as lithostathine-1-alpha or islet cell regeneration factor (ICRF) or islet of Langerhans regenerating protein (Reg) [80]. In the GI tract, the highest levels of expression of Reg1α have been observed in the small intestine and it is considered as a regulator of cell growth that is required to generate and maintain the villous structure [81]. A high level of the Reg1α may denote the effort of the small intestinal mucosa trying to compensate for the accelerated enterocyte injury/apoptosis/necrosis [82]. In patients with CeD where there is excessive apoptosis of enterocytes, there is a higher expression of the Reg1α gene in the intestinal crypts and the expression falls with GFD [83]. There is only one study showing elevated levels of Reg1α in patients with CeD (n = 40) compared to healthy controls (n = 35) and the levels declined after GFD [84]. There is a need for further study to prove whether Reg1α is a stable marker or not.

5. High-Throughput Technologies for Biomarker Discovery

Several studies have employed high throughput genomics, transcriptomics, and proteomics approaches to find out a panel of biomarkers to reveal the extent and status of small intestinal damage by CeD.

5.1. Transcriptomics Approaches

Since transcriptomics requires a lower amount of biological material such as intestinal mucosal biopsies, this approach has been used to explore various aspects of small intestinal biology including phenotypes and functions of T cells, as well as cytokine profiles within the small intestinal tissue [85]. In order to define the global cytokine gene expression network associated with CeD, one study demonstrated higher expression of interleukin (IL)-15, IL-18, and IL-21 with gluten ingestion, which could drive the inflammatory response in them [86]. In another study, a significant upregulation of 25 odd defense-related genes was observed, including IRF1, SPINK4, ITLN1, OAS2, CIITA, HLA-DMB, HLA-DOB, PSMB9, TAP1, BTN3A1, and CX3CL1 in intestinal epithelial cells of patients having active CeD in comparison with those treated with GFD [87]. Galatola M, et al. have explored the possibility of the development of a non-invasive biomarker obtainable from peripheral circulation by carrying out gene expression analysis using peripheral blood mono-nuclear cells (PBMCs) and they defined a 4 gene PBMC signature including NFKB, IL-21, LPP, and RGS1 for discriminating patients with CeD from non-CeD individuals [88]. Although these genes were significantly differentially expressed in the intestinal mucosa, their expression differences were much weaker in PBMCs. Subsequently the same group demonstrated a set of 9 genes including KIAA, TAGAP (T-cell Activation GTPase Activating Protein), and SH2B3 (SH2B Adaptor Protein 3), RGS1 (Regulator of G-protein signaling 1), TAGAP, TNFSF14 (Tumor Necrosis Factor Superfamily member 14), and SH2B3 which could differentiate patients with CeD from controls [89].

Two recent transcriptomics studies have made strides towards defining transcriptomics signatures in CeD. In one of the studies, we analyzed the transcriptomes in the intestinal mucosa of HLA DQ2/DQ positive asymptomatic first-degree relatives (FDRs) of patients with CeD and showed that pre-symptomatic FDRs harbored a transcriptomic signature that was distinct from controls in spite of the fact that these FDRs had no symptoms or enteropathy at the time of the study. This clearly suggests that there are phenotypic differences in individuals without active enteropathy, which may be exploited in order to develop a biomarker to predict intestinal damage. The second study demonstrated a CeD / no CeD diagnosis based on transcriptomic profiles of duodenal biopsies which revealed a potential biomarker subset consisting of CXCL10, GBP5, IFI27, IFNG, and UBD [90].

5.2. Proteomics Approach

Proteomics studies typically require a higher amount of biological material for studying the proteome profile in tissues. Recent advances in label-free quantitative approaches have enabled whole tissue proteomics of many tissues including small intestinal biopsies in patients with CeD [91]. In a recent study, biopsy specimens collected from patients with CeD before and after 1-year treatment with GFD showed differential expression of proteins such as Ig variable region IGHV5-51, which could serve as a specific marker of immune activation in patients with CeD.

Proteomics approaches have also been used to identify autoantigens in patients with CeD. Stulík J et al. used sera and intestinal biopsies from the patient with CeD and carried out 2D gel electrophoresis of the intestinal proteome followed by immunoblotting of matched patient sera in order to identify the repertoire of self-antigen in CeD patients [92]. This study detected 11 new self-antigen including Adenosine tri-phosphate (ATP) synthase β, enolase α, and several other unannotated proteins. A major limitation of this study was the limited use of proteomics to identify a very small number of autoantigens and the use of a very limited sample size. However, this study suggests that several autoantigens like tTG exist in patients with CeD against which serum antibodies may be developed.

5.3. Metabolomics Approaches

While there is a relative paucity of proteome-based studies, many metabolomic studies have been done in patients with CeD to find metabolic markers of CeD, presumably due to the fact that metabolites can be detected with greater sensitivity and with much lower requirement of biological material. Typically, mass spectrometric (MS) and nuclear magnetic resonance (NMR) methods are used for metabolomics [93]. Nuclear Magnetic Resonance studies that have been carried out with urine and sera of patients with CeD in comparison to those of healthy controls have revealed several metabolic differences between the two study groups [94]. Sera of CeD patients have demonstrated lower levels of amino acids, lipids, pyruvate, and choline and higher levels of glucose and 3-hydroxybutyric acid in comparison to the healthy controls. Differentiation of patients with CeD from healthy controls was done by ^{1}H NMR studies using serum and urine metabolomics, where a pattern of metabolites was observed [95].

Furthermore, using partial least squares-discriminant analysis of metabolites expressed in the small intestinal mucosa, we observed a clear distinction in the pattern of metabolites in the intestinal mucosa of patients with CeD and controls. There was a significantly higher concentration of isoleucine, leucine, aspartate, succinate, and pyruvate, and a lower concentration of glycerol-phosphocholine in the duodenal mucosa of patients with CeD patients compared with controls, suggesting abnormalities in glycolysis, Krebs cycle, and amino acid metabolism in patients with CeD.

While studies based on metabolomic approach have provided a distinctive pattern of metabolites which can differentiate patients with CeD from controls, such a pattern is based on a large panel of metabolites, rather than based on a few metabolites. Hence, it is less likely that such a pattern of metabolites can be tested individually in a clinical laboratory.

6. Biomarker to Predict Dietary Adherence

The mainstay of treatment of CeD is a life-long GFD with strict adherence. It is hard for the patient to achieve the high adherence rate because of widespread use of gluten in the food industry [96]. Approximately one-third of patients with CeD are not able to comply with GFD very well and even those who do, a persistence of enteropathy is observed in 20–40% of patients, which most likely attributable to inadvertent use of gluten by cross contamination [97,98]. It is therefore important to monitor the level of adherence to GFD by a biomarker which can detect ingestion of gluten by patients with CeD.

6.1. Gluten Immunogenic Peptide

Gluten immunogenic peptide (GIP) are fragments of gluten which are resistant to digestion and therefore eliminated in the urine and the stool [99]. The presence of gluten in the urine or stool indicates recent consumption of gluten-containing food [100]. The α-gliadin 33-mer is the main immunodominant toxic peptide that interacts with the immune system of patients with CeD and a proportion of this peptide is absorbed in the GI tract and makes it way from blood to and partly excreted in the stool [99].

The gluten peptide fraction has been detected in the stool of healthy subjects after consumption of not only a normal gluten-containing diet but even in those who have consumed even <100 mg gluten/day. The level of gluten peptides detected in the stool has been shown to be in proportionate with the amount of gluten ingestion [101]. Gluten Immunogenic Peptide is also detectable in urine, and a positive correlation was observed with the amount of gluten intake and amount excreted in the urine. Gluten Immunogenic Peptide can be detected in the urine even with 25 mg of gluten ingestion.

Gluten Immunogenic Peptide is detected by anti-GIP immunochromatographic strips and the conduct of the test is very simple and the test has high sensitivity and specificity [102]. The GIP detection kit is similar to the pregnancy test, where GIP present in the sample, react with specific antibody on the strips. As GIP is rapidly cleared through urine, the presence of GIP in the urine suggests the ingestion of gluten within 20 h. Since the GIP stays longer in the intestinal lumen before getting completely excreted, the detection of GIP in stool suggests the ingestion of gluten within 2–7 days. Approximately 17–80% of patients with CeD who are following GFD have been found to have GIP in their stool [102].

6.2. Mean Platelet Volume

Mean platelet volume (MPV) has been recognized as a marker of inflammation in various diseases such as ulcerative colitis, acute pancreatitis and myocardial infraction etc. [103–105]. Purnak et al. have shown significantly higher MPV in CeD compared to healthy subjects and significant decrease in MPV in those showing good compliance to GFD compared to non-compliant individuals [106].

7. Miscellaneous Biomarkers

7.1. MicroRNAs

MicroRNAs (miRNAs) are small, endogenous noncoding RNAs that act as post-transcriptional regulators of gene expression. Upon cell death, miRNAs are released into the surrounding environment and then reach peripheral blood circulation or body fluids, hence detection of tissue- specific or tissue-enriched miRNA in biofluids might be used as a biomarker for specific tissue damage and specific tissue event. In a study, including untreated adult CeD patients, treated CeD patients and control subjects without CeD showed dysregulation of seven miRNAs such as miR-31-5p, miR-192-3p, miR-194-5p, miR-551a, miR-551b-5p, miR-638 and miR-1290 in patients with CeD compared to those without CeD [107]. In another study, the expression pattern of miR-21 and miR-31 was assessed in pediatric patients with CeD using qRT-PCR where significant up-regulation of miR-21 and down-regulation of miR-31 was observed in the untreated celiac patients in comparison with the treated group (n = 25) and healthy controls (n = 20). Furthermore, there was a correlation between the expression of miR-21 and the titer of anti- tTG Ab [108]. Many miRNAs including specifically miR-21 and miR-31 require further exploration.

7.2. Biomarkers for Assessment of Intestinal Permeability

Assessment of intestinal permeability is performed to assess the overall function of transport through the intestinal epithelial paracellular route [109]. Urinary excretion of disaccharides and monosaccharides and the ratio of their excretion is a basis for the measurement of intestinal permeability. Intestinal permeability can be assessed using a variety of marker probes such as lactulose, mannitol, rhamnose and cellobiose, polyethylene glycol (PEG) 400, PEG 1000, ^{51}Cr-EDTA and ^{99m}Tc-DTPA. The lactulose and mannitol ratio is the most commonly used test for assessment of small intestinal permeability. The majority of treatment naïve patients with CeD have abnormal intestinal permeability [109]. While the withdrawal of gluten improves both clinical and histological abnormalities, it also normalizes the paracellular function and hence the intestinal permeability in them.

8. Conclusions

While many of the currently used biomarkers for the screening and diagnosis of CeD are quite reliable, there is need for blood biomarkers which can predict presence of villous abnormalities even without performing intestinal mucosal biopsies and biomarkers which can assist in the monitoring of the disease. While initial data on the performance of biomarkers such as plasma citrulline and plasma I-FABP in the prediction of the presence of villous abnormalities even without obtaining intestinal mucosal biopsies is very promising, there is a need for further validation of these biomarkers before they can be used reliably in the clinical practice. GIP detection in the stool or in the urine is now used in the clinical practice for detection of gluten ingestion; a positive test however, only reflects ingestion of gluten over the past few days, before the performance of the test. What really is required is a test which can tell us the adherence to gluten ingestion over a longer period of time. In order to understand the fundamental biology and in search of the clinically usable biomarker, a number of research laboratories are exploring various approaches such as transcriptomics, proteomics, and genetics, and we hope that these powerful technologies will provide us in the near future with clinically usable biomarkers for the diagnosis, treatment, and monitoring of the diseases.

Author Contributions: A.S; literature search, original draft preparation, manuscript writing, literature evaluation and interpretation, editing, A.P.; literature review, proof-reading, visualization, P.A.; review and editing, proof-reading, G.M.; conceptualization, critical revision of the manuscript, funding acquisition, overall study guarantor.

Funding: The financial grant for this study was provided by the Department of Science and Technology (DST), Government of India (SB/SO/HS/0097/2013) and Intra-mural grant from All India Institute of Medical Sciences, New Delhi, India.

Acknowledgments: We, all the authors, acknowledge the support of funding agency for providing the grant. We acknowledge the administrative and technical support.

Conflicts of Interest: We, all the authors, declare that there is no conflict of interest.

References

1. Ludvigsson, J.F.; Leffler, D.A.; Bai, J.C.; Biagi, F.; Fasano, A.; Green, P.H.; Hadjivassiliou, M.; Kaukinen, K.; Kelly, C.P.; Leonard, J.N.; et al. The Oslo definitions for coeliac disease and related terms. *Gut* **2013**, *62*, 43–52. [CrossRef] [PubMed]
2. Singh, P.; Arora, A.; Strand, T.A.; Leffler, D.A.; Catassi, C.; Green, P.H.; Kelly, C.P.; Ahuja, V.; Makharia, G.K. Global Prevalence of Celiac Disease: Systematic Review and Meta-analysis. *Clin. Gastroenterol. Hepatol.* **2018**, *16*, 823–836. [CrossRef] [PubMed]
3. Lohi, S.; Mustalahti, K.; Kaukinen, K.; Laurila, K.; Collin, P.; Rissanen, H.; Lohi, O.; Bravi, E.; Gasparin, M.; Reunanen, A.; et al. Increasing prevalence of coeliac disease over time. *Aliment. Pharmacol. Ther.* **2007**, *26*, 1217–1225. [CrossRef] [PubMed]
4. McMillan, S.A.; Watson, R.P.; McCrum, E.E.; Evans, A.E. Factors associated with serum antibodies to reticulin, endomysium, and gliadin in an adult population. *Gut* **1996**, *39*, 43–47. [CrossRef] [PubMed]
5. Werkstetter, K.J.; Korponay-Szabó, I.R.; Popp, A.; Villanacci, V.; Salemme, M.; Heilig, G.; Lillevang, S.T.; Mearin, M.L.; Ribes-Koninckx, C.; Thomas, A.; et al. Accuracy in Diagnosis of Celiac Disease Without Biopsies in Clinical Practice. *Gastroenterology* **2017**, *153*, 924–935. [CrossRef] [PubMed]
6. Aronson, J.K.; Ferner, R.E. Biomarkers-A General Review. *Curr. Protoc. Pharmacol.* **2017**, *76*, 1–9.
7. Cichewicz, A.B.; Mearns, E.S.; Taylor, A.; Boulanger, T.; Gerber, M.; Leffler, D.A.; Drahos, J.; Sanders, D.S.; Thomas Craig, K.J.; Lebwohl, B. Diagnosis and Treatment Patterns in Celiac Disease. *Dig. Dis. Sci.* **2019**. [CrossRef] [PubMed]
8. Kivel, R.M.; Kearns, D.H.; Liebowitz, D. Significance of antibodies to dietary proteins in the serums of patients with nontropical sprue. *N. Engl. J. Med.* **1964**, *271*, 769–772. [CrossRef]
9. Ladinser, B.; Rossipal, E.; Pittschieler, K. Endomysium antibodies in coeliac disease: An improved method. *Gut* **1994**, *35*, 776–778. [CrossRef]
10. Salmaso, C.; Ocmant, A.; Pesce, G.; Altrinetti, V.; Montagna, P.; Descalzi, D.; Martino, S.; Bagnasco, M.; Mascart, F. Comparison of ELISA for tissue trans-glutaminase autoantibodies with antiendomysium antibodies in pediatric and adult patients with celiac disease. *Allergy* **2001**, *56*, 544–547. [CrossRef]
11. Barcia, G.; Posar, A.; Santucci, M.; Parmeggiani, A. Autism and coeliac disease. *J. Autism Dev. Disord.* **2008**, *38*, 407–408. [CrossRef] [PubMed]
12. Villalta, D.; Tonutti, E.; Prause, C.; Koletzko, S.; Uhlig, H.H.; Vermeersch, P.; Bossuyt, X.; Stern, M.; Laass, M.W.; Ellis, J.H.; et al. IgG antibodies against deamidated gliadin peptides for diagnosis of celiac disease in patients with IgA deficiency. *Clin. Chem.* **2010**, *56*, 464–468. [CrossRef] [PubMed]
13. Volta, U.; Bellentani, S.; Bianchi, F.B.; Brandi, G.; De Franceschi, L.; Miglioli, L.; Granito, A.; Balli, F.; Tiribelli, C. High prevalence of celiac disease in Italian general population. *Dig. Dis. Sci.* **2001**, *46*, 1500–1505. [CrossRef] [PubMed]
14. Chorzelski, T.P.; Sulej, J.; Tchorzewska, H.; Jablonska, S.; Beutner, E.H.; Kumar, V. IgA class endomysium antibodies in dermatitis herpetiformis and coeliac disease. *Ann. N. Y. Acad. Sci.* **1983**, *420*, 325–334. [CrossRef] [PubMed]
15. Carroccio, A.; Cavataio, F.; Iacono, G.; Agate, V.; Ippolito, S.; Kazmierska, I.; Campagna, P.; Soresi, M.; Montalto, G. IgA antiendomysial antibodies on the umbilical cord in diagnosing celiac disease. Sensitivity, specificity, and comparative evaluation with the traditional kit. *Scand. J. Gastroenterol.* **1996**, *31*, 759–763. [CrossRef] [PubMed]

16. Chou, R.; Bougatsos, C.; Blazina, I.; Mackey, K.; Grusing, S.; Selph, S. Screening for Celiac Disease: Evidence Report and Systematic Review for the US Preventive Services Task Force. *JAMA* **2017**, *317*, 1258–1268. [CrossRef] [PubMed]
17. Carroccio, A.; Vitale, G.; Di Prima, L.; Chifari, N.; Napoli, S.; La Russa, C.; Gulotta, G.; Averna, M.R.; Montalto, G.; Mansueto, S.; et al. Comparison of anti-transglutaminase ELISAs and an anti-endomysial antibody assay in the diagnosis of celiac disease: A prospective study. *Clin. Chem.* **2002**, *48*, 1546–1550. [PubMed]
18. Dieterich, W.; Ehnis, T.; Bauer, M.; Donner, P.; Volta, U.; Riecken, E.O.; Schuppan, D. Identification of tissue transglutaminase as the autoantigen of celiac disease. *Nat. Med.* **1997**, *3*, 797–801. [CrossRef]
19. Candi, E.; Schmidt, R.; Melino, G. The cornified envelope: A model of cell death in the skin. *Nat. Rev. Mol. Cell Biol.* **2005**, *6*, 328–340. [CrossRef]
20. Eckert, R.L.; Kaartinen, M.T.; Nurminskaya, M.; Belkin, A.M.; Colak, G.; Johnson, G.V.; Mehta, K. Transglutaminase regulation of cell function. *Physiol. Rev.* **2014**, *94*, 383–417. [CrossRef]
21. Tursi, A.; Brandimarte, G.; Giorgetti, G.M. Prevalence of antitissue transglutaminase antibodies in different degrees of intestinal damage in celiac disease. *J. Clin. Gastroenterol.* **2003**, *36*, 219–221. [CrossRef] [PubMed]
22. Nardecchia, S.; Auricchio, R.; Discepolo, V.; Troncone, R. Extra-Intestinal Manifestations of Coeliac Disease in Children: Clinical Features and Mechanisms. *Front. Pediatr.* **2019**, *7*, 56. [CrossRef] [PubMed]
23. Seah, P.P.; Fry, L.; Hoffbrand, A.V.; Holborow, E.J. Tissue antibodies in dermatitis herpetiformis and adult coeliac disease. *Lancet* **1971**, *1*, 834–836. [CrossRef]
24. Jackson, J.R.; Eaton, W.W.; Cascella, N.G.; Fasano, A.; Kelly, D.L. Neurologic and psychiatric manifestations of celiac disease and gluten sensitivity. *Psychiatr. Q.* **2012**, *83*, 91–102. [CrossRef] [PubMed]
25. Hadjivassiliou, M.; Mäki, M.; Sanders, D.S.; Williamson, C.A.; Grünewald, R.A.; Woodroofe, N.M.; Korponay-Szabó, I.R. Autoantibody targeting of brain and intestinal transglutaminase in gluten ataxia. *Neurology* **2006**, *66*, 373–377. [CrossRef] [PubMed]
26. De Leo, L.; Aeschlimann, D.; Hadjivassiliou, M.; Aeschlimann, P.; Salce, N.; Vatta, S.; Ziberna, F.; Cozzi, G.; Martelossi, S.; Ventura, A.; et al. Anti-transglutaminase 6 Antibody Development in Children With Celiac Disease Correlates With Duration of Gluten Exposure. *J. Pediatr. Gastroenterol. Nutr.* **2018**, *66*, 64–68. [CrossRef] [PubMed]
27. Hadjivassiliou, M.; Aeschlimann, P.; Sanders, D.S.; Mäki, M.; Kaukinen, K.; Grünewald, R.A.; Bandmann, O.; Woodroofe, N.; Haddock, G.; Aeschlimann, D.P. Transglutaminase 6 antibodies in the diagnosis of gluten ataxia. *Neurology* **2013**, *80*, 1740–1745. [CrossRef] [PubMed]
28. Volta, U.; Granito, A.; Parisi, C.; Fabbri, A.; Fiorini, E.; Piscaglia, M.; Tovoli, F.; Grasso, V.; Muratori, P.; Pappas, G.; et al. Deamidated gliadin peptide antibodies as a routine test for celiac disease: A prospective analysis. *J. Clin. Gastroenterol.* **2010**, *44*, 186–190. [CrossRef]
29. Volta, U.; Granito, A.; Fiorini, E.; Parisi, C.; Piscaglia, M.; Pappas, G.; Muratori, P.; Bianchi, F.B. Usefulness of antibodies to deamidated gliadin peptides in celiac disease diagnosis and follow up. *Dig. Dis. Sci.* **2008**, *53*, 1582–1588. [CrossRef]
30. Lewis, N.R.; Scott, B.B. Meta-analysis: Deamidated gliadin peptide antibody and tissue transglutaminase antibody compared as screening tests for coeliac disease. *Aliment. Pharmacol. Ther.* **2010**, *31*, 73–81. [CrossRef]
31. Raivio, T.; Korponay-Szabó, I.; Collin, P.; Laurila, K.; Huhtala, H.; Kaartinen, T.; Partanen, J.; Mäki, M.; Kaukinen, K. Performance of a new rapid whole blood coeliac test in adult patients with low prevalence of endomysial antibodies. *Dig. Liver Dis.* **2007**, *39*, 1057–1063. [CrossRef] [PubMed]
32. Korponay-Szabó, I.R.; Raivio, T.; Laurila, K.; Opre, J.; Király, R.; Kovács, J.B.; Kaukinen, K.; Fésüs, L.; Mäki, M. Coeliac disease case finding and diet monitoring by point-of-care testing. *Aliment. Pharmacol. Ther.* **2005**, *22*, 729–737. [CrossRef] [PubMed]
33. Singh, P.; Wadhwa, N.; Chaturvedi, M.K.; Bhatia, V.; Saini, S.; Tandon, N.; Makharia, G.K.; Maki, M.; Not, T.; Phillips, A.; et al. Validation of point-of-care testing for coeliac disease in children in a tertiary hospital in north India. *Arch. Dis. Child.* **2014**, *99*, 1004–1008. [CrossRef]
34. Raivio, T.; Kaukinen, K.; Nemes, E.; Laurila, K.; Collin, P.; Kovács, J.B.; Mäki, M.; Korponay-Szabó, I.R. Self transglutaminase-based rapid coeliac disease antibody detection by a lateral flow method. *Aliment. Pharmacol. Ther.* **2006**, *24*, 147–154. [CrossRef] [PubMed]

35. Mooney, P.D.; Wong, S.H.; Johnston, A.J.; Kurien, M.; Avgerinos, A.; Sanders, D.S. Increased Detection of Celiac Disease with Measurement of Deamidated Gliadin Peptide Antibody Before Endoscopy. *Clin. Gastroenterol. Hepatol.* **2015**, *13*, 1278–1284. [CrossRef] [PubMed]
36. Singh, P.; Arora, A.; Strand, T.A.; Leffler, D.A.; Mäki, M.; Kelly, C.P.; Ahuja, V.; Makharia, G.K. Diagnostic Accuracy of Point of Care Tests for Diagnosing Celiac Disease: A Systematic Review and Meta-Analysis. *J. Clin. Gastroenterol.* **2018**. [CrossRef]
37. Castillo, N.E.; Theethira, T.G.; Leffler, D.A. The present and the future in the diagnosis and management of celiac disease. *Gastroenterol. Rep.* **2015**, *3*, 3–11. [CrossRef] [PubMed]
38. Rubio-Tapia, A.; Hill, I.D.; Kelly, C.P.; Calderwood, A.H.; Murray, J.A. American College of Gastroenterology. ACG clinical guidelines: Diagnosis and management of celiac disease. *Am. J. Gastroenterol.* **2013**, *108*, 656–676. [CrossRef]
39. Vilppula, A.; Kaukinen, K.; Luostarinen, L.; Krekelä, I.; Patrikainen, H.; Valve, R.; Mäki, M.; Collin, P. Increasing prevalence and high incidence of celiac disease in elderly people: A population-based study. *BMC Gastroenterol.* **2009**, *9*, 49. [CrossRef]
40. Sharma, M.; Singh, P.; Agnihotri, A.; Das, P.; Mishra, A.; Verma, A.K.; Ahuja, A.; Sreenivas, V.; Khadgawat, R.; Gupta, S.D.; et al. Celiac disease: A disease with varied manifestations in adults and adolescents. *J. Dig. Dis.* **2013**, *14*, 518–525. [CrossRef]
41. Singh, P.; Agnihotri, A.; Jindal, G.; Sharma, P.K.; Sharma, M.; Das, P.; Gupta, D.; Makharia, G.K. Celiac disease and chronic liver disease: Is there a relationship? *Indian J. Gastroenterol.* **2013**, *32*, 404–408. [CrossRef] [PubMed]
42. Murray, J.A.; Van Dyke, C.; Plevak, M.F.; Dierkhising, R.A.; Zinsmeister, A.R.; Melton, L.J., 3rd. Trends in the identification and clinical features of celiac disease in a North American community, 1950–2001. *Clin. Gastroenterol. Hepatol.* **2003**, *1*, 19–27. [CrossRef] [PubMed]
43. Singh, P.; Sharma, P.K.; Agnihotri, A.; Jyotsna, V.P.; Das, P.; Gupta, S.D.; Makharia, G.K.; Khadgawat, R. Coeliac disease in patients with short stature: A tertiary care centre experience. *Natl. Med. J. India* **2015**, *28*, 176–180. [PubMed]
44. Hill, I.D.; Dirks, M.H.; Liptak, G.S.; Colletti, R.B.; Fasano, A.; Guandalini, S.; Hoffenberg, E.J.; Horvath, K.; Murray, J.A.; Pivor, M.; et al. Guideline for the diagnosis and treatment of celiac disease in children: Recommendations of the North American Society for Pediatric Gastroenterology, Hepatology and Nutrition. *J. Pediatr. Gastroenterol. Nutr.* **2005**, *40*, 1–19. [CrossRef] [PubMed]
45. Verma, A.K.; Gatti, S.; Lionetti, E.; Galeazzi, T.; Monachesi, C.; Franceschini, E.; Balanzoni, L.; Scattolo, N.; Cinquetti, M.; Catassi, C. Comparison of Diagnostic Performance of the IgA Anti-tTG Test vs. IgA Anti-Native Gliadin Antibodies Test in Detection of Celiac Disease in the General Population. *Clin. Gastroenterol. Hepatol.* **2018**, *16*, 1997–1998. [CrossRef] [PubMed]
46. Vader, W.; Stepniak, D.; Kooy, Y.; Mearin, L.; Thompson, A.; van Rood, J.J.; Spaenij, L.; Koning, F. The HLA-DQ2 gene dose effect in celiac disease is directly related to the magnitude and breadth of gluten-specific T cell responses. *Proc. Natl. Acad. Sci. USA* **2003**, *100*, 12390–12395. [CrossRef] [PubMed]
47. Yates, B.; Braschi, B.; Gray, K.A.; Seal, R.L.; Tweedie, S.; Bruford, E.A. Genenames.org: The HGNC and VGNC resources in 2017. *Nucleic Acids Res.* **2017**, *45*, 619–625.
48. Ludvigsson, J.F.; Bai, J.C.; Biagi, F.; Card, T.R.; Ciacci, C.; Ciclitira, P.J.; Green, P.H.; Hadjivassiliou, M.; Holdoway, A.; van Heel, D.A.; et al. Diagnosis and management of adult coeliac disease: Guidelines from the British Society of Gastroenterology. *Gut* **2014**, *63*, 1210–1228. [CrossRef] [PubMed]
49. Wolters, V.M.; Wijmenga, C. Genetic background of celiac disease and its clinical implications. *Am. J. Gastroenterol.* **2008**, *103*, 190–195. [CrossRef]
50. Dubois, P.C.; Trynka, G.; Franke, L.; Hunt, K.A.; Romanos, J.; Curtotti, A.; Zhernakova, A.; Heap, G.A.; Adány, R.; Aromaa, A.; et al. Multiple common variants for celiac disease influencing immune gene expression. *Nat. Genet.* **2010**, *42*, 295–302. [CrossRef]
51. Diosdado, B.; Wapenaar, M.C.; Franke, L.; Duran, K.J.; Goerres, M.J.; Hadithi, M.; Crusius, J.B.; Meijer, J.W.; Duggan, D.J.; Mulder, C.J.; et al. A microarray screen for novel candidate genes in coeliac disease pathogenesis. *Gut* **2004**, *53*, 944–951. [CrossRef] [PubMed]
52. Bai, J.C.; Ciacci, C.; Melberg, J. World Gastroenterology Organisation Global Guidelines: Celiac Disease. *J. Clin. Gastroenterol.* **2017**, *51*, 755–768. [CrossRef] [PubMed]

53. Kaukinen, K.; Partanen, J.; Mäki, M.; Collin, P. HLA-DQ typing in the diagnosis of celiac disease. *Am. J. Gastroenterol.* **2002**, *97*, 695–699. [CrossRef] [PubMed]
54. Ramakrishna, B.S.; Makharia, G.K.; Chetri, K.; Dutta, S.; Mathur, P.; Ahuja, V.; Amarchand, R.; Balamurugan, R.; Chowdhury, S.D.; Daniel, D.; et al. Prevalence of Adult Celiac Disease in India: Regional Variations and Associations. *Am. J. Gastroenterol.* **2016**, *111*, 115–123. [CrossRef] [PubMed]
55. Lin, S.A.; Barker, N. Gastrointestinal stem cells in self-renewal and cancer. *J. Gastroenterol.* **2011**, *46*, 1039–1055. [CrossRef] [PubMed]
56. Cheng, H.; Leblond, C.P. Origin, differentiation and renewal of the four main epithelial cell types in the mouse small intestine. V. Unitarian Theory of the origin of the four epithelial cell types. *Am. J. Anat.* **1974**, *141*, 537–561. [CrossRef] [PubMed]
57. Bjerknes, M.; Cheng, H. Intestinal epithelial stem cells and progenitors. *Methods Enzymol.* **2006**, *419*, 337–383.
58. Stem, J.; Flickinger, J.C., Jr.; Merlino, D.; Caparosa, E.M.; Snook, A.E.; Waldman, S.A. Therapeutic targeting of gastrointestinal cancer stem cells. *Regen. Med.* **2019**. [CrossRef]
59. Potten, C.S. A comprehensive study of the radiobiological response of the murine(BDF1) small intestine. *Int. J. Radiat. Biol.* **1990**, *58*, 925–973. [CrossRef]
60. Shalimar, D.M.; Das, P.; Sreenivas, V.; Gupta, S.D.; Panda, S.K.; Makharia, G.K. Mechanism of villous atrophy in celiac disease: Role of apoptosis and epithelial regeneration. *Arch. Pathol. Lab. Med.* **2013**, *137*, 1262–1269. [CrossRef]
61. Kolars, J.C.; Lown, K.S.; Schmiedlin-Ren, P.; Ghosh, M.; Fang, C.; Wrighton, S.A.; Merion, R.M.; Watkins, P.B. CYP3A gene expression in human gut epithelium. *Pharmacogenetics* **1994**, *4*, 247–259. [CrossRef] [PubMed]
62. Lang, C.C.; Brown, R.M.; Kinirons, M.T.; Deathridge, M.A.; Guengerich, F.P.; Kelleher, D.; O'Briain, D.S.; Ghishan, F.K.; Wood, A.J. Decreased intestinal CYP3A in celiac disease: Reversal after successful gluten-free diet: A potential source of interindividual variability in first-pass drug metabolism. *Clin. Pharmacol. Ther.* **1996**, *59*, 41–46. [CrossRef]
63. Bragde, H.; Jansson, U.; Jarlsfelt, I.; Söderman, J. Gene expression profiling of duodenal biopsies discriminates celiac disease mucosa from normal mucosa. *Pediatr. Res.* **2011**, *69*, 530–537. [CrossRef] [PubMed]
64. Wu, G.; Knabe, D.A.; Flynn, N.E. Synthesis of citrulline from glutamine in pig enterocytes. *Biochem. J.* **1994**, *299*, 115–121. [CrossRef] [PubMed]
65. Crenn, P.; Coudray-Lucas, C.; Thuillier, F.; Cynober, L.; Messing, B. Postabsorptive plasma citrulline concentration is a marker of absorptive enterocyte mass and intestinal failure in humans. *Gastroenterology* **2000**, *119*, 1496–1505. [CrossRef] [PubMed]
66. Gondolesi, G.; Fishbein, T.; Chehade, M.; Tschernia, A.; Magid, M.; Kaufman, S.; Raymond, K.; Sansaricq, C.; LeLeiko, N. Serum citrulline is a potential marker for rejection of intestinal allografts. *Transplant. Proc.* **2002**, *34*, 918–920. [CrossRef]
67. Fragkos, K.C.; Forbes, A. Citrulline as a marker of intestinal function and absorption in clinical settings: A systematic review and meta-analysis. *United Eur. Gastroenterol. J.* **2018**, *6*, 181–191. [CrossRef]
68. Sarkar-Banerjee, S.; Chowdhury, S.; Sanyal, D.; Mitra, T.; Roy, S.S.; Chattopadhyay, K. The Role of Intestinal Fatty Acid Binding Proteins in Protecting Cells from Fatty Acid Induced Impairment of Mitochondrial Dynamics and Apoptosis. *Cell. Physiol. Biochem.* **2018**, *51*, 1658–1678. [CrossRef]
69. Ockner, R.K.; Manning, J.A.; Poppenhausen, R.B.; Ho, W.K. A binding protein for fatty acids in cytosol of intestinal mucosa, liver, myocardium, and other tissues. *Science* **1972**, *177*, 56–58. [CrossRef]
70. Chan, C.P.; Wan, T.S.; Watkins, K.L.; Pelsers, M.M.; Van der Voort, D.; Tang, F.P.; Lam, K.H.; Mill, J.; Yuan, Y.; Lehmann, M.; et al. Rapid analysis of fatty acid-binding proteins with immunosensors and immunotests for early monitoring of tissue injury. *Biosens. Bioelectron.* **2005**, *20*, 2566–2580. [CrossRef]
71. Guthmann, F.; Börchers, T.; Wolfrum, C.; Wustrack, T.; Bartholomäus, S.; Spener, F. Plasma concentration of intestinal- and liver-FABP in neonates suffering from necrotizing enterocolitis and in healthy preterm neonates. *Mol. Cell. Biochem.* **2002**, *239*, 227–234. [CrossRef] [PubMed]
72. Holmes, J.H., 4th; Lieberman, J.M.; Probert, C.B.; Marks, W.H.; Hill, M.E.; Paull, D.L.; Guyton, S.W.; Sacchettini, J.; Hall, R.A. Elevated intestinal fatty acid binding protein and gastrointestinal complications following cardiopulmonary bypass: A preliminary analysis. *J. Surg. Res.* **2001**, *100*, 192–196. [PubMed]
73. Kanda, T.; Fujii, H.; Fujita, M.; Sakai, Y.; Ono, T.; Hatakeyama, K. Intestinal fatty acid binding protein is available for diagnosis of intestinal ischaemia:immunochemical analysis of two patients with ischaemic intestinal diseases. *Gut* **1995**, *36*, 788–791. [CrossRef] [PubMed]

74. Kanda, T.; Fujii, H.; Tani, T.; Murakami, H.; Suda, T.; Sakai, Y.; Ono, T.; Hatakeyama, K. Intestinal fatty acid-binding protein is a useful diagnostic marker for mesenteric infarction in humans. *Gastroenterology* **1996**, *110*, 339–343. [CrossRef] [PubMed]
75. Edelson, M.B.; Sonnino, R.E.; Bagwell, C.E.; Lieberman, J.M.; Marks, W.H.; Rozycki, H.J. Plasma intestinal fatty acid binding protein in neonates with necrotizing enterocolitis: A pilot study. *J. Pediatr. Surg.* **1999**, *34*, 1453–1457. [CrossRef]
76. Adriaanse, M.P.; Tack, G.J.; Passos, V.L.; Damoiseaux, J.G.; Schreurs, M.W.; van Wijck, K.; Riedl, R.G.; Masclee, A.A.; Buurman, W.A.; Mulder, C.J.; et al. Serum I-FABP as marker for enterocyte damage in coeliac disease and its relation to villous atrophy and circulating autoantibodies. *Aliment. Pharmacol. Ther.* **2013**, *37*, 482–490. [CrossRef] [PubMed]
77. Adriaanse, M.P.; Leffler, D.A.; Kelly, C.P.; Schuppan, D.; Najarian, R.M.; Goldsmith, J.D.; Buurman, W.A.; Vreugdenhil, A.C. Serum I-FABP Detects Gluten Responsiveness in Adult Celiac Disease Patients on a Short-Term Gluten Challenge. *Am. J. Gastroenterol.* **2016**, *11*, 1014–1022. [CrossRef] [PubMed]
78. Kittaka, H.; Akimoto, H.; Takeshita, H.; Funaoka, H.; Hazui, H.; Okamoto, M.; Kobata, H.; Ohishi, Y. Usefulness of intestinal fatty acid-binding protein in predicting strangulated small bowel obstruction. *PLoS ONE* **2014**, *9*, e99915. [CrossRef]
79. Terazono, K.; Yamamoto, H.; Takasawa, S.; Shiga, K.; Yonemura, Y.; Tochino, Y.; Okamoto, H. A novel gene activated in regenerating islets. *J. Biol. Chem.* **1988**, *263*, 2111–2114. [PubMed]
80. Schiesser, M.; Bimmler, D.; Frick, T.W.; Graf, R. Conformational changes of pancreatitis-associated protein (PAP) activated by trypsin lead to insoluble protein aggregates. *Pancreas* **2001**, *22*, 186–192. [CrossRef]
81. Planas, R.; Pujol-Autonell, I.; Ruiz, E.; Montraveta, M.; Cabre, E.; Lucas-Martin, A.; Pujol-Borrell, R.; Martinez-Caceres, E.; Vives-Pi, M. Regenerating gene Iα is a biomarker for diagnosis and monitoring of celiac disease: A preliminary study. *Transl. Res.* **2011**, *158*, 140–145. [CrossRef] [PubMed]
82. Sekikawa, A.; Fukui, H.; Fujii, S.; Ichikawa, K.; Tomita, S.; Imura, J.; Chiba, T.; Fujimori, T. REG Ialpha protein mediates an anti-apoptotic effect of STAT3 signaling in gastric cancer cells. *Carcinogenesis* **2008**, *29*, 76–83. [CrossRef] [PubMed]
83. Rubio-Tapia, A.; Rahim, M.W.; See, J.A.; Lahr, B.D.; Wu, T.T.; Murray, J.A. Mucosal recovery and mortality in adults with celiac disease after treatment with a gluten-free diet. *Am. J. Gastroenterol.* **2010**, *105*, 1412–1420. [CrossRef] [PubMed]
84. Raine, T.; Liu, J.Z.; Anderson, C.A.; Parkes, M.; Kaser, A. Generation of primary human intestinal T cell transcriptomes reveals differential expression at genetic risk loci for immune-mediated disease. *Gut* **2015**, *64*, 250–259. [PubMed]
85. Garrote, J.A.; Gómez-González, E.; Bernardo, D.; Arranz, E.; Chirdo, F. Celiac disease pathogenesis: The proinflammatory cytokine network. *J. Pediatr. Gastroenterol. Nutr.* **2008**, *47* (Suppl. 1), S27–S32. [CrossRef] [PubMed]
86. Pietz, G.; De, R.; Hedberg, M.; Sjöberg, V.; Sandström, O.; Hernell, O.; Hammarström, S.; Hammarström, M.L. Immunopathology of childhood celiac disease-Key role of intestinal epithelial cells. *PLoS ONE* **2017**, *12*, e0185025.
87. Galatola, M.; Izzo, V.; Cielo, D.; Morelli, M.; Gambino, G.; Zanzi, D.; Strisciuglio, C.; Sperandeo, M.P.; Greco, L.; Auricchio, R. Gene expression profile of peripheral blood monocytes: A step towards the molecular diagnosis of celiac disease? *PLoS ONE* **2013**, *8*, e74747. [CrossRef] [PubMed]
88. Galatola, M.; Cielo, D.; Panico, C.; Stellato, P.; Malamisura, B.; Carbone, L.; Gianfrani, C.; Troncone, R.; Greco, L.; Auricchio, R. Presymptomatic Diagnosis of Celiac Disease in Predisposed Children: The Role of Gene Expression Profile. *J. Pediatr. Gastroenterol. Nutr.* **2017**, *65*, 314–320. [CrossRef]
89. Bragde, H.; Jansson, U.; Fredrikson, M.; Grodzinsky, E.; Söderman, J. Celiac disease biomarkers identified by transcriptome analysis of small intestinal biopsies. *Cell. Mol. Life Sci.* **2018**, *75*, 4385–4401.
90. Tutturen, A.E.V.; Dørum, S.; Clancy, T.; Reims, H.M.; Christophersen, A.; Lundin, K.E.A.; Sollid, L.M.; de Souza, G.A.; Stamnaes, J. Characterization of the Small Intestinal Lesion in Celiac Disease by Label-Free Quantitative Mass Spectrometry. *Am. J. Pathol.* **2018**, *188*, 1563–1579. [CrossRef]
91. Stulík, J.; Hernychová, L.; Porkertová, S.; Pozler, O.; Tucková, L.; Sánchez, D.; Bures, J. Identification of new celiac disease autoantigens using proteomic analysis. *Proteomics* **2003**, *3*, 951–956. [CrossRef] [PubMed]

92. Gundamaraju, R.; Vemuri, R.; Eri, R.; Ishiki, H.M.; Coy-Barrera, E.; Yarla, N.S.; Dos Santos, S.G.; Alves, M.F.; Barbosa Filho, J.M.; Diniz, M.F.F.M.; et al. Metabolomics as a Functional Tool in Screening Gastro Intestinal Diseases: Where are we in High Throughput Screening? *Comb. Chem. High Throughput Screen.* **2017**, *20*, 247–254. [CrossRef] [PubMed]
93. Bertini, I.; Calabrò, A.; De Carli, V.; Luchinat, C.; Nepi, S.; Porfirio, B.; Renzi, D.; Saccenti, E.; Tenori, L. The metabonomic signature of celiac disease. *J. Proteome Res.* **2009**, *8*, 170–177. [CrossRef] [PubMed]
94. Bernini, P.; Bertini, I.; Calabrò, A.; la Marca, G.; Lami, G.; Luchinat, C.; Renzi, D.; Tenori, L. Are patients with potential celiac disease really potential? The answer of metabonomics. *J. Proteome Res.* **2011**, *10*, 714–721. [CrossRef] [PubMed]
95. Bernardo, D.; Peña, A.S. Developing strategies to improve the quality of life of patients with gluten intolerance in patients with and without coeliac disease. *Eur. J. Intern. Med.* **2012**, *23*, 6–8. [CrossRef] [PubMed]
96. Bethune, M.T.; Crespo-Bosque, M.; Bergseng, E.; Mazumdar, K.; Doyle, L.; Sestak, K.; Sollid, L.M.; Khosla, C. Noninflammatory gluten peptide analogs as biomarkers for celiac sprue. *Chem Biol.* **2009**, *16*, 868–881. [CrossRef] [PubMed]
97. Tye-Din, J.A.; Stewart, J.A.; Dromey, J.A.; Beissbarth, T.; van Heel, D.A.; Tatham, A.; Henderson, K.; Mannering, S.I.; Gianfrani, C.; Jewell, D.P.; et al. Comprehensive, quantitative mapping of T cell epitopes in gluten in celiac disease. *Sci. Transl. Med.* **2010**, *2*, 41ra51. [CrossRef] [PubMed]
98. Costa, A.F.; Sugai, E.; Temprano, M.P.; Niveloni, S.I.; Vázquez, H.; Moreno, M.L.; Domínguez-Flores, M.R.; Muñoz-Suano, A.; Smecuol, E.; Stefanolo, J.P.; et al. Gluten immunogenic peptide excretion detects dietary transgressions in treated celiac disease patients. *World J. Gastroenterol.* **2019**, *25*, 1409–1420. [CrossRef] [PubMed]
99. Gerasimidis, K.; Zafeiropoulou, K.; Mackinder, M.; Ijaz, U.Z.; Duncan, H.; Buchanan, E.; Cardigan, T.; Edwards, C.A.; McGrogan, P.; Russell, R.K. Comparison of Clinical Methods with the Faecal Gluten Immunogenic Peptide to Assess Gluten Intake in Coeliac Disease. *J. Pediatr. Gastroenterol. Nutr.* **2018**, *67*, 356–360. [CrossRef]
100. Comino, I.; Real, A.; Vivas, S.; Síglez, M.Á.; Caminero, A.; Nistal, E.; Casqueiro, J.; Rodríguez-Herrera, A.; Cebolla, A.; Sousa, C. Monitoring of gluten-free diet compliance in celiac patients by assessment of gliadin 33-mer equivalent epitopes in feces. *Am. J. Clin. Nutr.* **2012**, *95*, 670–677. [CrossRef]
101. Moreno, M.L.; Cebolla, Á.; Muñoz-Suano, A.; Carrillo-Carrion, C.; Comino, I.; Pizarro, Á.; León, F.; Rodríguez-Herrera, A.; Sousa, C. Detection of gluten immunogenic peptides in the urine of patients with coeliac disease reveals transgressions in the gluten-free diet and incomplete mucosal healing. *Gut* **2017**, *66*, 250–257. [CrossRef] [PubMed]
102. Comino, I.; Fernández-Bañares, F.; Esteve, M.; Ortigosa, L.; Castillejo, G.; Fambuena, B.; Ribes-Koninckx, C.; Sierra, C.; Rodríguez-Herrera, A.; Salazar, J.C.; et al. Fecal Gluten Peptides Reveal Limitations of Serological Tests and Food Questionnaires for Monitoring Gluten-Free Diet in Celiac Disease Patients. *Am. J. Gastroenterol.* **2016**, *111*, 1456–1465. [CrossRef] [PubMed]
103. Yüksel, O.; Helvaci, K.; Başar, O.; Köklü, S.; Caner, S.; Helvaci, N.; Abayli, E.; Altiparmak, E. An overlooked indicator of disease activity in ulcerative colitis: Mean platelet volume. *Platelets* **2009**, *20*, 277–281. [CrossRef] [PubMed]
104. Ghaffari, S.; Pourafkari, L.; Javadzadegan, H.; Masoumi, N.; Jafarabadi, M.A.; Nader, N.D. Mean platelet volume is a predictor of ST resolution following thrombolysis in acute ST elevation myocardial infarction. *Thromb. Res.* **2015**, *136*, 101–106. [PubMed]
105. Purnak, T.; Efe, C.; Yuksel, O.; Beyazit, Y.; Ozaslan, E.; Altiparmak, E. Mean platelet volume could be a promising biomarker to monitor dietary compliance in celiac disease. *Ups. J. Med. Sci.* **2011**, *116*, 208–211. [CrossRef] [PubMed]
106. Bascuñán-Gamboa, K.A.; Araya-Quezada, M.; Pérez-Bravo, F. MicroRNAs: An epigenetic tool to study celiac disease. *Rev. Esp. Enferm. Dig.* **2014**, *106*, 325–333.
107. Amr, K.S.; Bayoumi, F.S.; Eissa, E.; Abu-Zekry, M. Circulating microRNAs as potential non-invasive biomarkers in pediatric patients with celiac disease. *Eur. Ann. Allergy Clin. Immunol.* **2019**. [CrossRef]

108. Mishra, A.; Makharia, G.K. Techniques of functional and motility test: How to perform and interpret intestinal permeability. *J. Neurogastroenterol. Motil.* **2012**, *18*, 443–447. [CrossRef]
109. Mishra, A.; Prakash, S.; Sreenivas, V.; Das, T.K.; Ahuja, V.; Gupta, S.D.; Makharia, G.K. Structural and Functional Changes in the Tight Junctions of Asymptomatic and Serology-negative First-degree Relatives of Patients with Celiac Disease. *J. Clin. Gastroenterol.* **2016**, *50*, 551–560. [CrossRef]

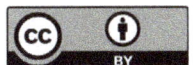

© 2019 by the authors. Licensee MDPI, Basel, Switzerland. This article is an open access article distributed under the terms and conditions of the Creative Commons Attribution (CC BY) license (http://creativecommons.org/licenses/by/4.0/).

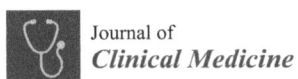

Review

Use of Hyperspectral/Multispectral Imaging in Gastroenterology. Shedding Some–Different–Light into the Dark

Samuel Ortega [1,*], Himar Fabelo [1], Dimitris K. Iakovidis [2], Anastasios Koulaouzidis [3] and Gustavo M. Callico [1]

1. Institute for Applied Microelectronics (IUMA), University of Las Palmas de Gran Canaria (ULPGC), Las Palmas de Gran Canaria 35017, Spain; hfabelo@iuma.ulpgc.es (H.F.); gustavo@iuma.ulpgc.es (G.M.C.)
2. Dept. of Computer Science and Biomedical Informatics, University of Thessaly, 35131 Lamia, Greece; diakovidis@dib.uth.gr
3. Endoscopy Unit, The Royal Infirmary of Edinburgh, Edinburgh EH16 4SA, UK; akoulaouzidis@hotmail.com
* Correspondence: sortega@iuma.ulpgc.es; Tel.: +34-928-451-220

Received: 26 November 2018; Accepted: 26 December 2018; Published: 1 January 2019

Abstract: Hyperspectral/Multispectral imaging (HSI/MSI) technologies are able to sample from tens to hundreds of spectral channels within the electromagnetic spectrum, exceeding the capabilities of human vision. These spectral techniques are based on the principle that every material has a different response (reflection and absorption) to different wavelengths. Thereby, this technology facilitates the discrimination between different materials. HSI has demonstrated good discrimination capabilities for materials in fields, for instance, remote sensing, pollution monitoring, field surveillance, food quality, agriculture, astronomy, geological mapping, and currently, also in medicine. HSI technology allows tissue observation beyond the limitations of the human eye. Moreover, many researchers are using HSI as a new diagnosis tool to analyze optical properties of tissue. Recently, HSI has shown good performance in identifying human diseases in a non-invasive manner. In this paper, we show the potential use of these technologies in the medical domain, with emphasis in the current advances in gastroenterology. The main aim of this review is to provide an overview of contemporary concepts regarding HSI technology together with state-of-art systems and applications in gastroenterology. Finally, we discuss the current limitations and upcoming trends of HSI in gastroenterology.

Keywords: hyperspectral imaging; multispectral imaging; clinical diagnosis; biomedical optical imaging; gastroenterology; medical diagnostic imaging

1. Introduction

Hyperspectral/Multispectral (HS/MS) imaging (HSI/MSI), also known as Imaging Spectroscopy, is a technology capable of overcoming the imaging limitations of the human vision based in white light (WL). In fact, HSI combines the features provided by two technologies that have been, for decades now, used separately i.e., digital imaging and spectroscopy. Digital imaging allows recording of the morphological features of a given scene, extracting information of different objects in regards to shape and textures. Spectroscopy deals with the interaction between the electromagnetic (EM) radiation and matter. While the capabilities of the human vision are restricted to a certain region of the EM spectrum (EMS), the visible spectrum that spans from 400 to 700 nm, most common HS commercial systems expand this spectral range from 400 to 2500 nm. Although there are HS cameras able to cover the EM up to 12 microns, such systems are restricted to certain applications that are out of the scope of this manuscript. HSI provides information in regions of the EMS that the human eye cannot see, revealing therefore substance properties that are normally unavailable to human beings. Furthermore, while the human eye is only capable of distinguishing three different wavelengths associated with the opsins of the retina (Cianopsin sensitive to 430 nm -*blue light*-; Cloropsin sensitive to 530 nm -*green light*-; and, Eritropsin sensitive to 650 nm -*red light*-), HS cameras can capture the EMS in hundreds of different narrow wavelengths, largely increasing the resolution to over what humans can see. On the other hand, MSI is based on the same principle of HSI with the main difference being that MSI is generally characterized by a lower number of spectral channels [1].

An HS image is recorded in a data structure called HS cube, which contains both spatial and spectral information from a given image. The information inside the HS cube can be visualized in several different ways. If a single pixel from an HS image is selected, the spectrum related to this pixel can be examined. Likewise, it is possible to visualize the entire spatial information for a given wavelength. The observed information at various wavelengths represents different properties of the matter. Figure 1 shows an HS cube, where both types of representations can be observed.

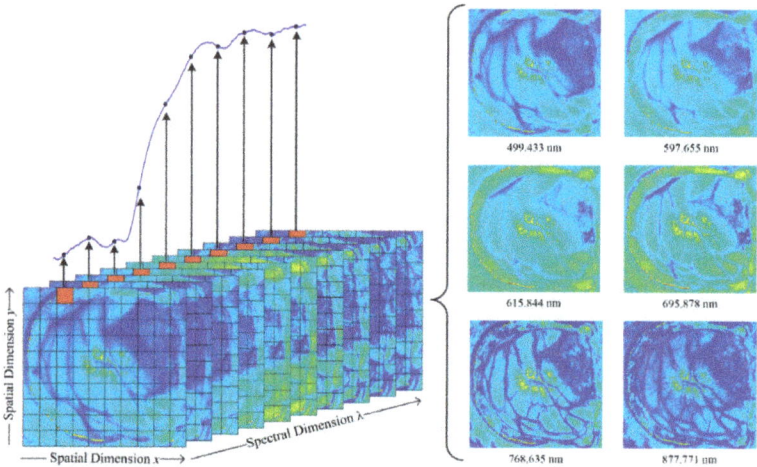

Figure 1. Example of an HS cube from in-vivo human brain surface and spectrum from the pixel in red (**left**). Several images at different wavelengths obtained from the HS datacube (**right**).

The spectral signature (also called spectral fingerprint) is the curve that links the EM radiation with a certain material. The key point of this concept is that each material has its own interaction with the EMS, hence the spectral signature of any given material is unique. By analyzing the spectral signatures contained in an HS image, it is possible to distinguish between the different substances that are present in the captured image. Nevertheless, to properly differentiate materials by using the spectral signature information, some issues have to be addressed. First, the measured spectral signature from the same material can present subtle variations, i.e., inter-sample variability. Second, there are materials that present spectral similarities among them, being extremely challenging to perform an automatic differentiation of such materials based only on their spectral signatures.

Many researchers have employed HSI technology for different applications [1] such as non-invasive food quality inspection [2,3], improving recycling processes [4], or examining paintings for accurate identification of the pigments used in order to refine their restoration [5,6]. Geologists use HSI to identify the location of different minerals [7]. Furthermore, in agriculture this technology has been used to quantitatively characterize the soil [8] or to identify the stress levels of plants [9].

Figure 2 presents an example of the spectral signatures of different tissues [10], where the differences between the spectral signatures of primary (glioblastoma and oligodendroglioma grade III) and secondary brain tumors (metastatic lung, renal and breast) are evident. Just a visual inspection of the shape of the reflectance curve reveals that it is possible to identify the type of tissue present at each pixel of the image. The measured spectral signatures are mainly affected by illumination, the mixture of different substances, and/or by noise.

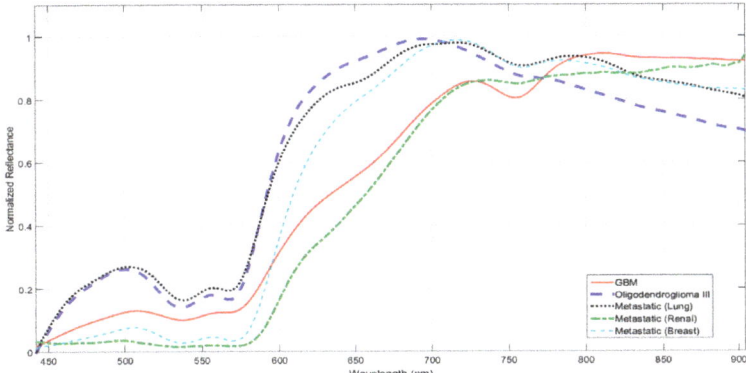

Figure 2. Spectral signatures of different brain tumor tissues in the VNIR (Visible and Near Infrared) range [10]. The abscissa axis represents the different wavelengths, and the ordinate axis represents the normalized reflectance. The continuous red line corresponds to Glioblastoma (GBM); the dashed blue line corresponds to Oligodendroglioma grade III; the dashed black, green and cyan lines correspond to a metastatic lung, renal and breast tumors, respectively.

In biomedical applications, the spectral signature is employed as an indicator of the different biochemical constituents of different tissues [11]. The spectral signature is a useful tool to differentiate among different tissues, and also to provide information useful to discriminate healthy from diseased tissue [12]. Nevertheless, spectral signatures of the same tissue from different subjects present differences due to biological variability. This fact is called inter-patient variability of data. Furthermore, the spectral signatures measures from different parts of the same tissue also present subtle differences. This is called intra-patient variability of data. Handling the intra- and inter-patient variability of data is one of the most important challenges in biomedical HS image analysis.

Due to the large amount of information that HSI provides, it is necessary to process and analyze the acquired HS images by using high-performance computational techniques, thus focusing on the information that is more useful for a particular application. In this review, we briefly discuss the different applications of HSI in the medical field and the HS systems and algorithms more commonly used as well as the current investigations performed in the application of HSI to study and diagnostic gastrointestinal (GI) diseases using in-vitro, ex-vivo and in-vivo samples.

2. Medical Hyperspectral Imaging

This section is intended to provide some context on the use of HS technology in the medical field prior to analyzing details of the use on HS in GI medicine. However, for a deeper introduction about the use of HSI in biomedical applications we strongly recommend the review articles published by Li et al. [13], Lu et al. [14] and Calin et al. [15]. Furthermore, for a better understating about light tissue interactions and how this information can be used in diagnostic applications, we recommend the studies performed in [11,12].

In the first decade of the 21st century, HSI has attracted the interest of researchers in the medical field for two main reasons. First, it has been proven that the interaction between the EM radiation and tissues carries quantitative diagnostic information about tissue pathology [11,12]; and second, because of the non-invasive nature of this technology. Recently, clinicians have started to use HSI in a number of situations. Some aim to detect cholesterol by analyzing HSI of the face [16] or arthritis by studying the skin reflectance [17]. HSI has also been used for detecting peripheral arterial disease [18], to enhance the visualization of blood vessels [19] or to achieve automatic differentiation between veins and arteries during surgery [20]. This technology has also been used to measure the oxygenation levels of retina [21], brain [22], or kidney [23].

In detection of neoplasia, the main aim of using HSI is to develop aid-visualization tools able to accurately delineate the boundaries of the tumor in order to improve resection of cancerous lesions, hence avoiding the unnecessary resection of healthy tissue. This technology has been successfully applied in detecting prostate cancer [24], head and neck cancer [25,26] or breast cancer [27] in animal models. In humans, this technology has been employed for the detection of tongue cancer [28], oral cancer [29], skin tumors [30–32] or brain cancer [10,33].

In the field of histopathology, where the current diagnostic techniques are based on the morphological analysis of tissue specimen slides, HSI can be employed as a complementary source of information that may unburden the workload of the pathologists. Researchers have proven the capabilities in detecting several diseases using this technology, such as examining retina sections for the quantitative assessment and evaluation of the effect of medication [34], detecting cancer metastasis in lung and lymph nodes tissue [35], identifying brain tumors [36] or lung cancer [37].

In the following sections, we briefly introduce the main concepts involved in medical HSI and the use of HSI as a new technology for assessing the detection of GI diseases.

3. Hyperspectral Systems

HS acquisition systems present a challenge to engineers, who have to handle sophisticated optical and electronic systems to generate an HS cube. There are several types of HS cameras, however depending on how data are acquired the main categorization is in spatial scanning cameras and spectral scanning cameras [38].

Spatial scanning cameras, based on the push-broom technique, are capable of acquiring simultaneously a single spatial dimension (a narrow line of an image) and the whole spectral information for a given scene. To capture an HS cube in this manner, it is necessary to perform a spatial scanning, where either the camera or the captured object(s) shift their position while the camera is capturing frames. The scanning can be also performed by using a mirror in front of the fore optic, and moving the mirror to image the whole object. Although the use of mirrors allows developing more compact instrumentation (hence more appealing in clinical circumstances), it is necessary to take care regarding the geometric distortions mirrors can produce in the captured image. The core of these cameras is an optical element that splits the incoming radiation into specific wavelengths values [39].

This type of camera has the advantage of capturing images with high spectral resolution, offering also an excellent trade-off between spatial and spectral resolutions, compared to other HS cameras, in the expense of performing scanning in order to acquire an HS cube. For this reason, in the medical field these types of cameras are used in open surgical procedures, for in-vivo surface inspection or for ex-vivo tissue analysis. It is not possible to directly attach this type of camera to medical apparatus, like laparoscopes or intraoperative microscopes, due to their inability to perform spatial scanning. Some examples of HS acquisition systems, based on push-broom cameras, can be found in Figure 3A,B, while the intraoperative use of these systems are presented in [20,40]. Furthermore, it is possible to use this kind of camera for registering pathological slides [41], as can be observed in Figure 3C.

On the other hand, *spectral scanning* cameras employ an optical element that filters the incoming radiation, registering the entire spatial information of a single wavelength at each and every moment. Capturing an HS cube requires change of the tuned wavelength of the filter in order to perform spectral scanning. There are several types of spectral scanning cameras. The filter wheel cameras require the manual shift of the optical filter, while the Liquid Crystal Tunable Filter (LCTF) or the Acousto-Optic Tunable Filter (AOTF) are devices where the spectral transmission can be electronically controlled [42]. These cameras have lower spectral resolution than the push-broom cameras, and are not suitable for applications where the captured object is moving, because the spatial information may vary for different wavelengths. Nevertheless, these cameras can be easily attached to medical instruments and can offer high spatial resolutions. An example of HS acquisition system for medical applications using these cameras is shown in Figure 3D [43].

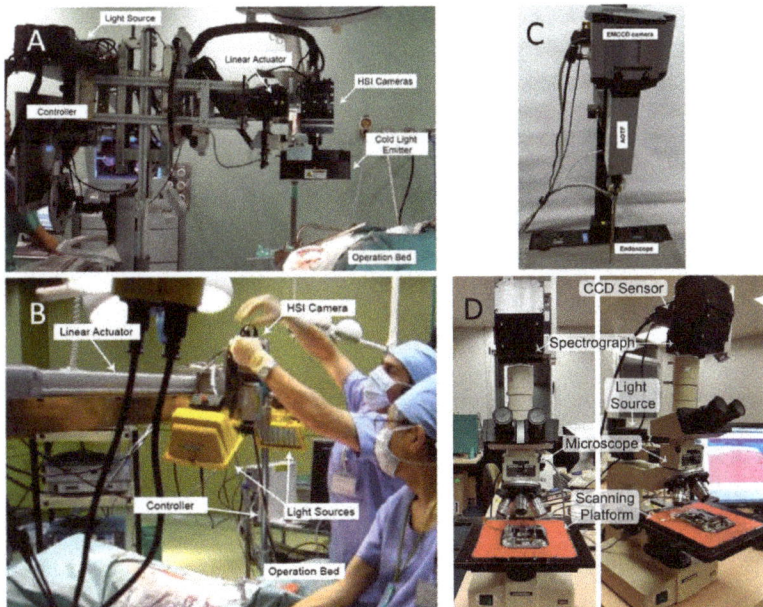

Figure 3. HS acquisition system used in medical applications. (**A,B**) HSI acquisition systems based on push-broom cameras for in-vivo human brain tumor detection [40] and in-vivo pig abdominal surgery [20]; (**C**) Liquid crystal tunable filter camera attached to an endoscope for cancerous tissue detection [43]; (**D**) Microscope coupled to an HSI push-broom camera for pathological slides registration [36].

The remaining type of HS cameras is called snapshot [44]. Snapshot technology is intended to deal with the main limitation imposed by the previously described HS technologies: real-time acquisition. It is not possible to collect HS or MS data in real-time using the above-mentioned HS technologies for the requirement of performing a scan (either spatial or spectral). These technologies are restricted to static situations, or scenarios where the object that is moving has a slightly lower speed compared to the scan speed. For these reasons, where necessary to obtain HS data of non-static scenes (e.g., living cell imaging) a snapshot camera must be employed. Furthermore, snapshot cameras can be directly attached to clinical instrumentation, such as endoscopes or laparoscopes. Nevertheless, both the spectral and the spatial resolution of the snapshot cameras are lower compared to the other HS technologies. To the best of our knowledge, there is no current research in GI using snapshot cameras, mainly because all preliminary exploration of HS technology in GI is focused to prove the capabilities of the technology for diagnosis, and hence it is necessary to evaluate each scenario using high performance spectral and spatial instrumentation.

4. Hyperspectral Image Analysis

As mentioned in the previous sections, HSI data facilitates the identification of different materials. However, to successfully retrieve useful information from HS images, the application of appropriate image analysis techniques is necessary. In this section, a brief overview of such techniques is provided. They include pre-processing algorithms, e.g., for noise removal (HS images carry noise that may affect information extraction) [45,46], HSI system calibration (with respect to the camera spectral range and resolution) [47], feature extraction [48], dimensionality reduction [49], classification [50], spectral unmixing [51], and Normalized Difference Index (NDI) estimation [52,53].

Data acquired using HS instrumentation is highly biased by both the instrumentation and the environmental conditions. In order to remove the influence of instrumentation (mostly the wavelength dependencies of the sensor and grating efficiency and transmission of the lens), is common to perform a calibration. The typical calibration procedure in HS and MS imagery consist of capturing a reference image using a material that has a flat spectral response (e.g., Spectralon). This reference image captures the spectral dependencies of the instrumentation and is used to remove the influence of the instrumentation in the captured HS images.

To ameliorate the challenges imposed by the high dimensionality of HS data, feature extraction and dimensionality reduction approaches are usually employed. Firstly, feature extraction (or band selection) methods are used to select a subset of the original spectral data that contains the most useful information for data exploitation. This reduced set of spectral bands strongly depends on the nature of the specimens under study. Secondly, dimensionality reduction approaches aim to find a representation of HS image data with a lower dimensionality than the original data, while maintaining the most significant information. In HSI, data reduction techniques are widely used for finding new data representations prior to the application of other data analysis techniques (such as classification). This procedure reduces the complexity of the classification task, and it can also contribute to better data visualization or compression [54,55].

One of the key topics in HS image analysis is classification, which aims for the identification of the materials depicted within an HS image. HS data classification methods can be categorized into supervised and unsupervised. Supervised classifiers require training using prior information on the materials to be classified; hence, a mathematical model is optimized using this information. Then, this model is able to infer predictions about new data. A recent review article by Ghamisi et al. [56] analyzes the mostly extended supervised classifiers employed by the HS community. Unsupervised classification methods (also known as clustering methods [57]) have the goal of grouping pixels according to some spectral similarity criteria. Although these kinds of algorithms provide useful information about the materials that are present in a scene, it is not possible to relate these groups of similar pixels with their class membership. Recent studies have shown that the joint exploitation of the spectral and the spatial information in HS images improves the classification performance [58].

Finally, spectral unmixing and NDI estimation have been used for HS image analysis. On the one hand, spectral unmixing techniques, such as those based on Linear Mixture Models (LMMs), make the assumption that each pixel of an HS image can be modeled as the weighted sum of pure spectra elements (called endmembers). This technique tries to overcome the limited spatial resolution that generally characterizes MS and HS imaging compared to the traditional RGB imaging. Unmixing algorithms first find the endmembers and then estimate the abundance (proportion) of each endmember in a single pixel [51]. On the other hand, NDI-based approaches try to establish a combination of spectral channels that reveal some characteristics of the subject under study. For example, the Normalized Difference Vegetation Index (NDVI) aims to assess the presence of live vegetation in HS satellite images [52]. In the context of medical applications, a Melanoma Identification Index has been proposed in [53] for identification of skin lesions in dermoscopic HS images. Additionally, there are some researches that make use of Light Transport Models in tissue to retrieve useful information about tissue diagnosis [16,17,59,60].

5. Hyperspectral Imaging in GI Diagnosis

HSI is an emerging technology still at an early application stage in the medical field. Therefore, the number of publications regarding the use of this technology in gastroenterology is limited. This section summarizes the main research works performed in this field, structured following the taxonomy presented in Figure 4. This taxonomy divides the gastrointestinal HSI applications categorized by the type of application, the type of subject to study and the type of sample (i.e., the organ where this technology is applied).

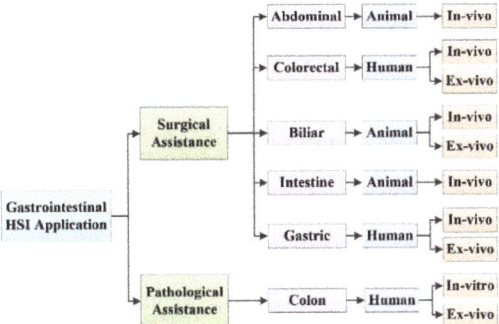

Figure 4. Taxonomy of the current gastrointestinal HSI applications.

5.1. Surgical Assistance in Real-Time

One of the current target applications of medical HSI is in the field of surgical guidance. Such applications are motivated by the non-invasive nature of HSI technology, and for its capability of generating an alternative visualization of tissues, that can assist in the identification of several GI diseases. In this section, we present the most important surgical guidance tools based on HSI developed for GI use.

5.1.1. Abdominal Organs Differentiation

An illustrative use of HSI as a visual guide tool during surgery can be found in [61]. In this research work, the authors collected and processed spectral signatures from various abdominal organs. The experiment was performed during an open abdominal surgery on a pig. By processing the spectral signatures of the small intestine, colon, peritoneum, bladder and spleen, a thematic map where each organ is identified was generated. The results of this thematic map can be found in Figure 5, where each organ is represented with a different color. The automatic identification of different tissues during surgery may extend the surgeon's visual capabilities, making possible examining larger areas of tissue, and therefore saving surgical time.

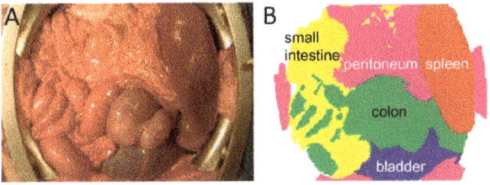

Figure 5. Use of HSI for organs identification in pig's abdominal surgery performed in [61]. (**A**) RGB image from pig's abdominal cavity and organs; (**B**) Segmentation map obtained after HS image processing and analysis, where the different organs are identified using different colors.

5.1.2. Colorectal Surgery

Colorectal surgeries have also been studied using HSI as a guidance tool during tissue resections. Schols et al. [62] presented an explorative study aiming to collect and automatically differentiate five different tissue types within the human abdomen: colon, muscle, artery, vein and mesenteric adipose tissue (Figure 6). This tool could help surgeons to avoid ureteral injuries, which may lead to severe complications such as intra-abdominal sepsis, renal failure or loss of renal functions. Near-infrared

(NIR) fluorescence imaging has been also used to enhance the visualization of the ureters and arteries. However, this technique requires the use of a contrast agent. HS images from 10 human patients were collected and analyzed to verify whether HS images were a suitable tool for identifying arteries and ureters intraoperatively. Although the spectral signatures collected from various organs presented similarities, the authors reached promising results in the automatic discrimination between different tissues. Therefore, the foundations for a non-invasive optical guidance tool that could be used during colorectal surgery, enhancing the visualization of critical anatomy, have been laid. The same research group also studied an approach to automatically identify different tissue types that can be observed during laparoscopic colorectal surgery procedures [63]. Five types of tissue were recorded from ex-vivo human resected specimens, i.e., mesenteric fat, blood vessels, ureter, colonic tissue and tumorous colonic tissue. The data acquisition was carried out by using a spectrometer working in the spectral range 440–1830 nm. Based on the measured spectral signatures, the authors posed that the differentiation between tissues is possible by exploiting the spectral fingerprints of each tissue.

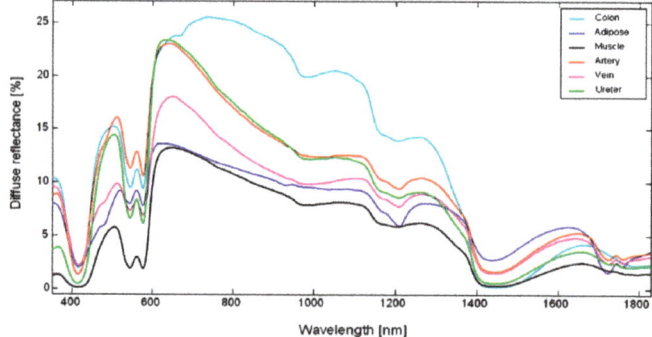

Figure 6. Mean spectra per tissue type acquired during colorectal surgery in [62]. Average tissue spectra for ureter (green), mesenteric adipose tissue (dark blue), artery (red), colon (light blue), muscle (black), and vein (purple).

The above-mentioned research consisted on analyzing the capabilities of HSI to differentiate between different types of tissue. Nevertheless, this technology has been also used for colon diagnosis applications. Malignant colorectal tumors, adenomatous polyps and different types of colorectal normal mucosa were analyzed in [64]. To collect in-vivo HS data, a contactless endoscopic diagnosis support system was attached to an HS camera. The endoscopic system was able to capture HS images in the wavelength range from 405 to 665 nm, acquiring 27 spectral bands using a filter wheel. A total of 21 HS cubes from 12 different patients were employed to assess an innovative band selection algorithm based on Recursive Divergence Method (RDFS). In order to evaluate the performance of the proposed algorithm, a supervised classification method based on a Support Vector Machine (SVM) classifier was used, with the manually labeled spectral samples of the different types of tissue acquired, to serve as a training set. Using only five bands from the original 27, the HSI system was able to identify in real-time the colorectal tumors and outlining the region affected by the tumor with an average accuracy of $92.9 \pm 5.4\%$. Furthermore, only these five bands were sufficient for the enhancement of the visualization of the microvascular network on the mucosa surface. Another approach for colonic cancer detection using HSI can be found in [65], where the authors study the identification of esophageal squamous neoplasm by using an HS endoscopic imaging system.

Finally, although the work performed by Beaulieu et al. [66] cannot be considered strictly as HSI (they use a spectrometer, so there is no spatial information), they present an interesting discussion about which spectral range provides a better discrimination between tumor and normal colon tissues. After the analysis, they concluded that the inclusion of SWIR (Short-Wave InfraRed) spectral bands contribute to a better discrimination of malignant and normal tissue.

5.1.3. Bowel Anastomosis

The correct monitorization of oxygenation and blood volume fractions are key for success in colorectal surgery. For this reason, some researchers have focused their attention on imaging visualization tools that can prevent surgical complications such as intestinal anastomosis. In [67,68] the authors proposed methods to derive both the oxygenation of tissue and the blood volume fraction by using models for light transportation in tissue. The results are shown to surgeons as thematic maps where these physiological parameters are presented (Figure 7A). The work presented in [69] go beyond, and propose a method to suggest the optimal location of sutures for a better surgical outcome. To generate such map (Figure 7B), the authors made use of the information about the blood-vessels location and the tissue thickness (measured from a MS image). Although these research works have been only tested in swine models, they show a promising methodology for improving colorectal surgeries. Another interesting application of MSI in bowel anastomosis can be found on [70]. In this research, authors noticed that the variations in the measured reflectance spectra using an MSI laparoscope are coherent with biophysical changes during small bowel radiofrequency fusions.

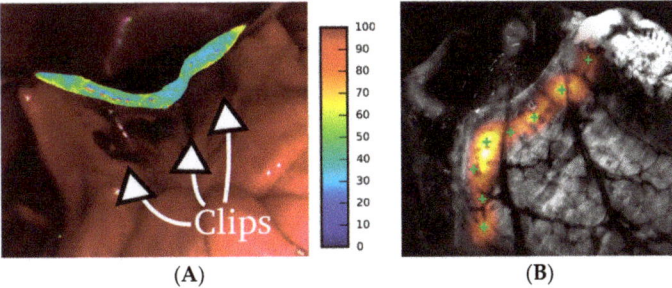

Figure 7. HSI application in Bowel anastomosis. (**A**) Small bowel oxygenation estimation shown in [68]; (**B**) Suture map and recommendations about the location of the suture provided in [69].

5.1.4. Biliary Anatomy Identification

Currently, the technologies used to delineate the anatomy of the biliary tree, such as the Intraoperative Cholangiography (IOC) or the routine intraoperative ultrasonography, are not sufficiently accurate. For this reason, the biliary anatomy has been also investigated using HSI to accurately identify the different parts of the anatomic structure. Concretely, in [71] and [55], Zuzak et al. proposed to use HSI to develop a visualization system capable of identifying the biliary trees that do not depend on any prior dissection. The authors developed an acquisition system consisting of an HS camera coupled with a conventional laparoscope that was intended to enhance the visualization of the biliary anatomy. The spectral range of this device covers the EM spectrum from 650 to 1100 nm. This technology may achieve a reduction of bile duct injuries during surgery. In order to test the ability of HSI in detecting the bile tree, a study visualizing intraoperatively the abdominal organs of pigs during close cholecystectomy procedures was carried out. The authors found that the measured spectra of several anatomic structures are unique, allowing the differentiation of arterial vessels, venous structures and bile duct. In [55], the HS images were processed using PCA (Principal Component Analysis), which proves a visual enhancement of the different observed anatomical structures, i.e., the gall bladder and the liver. The correct identification of the tissue types was assessed by using the morphological structures of each tissue. This research work shows that the visualization of the biliary tree could be safely performed during surgical procedures without the need for prior imaging. The inclusion of this technology may lead to eliminating the risk of the bile duct injury during cholecystectomy, avoiding also the current need of injecting radioactive contrast agents.

In addition, dual-mode imaging systems have been using for this goal. Mitra et al. [72] used a system composed by a Indocyanine-green-loaded (IGC) micro-balloon and an HS camera. The goal of this study was to identify the surrounding anatomy during IOC in real-time. This imaging technique was tested over ex-vivo swine tissues, showing an accurate identification of the biliary anatomy. The advantages of this imaging modality over IOC are its low cost, its real-time response, and its independence of radiation agents. This type of visualization tool can be used for guidance during surgical procedures. Furthermore, it can be used as an additional input to surgical robots, such as the Da Vinci robot [73].

5.1.5. Intestinal Ischemia Identification

The intestinal ischemia can be defined as an inadequate blood flow to the intestine, causing an inability to absorb food and nutrients, bloody diarrheal, infection and gangrene. In this sense, HS technology has been also used for this application. Akbari et al. [74] developed a intraoperative HSI tool capable of obtaining spectral signatures of intestinal ischemia acquired during a pig abdominal surgery. Two cameras were used, covering from 400 to 1700 nm. The methodology followed in this paper to process the HSI data consisted in finding an optimal NDI that allows the discrimination of intestinal ischemia over other kind of tissue. This article demonstrated that the HS image analysis is suitable for visualizing intestinal ischemia during surgical procedures. However, although this study was performed with a wide spectral range and presents good analysis of the capabilities of HSI technology, the instrumentation based on push-broom cameras is extremely outsized, being inappropriate for clinical environments.

5.1.6. Gastric Cancer Identification

Other relevant research where HSI is used to study GI diseases can be found in [75], where the authors describe the use of HSI for detecting human gastric cancer. This study was carried out over ten patients who underwent a total gastrectomy. The HS images were captured ex-vivo after the resection of a tumor using an HS camera covering the range from 1000 to 2500 nm. After pathologic diagnosis, the real diagnosis was compared with the image processing results. Although the data acquisition system was not appropriate to be used for endoscopic diagnosis (it consisted on a proof-of-concept demonstrator), the data analysis enabled the identification of wavelengths improving the differentiation between healthy and tumor tissues. These wavelengths can be employed as specifications in the development of future laparoscopic HSI systems optimized for gastric cancer detection.

Another application of HSI as a guidance tool during surgical procedures can be found in [76]. In this research work, the authors processed the HS data aiming to determine a combination of wavelengths, highlighting the presence of ulcer regions in gastric tissue. Using different spectral components from different types of tissue, the authors generated a thematic map where the visualization of ulcer and erythematous regions of the image were able to be differentiated with respect to the surrounding tissue. Other research works have also studied the in-vivo identification of gastric ulcers using HSI [77] or gastric cancer employing a customized MSI video endoscopy system capable of capturing multispectral video composed by six bands located in the visual spectral range [78]. These research works suggest that HSI and MSI can be used as a guidance tool both for diagnosing, and for delimitating the gastric tumor margins accurately.

5.2. Pathological Assistance

The research works previously presented investigate methods aiming to automatic identification and visualization of different types of tissues, in the context of clinical diagnosis, mainly to facilitate surgical procedures in real-time. Nevertheless, HS images have been also applied to the pathological diagnosis of colonic diseases. The following papers describe the use of HSI for the identification of tumorous tissues from in-vitro and ex-vivo human colon pathology samples.

The work described in [79] presents a study performed on biopsy slides of colon tissue aiming to distinguish between normal and malignant cells through exploiting HSI. A morphological analysis of the HS images of biopsy slides with several microdots belonging to different patients was performed employing a dimensionality reduction and cellular segmentation to describe the shape, orientation and other geometrical attributes, using ICA (Independent Component Analysis) and the k-Means algorithm. The segmentation maps obtained after the application of k-Means clustering algorithm allow differentiating the malignant and benign cells by their morphological features. These morphological features were then used as input to a classification process that differentiates between normal and malignant cells. For this purpose, LDA (Linear Discriminant Analysis) algorithm was used due to its reduced computational cost and acceptable performance. The images were captured with an HSI system based on a tunable light source and a CCD (Charge-Coupled Device) camera coupled to a microscope with a magnification of 400×, covering the spectral range between 450 and 850 nm. An accuracy of up to 84% was obtained in the classification experiments, demonstrating that the use of HSI facilitates the discrimination between normal and malignant cells of colon tissue by using its morphological features.

Furthermore, Rajpoot et al. [80] employed an SVM to classify in-vitro samples of normal and malignant human colon cells. Archival Hematoxylin and Eosin (H&E) stained micro-array tissue sections of normal and malignant (adenocarcinoma) colonic tissue image data cubes were acquired at microscopic level. The spatial dimensions of each HS cube were 1024 × 1024 pixels, having 20 spectral bands covering the wavelength range from 450 to 640 nm. Multiscale morphological features such as area, eccentricity, equivalent diameter, Euler number, extent, orientation, solidity, major axis length, and minor axis length, were obtained from the segmented maps to be used in the SVM classification procedure. The experiments carried out in this study reveal that an accurate discrimination (99.72%) between normal and malignant tissue can be achieved.

Colon biopsy samples have also been studied by Masood et al. [81], where the authors propose an algorithm for the automatic classification of colon biopsies based on spatial analysis of HS images captured from colon biopsy samples. The aim of their work was to distinguish between benign and malignant tissue. Although the authors collected HS cubes with 128 bands, they only use a single spectral band. To this end, the processing framework consisted on selecting a single band and performing a spatial analysis of this image by using Circular Local Binary Patterns (CLBPs). Then this information is used by different supervised classifiers in order to retrieve diagnostic information from colon biopsies. The maximum accuracy obtained was 90.6% for the SVM classification, with 87.5% sensitivity and 93.7% specificity. A clear advantage of performing the spatial analysis on a single band is to save acquisition, storage, and computational costs, but it is difficult to state that this algorithm really makes use of the richness of information contained in the HS images. Although authors reached good discrimination between malignant and benign tissue, the discrimination capabilities may increase if more spectral channels are used.

HSI technology was also evaluated for differentiating normal and cancerous gastric cells in H&E stained pathological slides [82]. In this case, the main motivation to perform the study was to analyze the differences in pH levels between cancerous and normal cells. These pH differences were reflected in the spectral signature of the different cells, providing good discrimination between malignant and normal cells using only the spectral information of cell nuclei. Conversely, the work presented by Hidovic-Rowe et al. [59,60] aimed to extract histological parameters from ex-vivo colon tissues using HSI. The measured parameters were the blood volume fractions, the hemoglobin saturation levels and the size of collagen fibers or the thickness of the mucosa layer. These parameters were computationally estimated by using a light transportation model over colon tissue, identifying both normal and tumor tissues.

Some current technologies used to improve colorectal exams are the White Light Endoscopy (WLE), the Chomoendoscopy, Autofluorescence Imaging and Narrow Band Imaging. Nevertheless, these technologies present limitations that motivate the finding of new technologies to this end. Motivated by this fact, the work presented in [83] evaluated the initial feasibility of using HSI for colonic adenocarcinoma identification using HSI fluorescence excitation-scanning for measuring changes in fluorescence excitation spectrum. To this end, an ex-vivo and in-vitro analysis of colonic tissue was carried out, in order to determinate if HSI fluorescence can be used as an additional endoscopy technology. A total number of eight patients were enrolled in that study. Specimens were imaged using a custom HSI fluorescence excitation-scanning microscope system. As it can be seen in Figure 8A, at short excitation wavelengths, the fluorescence total intensity of adenocarcinomas was lower than normal tissue. However, fluorescence resulting from excitation at higher wavelengths was increased, and in the S4 sample was higher than normal tissue, Figure 8B,C. Transmission and absorbance spectral data indicate that adenocarcinoma displayed increased optical absorbance, as compared to surrounding normal tissue (Figure 8D,E). These preliminary data suggest that there are significant differences in the spectral signature of cancerous and normal tissue. In this sense, the same research group continued the investigations and presented new results in [84,85]. These results could pave the way towards advanced classification systems than can automatically identify tissues attending to their spectral signatures.

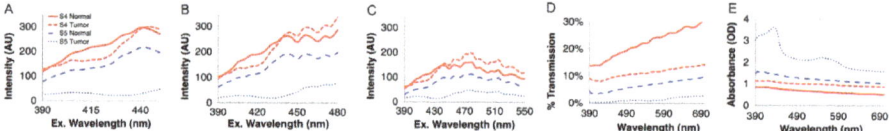

Figure 8. Spectral differences between normal and cancerous tissue for two specimen pairs: S4 and S5 presented in [83]. Preliminary data demonstrate the differences in spectral signature between cancerous and normal tissue. Transmission and absorbance spectral data indicate that adenocarcinoma displays increased optical absorbance, as compared to surrounding normal tissue, with additional spectral differences that could be exploited to increase sensitivity and specificity for tumor detection. Spectral scan types are as follows: (**A**) Fluorescence excitation scan from 390 to 450 nm; (**B**) Fluorescence excitation scan from 390 to 480 nm; (**C**) Fluorescence excitation scan from 390 to 550 nm; (**D**) Transmission scan from 390 to 700 nm; (**E**) Absorbance scan from 390 to 700 nm.

In addition to the studies presented before, there are other interesting and novel applications of pathological assistance using MSI/HSI. For example, authors in [86] collected MS images from four types of colorectal cells: viz. normal, hyperplastic polyps, tabular adenoma with low grade dysplasia and carcinoma. After MSI analysis of different colorectal tissues, an accurate discrimination using colorectal cells was achieved.

Finally, another less conventional approach, investigated in the context of HSI for GI pathological assistance, presents a vocal synthesis model and its application to sonification of HS colonic tissue images [87,88]. The authors state that sonification could be used as an intuitive means of representing and analyzing high-dimensional and complex data. The high-dimensional data for sonification have been obtained from HS scans of normal and abnormal colon tissue, the abnormal tissue being potentially cancerous. The tissue images were collected in cooperation with the Department of Applied Mathematics at Yale University. A series of slides were prepared from distinct patients, containing more than 300 microdots each slide, and each microdot corresponding to a slice of colon tissue (roughly 0.5 × 0.5 mm in size). Each microdot may contain either normal or malignant colon tissue. A slide was chosen and illuminated with a tuned light source (capable of emitting any combination of light frequencies in the range of 450 to 850 nm), and the transmitted image was magnified 400× by a Nikon Biophot microscope. An amount of 15 data cubes of normal colonic tissue and 46 data cubes of abnormal colonic tissue were collected. Examples of pre-processed specimens are illustrated in Figure 9. Initial experiments with a variety of vocal tract models suggest that human ability to easily identify vowel-like sounds is promising for intuitive sonification.

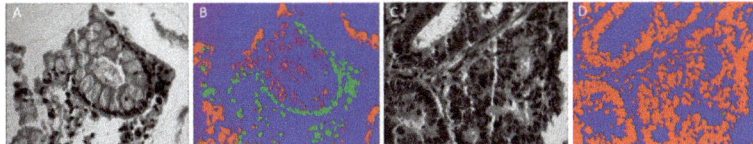

Figure 9. Samples of HS normal and abnormal colonic tissue images and the results obtained after applying the pre-processing sonification presented in [87]. (**A**) Sample specimen showing normal colonic tissue in gray-scale image; (**B**) Final three-dimension image that gives the probabilities that the point in the specimen belongs to normal colon tissue; (**C**) Sample specimen showing abnormal colonic tissue in gray-scale image; (**D**) Final three-dimension image that gives the probabilities that the point in the specimen belongs to abnormal colon tissue.

5.3. HSI Application Summary

Finally, in Table 1 we provide a summary of the most relevant research work in the field of gastroenterology using HSI. This table is organized attending to: (1) the disease that has been investigated; (2) the type of tissue involved in each study; (3) the subject of the research; (4) the HSI technology employed to acquire the images; and (5) the data processing methods applied to extract useful information from HS data.

Table 1. Summary of HSI applications in gastroenterology.

Application/Disease	Spectral Range (nm)	HSI Technology	Experiment Type	Study Subjects	Data Analysis Methods (Category */Method †)	Reference(s)
Biliary tree visualization	650–1050	LCTF	In-vivo	Swine	D, E/PCA	[35]
Colon cancer detection	400–700	LCTF	Ex-vivo	Humans	F, E/LPM	[59,60]
Organs identification during surgery	900–1700	Push-broom	In-vivo	Swine	SA, P/DWT; C/SOM	[61]
Identifying tissues during surgery	350–1830	DRS	In-vivo	Humans	SA, F/SGAD; C/SVM	[62]
Tissue identification during colorectal surgery	440–1830	DRS	Ex-vivo	Humans	SA, C/TPCR	[63]
Malignant colorectal tumors and adenomatous polyps	405–665	Filter Wheel	In-vivo	Humans	R/RDFS; C/SVM	[64]
Colon cancer detection	300–1800	Spectroscopy	Ex-vivo	Humans	C/LDA; C/SVM	[66]
Oxygenation measurement (small bowel)	400–720	LCTF	In-vivo	Swine	Ex/Linear light model	[67]
Oxygenation measurement (small bowel)	470–700	Filter-based	In-vivo	Swine	Ex/Non-linear light model	[68]
Suture recommendation (intestinal anastomosis)	470–770	LED-based	Ex-vivo	Swine	Ex/2D-filtering, SAM and composite images from the multispectral image	[69]
Monitoring radiofrequency fusions in small bowel	460–700	LCTF	In-vivo	Swine	Ex/Linear light model	[70]
Biliary trees identification	650–1100	LCTF	In-vivo	Swine	D, E/PCA	[71]
Biliary anatomy visualization	650–700	LCTF	Ex-vivo	Swine	S/LMM, R/PCA	[72]
Intestinal ischemia identification	400–1700	Push-broom	In-vivo	Swine	I/Ischemia Index; C/SVM	[74]
Gastric cancer detection	1000–2500	Push-broom	Ex-vivo	Humans	I/Cancer Index; C/SVM	[75]
Gastric ulcers	405–665	Filter Wheel	In-vivo	Humans	R, E/DI	[76]
Gastric cancer	400–800	N/A	Ex-vivo	Humans	C/MDC	[77,89]
Gastric cancer	400–650	Tunable Light Source	In-vivo	Humans	C/SVM; C/RF; C/RobustBoost; C/AdaBoost	[78]
Colon cancer detection	450–850	Tunable Light Source	In-vitro	Humans	R/ICA; R/PCA; C/k-Means; C/LDA; C/SVM	[79,80]
Colon cancer detection	440–700	Tunable Light Source	In-vitro	Humans	F/CLBP; R/PCA; C/LDA; C/SVM	[81]
Gastric cancer cell identification	420–720	LCTF	In-vitro	Humans	R/Manual band selection; C/ANNs	[82]
Colonic adenocarcinoma identification	390–700	LCTF	Ex-vivo	Humans	SA	[83]
Colon cancer detection	360–550	LCTF	In-vivo	Humans	S/LMM; R/PCA	[84,85]
Colorectal cell differentiation	400–1700	LCTF	In-vitro	Humans	F/LBP, C/RF	[86]
Colon cancer detection	400–1000	Push-broom	Ex-vivo	Humans	DR/SPA; C/LDA	[90]

* Categories of data analysis methods: (P) Preprocessing; (F) Feature extraction; (C) Classification; (R) Data Reduction; (S) Spectral Unmixing; (I) Normalized Difference Index; (E) Tissue Visualization Enhancement; (SA) Spectral Signature Analysis; (Ex) Exploratory Data Analysis. † Data analysis methods: (SGAD) Spectral Gradients and Amplitude Differences; (SVM) Support Vector Machines; (DWT) Discrete Wavelet Transformation; (SOM) Self-Organizing Maps; (CLBP) Circular Local Binary Patterns; (PCA) Principal Component Analysis; (LDA) Linear Discriminant Analysis; (LPM) Light Propagation Modeling; (LMM) Linear Mixture Model; (ICA) Independent Component Analysis; (RDFS) Recursive Divergence Feature Selection; (DI) Dependence of Information; (MDC) Minimum Distance Classifiers; (TPCR) Total Principal Component Regression; (RF) Random Forest; (SAM) Spectral Angle Mapper; (SPA) Successive Projection Algorithm; (LBP) Local Binary Pattern; (ANNs) Artificial Neural Networks.

6. Discussion

Although HSI technology has shown its potential to be used as a diagnostic tool, the roadmap for a new generation of HS medical devices is not clear yet. One of the most relevant challenges holds in the acquisition system. The most appropriate technology to be used in the GI tract is not clear. Although most of the state-of-art studies employ systems based on LCTF, acquisition systems based on push-broom or tunable light sources have also been successfully employed to this end. Despite the fact that higher spectral resolution is achieved using push-broom cameras, the spatial scanning required to obtain an HS cube makes difficult the integration of such kind of cameras with standard medical instrumentation, such as gastroscopes, colonoscopes, and laparoscopes. For this reason, LCTF can be regarded as the most extended technology for the GI tract. On the other hand, a novel study has been recently performed to identify in-vivo esophageal squamous neoplasia in human patients by using a RGB-HSI combined system [65]. In this study, authors developed a system capable of artificially generating an in-vivo HS image in the visual range by merging the information of a RGB endoscopic image with the spectral information obtained from a 30 Macbeth color checker tile measured with a spectrometer.

Concerning the optimal spectral range for GI diagnosis, the answer is still unclear. Although most of the studies in the state-of-art use images in the VNIR spectral range, there are several research works reporting successful detection of diseases using a spectral range beyond 1000 nm. In the upcoming years, the research community should assess the optimal spectral range for diagnostic applications. Depending on this spectral range, the directions on medical HS acquisition systems will possibly vary. On the one hand, if the VNIR spectral range is optimal for disease detection in the GI tract, the future medical HS images will be probably based on LCTF or snapshot cameras, that provide lower spectral resolution and a limited spectral range compared with push-broom cameras, but they are easily adapted to conventional medical instrumentation. On the other hand, if the spectral range increases beyond 1000 nm, the identification of diseases will probably improve due to the richer amount of available spectral information. However, push-broom cameras have to be used, and the engineering challenge will be the adaptation of the push-broom cameras to conventional medical instrumentation.

Recently, pioneering HSI-enabled flexible endoscopes and concept capsule endoscopes have been proposed [47,91,92], indicating the feasibility of incorporating HSI in clinical practice for colorectal cancer detection. Future challenges of HSI in gastrointestinal endoscopy are mainly associated with its application for the detection and characterization of various different kinds of abnormalities.

There are other interesting applications of MSI/HSI that are closely related to gastroenterology, but they are out of the scope of this manuscript. For example, in a recent study performed by Bhutiani et al. [93], the authors studied the in-vivo detection of AF-680 dye encapsulated PLA (Polylactic Acid) using an MSI laparoscope. The exploitation of such type of information has a potential use for in-vivo characterization of drug delivery.

Besides, on a recent review regarding current trends in endoscopic imaging, Joshi et al. [94] mentioned two novel applications of MSI that are relevant to be mentioned in this review. The first application is related to the use of dual-channel fluorescence images from in-vivo cross sections using a confocal microendoscope [95]. This research points out that in-vivo cross section images can be captured with a similar orientation as the corresponding histological sample. The same methodology could be applied with MSI/HSI instead of fluorescence. The second application presented by Joshi et al. [96] used a multispectral endoscope to simultaneously collect three fluorescence images (DEAC, 6-TAMRA and CF633). They were able to acquire images from colonic adenoma stained with two different peptides at the same time, providing sharp visualization of the lesion margins.

Structured light and MSI were used to simultaneously extract information about reflectance and surface structure of tissue during small bowel surgery [97]. Although this research was just a proof-of-concept, the incorporation of an additional spatial dimension to MSI/HSI can lead to better discrimination among different tissues.

Other spectral technologies based on Raman spectroscopy and Quantum Cascade Lasers (QCL) have been applied to assist pathological analysis. First, Raman spectroscopy has been employed to detect alterations in the biomedical composition of intestinal tissue biopsies, which can reveal coeliac disease [98]. Although more research is needed to confirm the hypothesis, Raman spectroscopy is also presented as a promising alternative for coeliac disease detection. Furthermore, several research works have been performed in the literature with the goal of diagnosing histological slides without requiring stains using QCL acquisition systems. These systems are able to acquire hyperspectral images beyond five microns. Firstly, in [99], Kröger-Lui et al. had the goal of detecting goblet cell regions in colonic epithelium using unstained histological sections, instead of conventional H&E stained samples. They demonstrated a strong correlation between the contents obtained with HS unstained images and the corresponding stained section using H&E. Secondly, in [100], Petersen et al. presented a proof-of-concept following a similar methodology, demonstrating that the mid-infrared information could be also useful for diagnosis purposes. In this pilot study, the authors found valuable information about protein rich amide regions of colonic crypts, the musin secretions and the surface epithelium walls that could be extracted from unstained colon sections using this spectral range (beyond 2500 nm).

As far as the data analysis techniques are concerned, there is not a generalized framework for processing HS data. Table 1 summarizes the data analysis methods currently used in GI HS applications. Actually, most techniques aim to get an enhanced visualization of tissues, with dimensional reduction techniques, such as PCA, LDA or ICA, being the most popular HS data processing methods. Another interesting trend is the definition of some normalized difference indexes to retrieve some characteristics of tissues, such as the proposed Normalized Difference Ischemia Index (NDII) or the Normalized Difference Cancer Index (NDCI). Although the use of such types of indices is handy, their use is still limited. As far as classification methods are concerned, in contrast to other HSI applications (such as precision agriculture or food quality analysis) the classification approaches used in the context of GI endoscopy imaging are limited, mainly based on SVMs. Maybe the slow raise of HS data classifiers for GI HS data is motivated by the difficulties to collect sufficiently large labeled datasets, allowing the generation and evaluation of reliable classification models. A relevant challenge for the analysis of medical HS data would be to investigate adaptation or enhancements of the current state-of-art HS data classification approaches (mainly coming from the Remote Sensing community) for the analysis of GI endoscopy data.

7. Conclusions

This survey is intended to provide a useful introduction to HSI in the medical field, paying special attention to the applications in gastroenterology. HSI has been limitedly explored for clinical purposes in GI endoscopy; moreover, the study of the literature indicates that it is a novel imaging modality with a high potential to improve several current medical procedures. For instance, HSI can contribute to make gastric surgical procedures safer by avoiding bile duct injury or ureteral injuries. Furthermore, it can contribute in a more accurate determination of tumor boundaries, facilitating a complete resection of the tumor tissue. Detection of malignant tissue, beyond the limitations of the contemporary white light imaging remains an area where properly employed HSI could lead to precision diagnosis. Further use of HSI technology has to face limitations of space and applicability [101].

Author Contributions: conceptualization, S.O., A.K. and G.M.C.; writing—original draft preparation, S.O., H.F. and D.K.I; writing—review and editing, A.K. and G.M.C.; supervision, A.K. and G.M.C.; funding acquisition, G.M.C.

Funding: This work has been supported in part by the Canary Islands Government through the ACIISI (Canarian Agency for Research, Innovation and the Information Society), ITHACA project "Hyperspectral Identification of Brain Tumors" under Grant Agreement ProID2017010164. This work has been also supported in part by the European Commission through the FP7 FET (Future Emerging Technologies) Open Programme ICT-2011.9.2, European Project HELICoiD "HypErspectral Imaging Cancer Detection" under Grant Agreement 618080. Additionally, this work was completed while Samuel Ortega was beneficiary of a pre-doctoral grant given by the "*Agencia Canaria de Investigacion, Innovacion y Sociedad de la Información (ACIISI)*" of the "*Consejería de Economía,*

Industria, Comercio y Conocimiento" of the "*Gobierno de Canarias*", which is part-financed by the European Social Fund (FSE) (POC 2014-2020, *Eje 3 Tema Prioritario 74* (85%)). Finally, this work has been supported in part by the 2016 PhD Training Program for Research Staff of the University of Las Palmas de Gran Canaria.

Conflicts of Interest: The authors declare no conflict of interest. The funders had no role in the design of the study; in the collection, analyses, or interpretation of data; in the writing of the manuscript, or in the decision to publish the results.

References

1. Grahn, H.F.; Geladi, P. (Eds.) *Techniques and Applications of Hyperspectral Image Analysis*; John Wiley & Sons, Ltd.: Chichester, UK, 2007; ISBN 9780470010884.
2. Feng, Y.-Z.; Sun, D.-W. Application of Hyperspectral Imaging in Food Safety Inspection and Control: A Review. *Crit. Rev. Food Sci. Nutr.* **2012**, *52*, 1039–1058. [CrossRef] [PubMed]
3. Lorente, D.; Aleixos, N.; Gómez-Sanchis, J.; Cubero, S.; García-Navarrete, O.L.; Blasco, J. Recent Advances and Applications of Hyperspectral Imaging for Fruit and Vegetable Quality Assessment. *Food Bioprocess Technol.* **2011**, *5*, 1121–1142. [CrossRef]
4. Tatzer, P.; Wolf, M.; Panner, T. Industrial application for inline material sorting using hyperspectral imaging in the NIR range. *Real-Time Imaging* **2005**, *11*, 99–107. [CrossRef]
5. Kubik, M. Chapter 5 Hyperspectral Imaging: A New Technique for the Non-Invasive Study of Artworks. *Phys. Tech. Study Art, Archaeol. Cult. Herit.* **2007**, *2*, 199–259. [CrossRef]
6. Cucci, C.; Delaney, J.K.; Picollo, M. Reflectance Hyperspectral Imaging for Investigation of Works of Art: Old Master Paintings and Illuminated Manuscripts. *Acc. Chem. Res.* **2016**, *49*, 2070–2079. [CrossRef] [PubMed]
7. Brossard, M.; Marion, R.; Carrére, V. Deconvolution of SWIR reflectance spectra for automatic mineral identification in hyperspectral imaging. *Remote Sens. Lett.* **2016**, *7*, 581–590. [CrossRef]
8. Ben-Dor, E. Quantitative remote sensing of soil properties. In *Advances in Agronomy*; Elsevier BV: Amsterdam, The Netherlands, 2002; pp. 173–243.
9. Behmann, J.; Steinrücken, J.; Plümer, L. Detection of early plant stress responses in hyperspectral images. *ISPRS J. Photogramm. Remote Sens.* **2014**, *93*, 98–111. [CrossRef]
10. Fabelo, H.; Ortega, S.; Lazcano, R.; Madroñal, D.; MCallicó, G.; Juárez, E.; Salvador, R.; Bulters, D.; Bulstrode, H.; Szolna, A.; et al. An intraoperative visualization system using hyperspectral imaging to aid in brain tumor delineation. *Sensors* **2018**, *18*. [CrossRef]
11. *Handbook of Biomedical Optics*; CRC Press: Boca Raton, FL, USA, 2016; ISBN 9781420090369.
12. Jacques, S.L. Optical properties of biological tissues: A review. *Phys. Med. Biol.* **2013**, *58*, R37–R61. [CrossRef]
13. Li, Q.; He, X.; Wang, Y.; Liu, H.; Xu, D.; Guo, F. Review of spectral imaging technology in biomedical engineering: Achievements and challenges. *J. Biomed. Opt.* **2013**. [CrossRef]
14. Lu, G.; Fei, B. Medical hyperspectral imaging: A review. *J. Biomed. Opt.* **2014**, *19*, 10901. [CrossRef] [PubMed]
15. Calin, M.A.; Parasca, S.V.; Savastru, D.; Manea, D. Hyperspectral Imaging in the Medical Field: Present and Future. *Appl. Spectrosc. Rev.* **2013**, *49*, 435–447. [CrossRef]
16. Milanic, M.; Bjorgan, A.; Larsson, M.; Strömberg, T.; Randeberg, L.L. Detection of hypercholesterolemia using hyperspectral imaging of human skin. In *Clinical and Biomedical Spectroscopy and Imaging IV, Proceedings of SPIE—The International Society for Optical Engineering*; Brown, J.Q., Deckert, V., Eds.; SPIE: Washington, DC, USA, 2015.
17. Milanic, M.; Paluchowski, L.A.; Randeberg, L.L. Hyperspectral imaging for detection of arthritis: Feasibility and prospects. *J. Biomed. Opt.* **2015**, *20*, 96011. [CrossRef] [PubMed]
18. Chin, J.A.; Wang, E.C.; Kibbe, M.R. Evaluation of hyperspectral technology for assessing the presence and severity of peripheral artery disease. *J. Vasc. Surg.* **2011**, *54*, 1679–1688. [CrossRef] [PubMed]
19. Bjorgan, A.; Denstedt, M.; Milanič, M.; Paluchowski, L.A.; Randeberg, L.L. Vessel contrast enhancement in hyperspectral images. In *Optical Biopsy XIII: Toward Real-Time Spectroscopic Imaging and Diagnosis, Proceedings of SPIE—The International Society for Optical Engineering*; Alfano, R.R., Demos, S.G., Eds.; SPIE: Washington, DC, USA, 2015.
20. Akbari, H.; Kosugi, Y.; Kojima, K.; Tanaka, N. Blood vessel detection and artery-vein differentiation using hyperspectral imaging. In Proceedings of the 31st Annual International Conference of the IEEE Engineering in Medicine and Biology Society: Engineering the Future of Biomedicine, EMBC 2009, Minneapolis, MN, USA, 3–6 September 2009; pp. 1461–1464.

21. Mordant, D.J.; Al-Abboud, I.; Muyo, G.; Gorman, A.; Sallam, A.; Ritchie, P.; Harvey, A.R.; McNaught, A.I. Spectral imaging of the retina. *Eye* **2011**, *25*, 309–320. [CrossRef] [PubMed]
22. Mori, M.; Chiba, T.; Nakamizo, A.; Kumashiro, R.; Murata, M.; Akahoshi, T.; Tomikawa, M.; Kikkawa, Y.; Yoshimoto, K.; Mizoguchi, M.; et al. Intraoperative visualization of cerebral oxygenation using hyperspectral image data: A two-dimensional mapping method. *Int. J. Comput. Assist. Radiol. Surg.* **2014**, *9*, 1059–1072. [CrossRef] [PubMed]
23. Olweny, E.O.; Faddegon, S.; Best, S.L.; Jackson, N.; Wehner, E.F.; Tan, Y.K.; Zuzak, K.J.; Cadeddu, J.A. First Place: Renal Oxygenation During Robot-Assisted Laparoscopic Partial Nephrectomy: Characterization Using Laparoscopic Digital Light Processing Hyperspectral Imaging. *J. Endourol.* **2013**, *27*, 265–269. [CrossRef]
24. Akbari, H.; Halig, L.V.; Schuster, D.M.; Osunkoya, A.; Master, V.; Nieh, P.T.; Chen, G.Z.; Fei, B. Hyperspectral imaging and quantitative analysis for prostate cancer detection. *J. Biomed. Opt.* **2012**, *17*, 0760051. [CrossRef]
25. Lu, G.; Qin, X.; Wang, D.; Chen, Z.G.; Fei, B. Quantitative wavelength analysis and image classification for intraoperative cancer diagnosis with hyperspectral imaging. In *Progress in Biomedical Optics and Imaging—Proceedings of SPIE*; SPIE: Washington, DC, USA, 2015; Volume 9415.
26. Lu, G.; Wang, D.; Qin, X.; Halig, L.; Muller, S.; Zhang, H.; Chen, A.; Pogue, B.W.; Chen, Z.G.; Fei, B. Framework for hyperspectral image processing and quantification for cancer detection during animal tumor surgery. *J. Biomed. Opt.* **2015**, *20*, 126012. [CrossRef]
27. Panasyuk, S.V.; Yang, S.; Faller, D.V.; Ngo, D.; Lew, R.A.; Freeman, J.E.; Rogers, A.E. Medical hyperspectral imaging to facilitate residual tumor identification during surgery. *Cancer Biol. Ther.* **2007**, *6*, 439–446. [CrossRef]
28. Liu, Z.; Wang, H.; Li, Q. Tongue tumor detection in medical hyperspectral images. *Sensors* **2012**, *12*, 162–174. [CrossRef] [PubMed]
29. Duann, J.-R.; Jan, C.-I.; Ou-Yang, M.; Lin, C.-Y.; Mo, J.-F.; Lin, Y.-J.; Tsai, M.-H.; Chiou, J.-C. Separating spectral mixtures in hyperspectral image data using independent component analysis: Validation with oral cancer tissue sections. *J. Biomed. Opt.* **2013**, *18*, 126005. [CrossRef] [PubMed]
30. Martin, J.; Krueger, J.; Gareau, D. Hyperspectral imaging for melanoma screening. In *Photonic Therapeutics and Diagnostics X, Proceedings of SPIE—The International Society for Optical Engineering*; Choi, B., Kollias, N., Zeng, H., Eds.; SPIE: Washington, DC, USA, 2014.
31. Nagaoka, T.; Kiyohara, Y.; Koga, H.; Nakamura, A.; Saida, T.; Sota, T. Modification of a melanoma discrimination index derived from hyperspectral data: A clinical trial conducted in 2 centers between March 2011 and December 2013. *Ski. Res. Technol.* **2015**, *21*, 278–283. [CrossRef] [PubMed]
32. Song, E.; Grant-Kels, J.M.; Swede, H.; D'Antonio, J.L.; Lachance, A.; Dadras, S.S.; Kristjansson, A.K.; Ferenczi, K.; Makkar, H.S.; Rothe, M.J. Paired comparison of the sensitivity and specificity of multispectral digital skin lesion analysis and reflectance confocal microscopy in the detection of melanoma in vivo: A cross-sectional study. *J. Am. Acad. Dermatol.* **2016**, *75*, 1187–1192.e2. [CrossRef] [PubMed]
33. Fabelo, H.; Ortega, S.; Ravi, D.; Kiran, B.R.; Sosa, C.; Bulters, D.; Callicó, G.M.; Bulstrode, H.; Szolna, A.; Piñeiro, J.F.; et al. Spatio-spectral classification of hyperspectral images for brain cancer detection during surgical operations. *PLoS One* **2018**, *13*, 1–27. [CrossRef] [PubMed]
34. Li, Q.; Xue, Y.; Xiao, G.; Zhang, J. Study on microscope hyperspectral medical imaging method for biomedical quantitative analysis. *Sci. Bull.* **2008**, *53*, 1431–1434. [CrossRef]
35. Akbari, H.; Halig, L.V.; Zhang, H.; Wang, D.; Chen, Z.G.; Fei, B. Detection of Cancer Metastasis Using a Novel Macroscopic Hyperspectral Method. *Proc. SPIE* **2012**, *8317*, 831711. [CrossRef]
36. Ortega, S.; Fabelo, H.; Camacho, R.; de la Luz Plaza, M.; Callicó, G.M.; Sarmiento, R. Detecting brain tumor in pathological slides using hyperspectral imaging. *Biomed. Opt. Express* **2018**, *9*, 818. [CrossRef]
37. Akalin, A.; Mu, X.; Kon, M.A.; Ergin, A.; Remiszewski, S.H.; Thompson, C.M.; Raz, D.J.; Diem, M. Classification of malignant and benign tumors of the lung by infrared spectral histopathology (SHP). *Lab. Investig.* **2015**, *95*, 406–421. [CrossRef]
38. Wu, D.; Sun, D.-W. Advanced applications of hyperspectral imaging technology for food quality and safety analysis and assessment: A review—Part I: Fundamentals. *Innov. Food Sci. Emerg. Technol.* **2013**, *19*, 1–14. [CrossRef]
39. Holt, E.E.; Aikio, M.; Tutkimuskeskus, V.T. Hyperspectral Prism-grating-prism Imaging Spectrograph. In *Hyperspectral Prism-grating-prism Imaging Spectrograph*; VTT julkaisuja; Technical Research Centre of Finland: Espoo, Finland, 2001; ISBN 9789513858506.

40. Fabelo, H.; Ortega, S.; Kabwama, S.; Callico, G.M.; Bulters, D.; Szolna, A.; Pineiro, J.F.; Sarmiento, R. HELICoiD project: A new use of hyperspectral imaging for brain cancer detection in real-time during neurosurgical operations. In *Hyperspectral Imaging Sensors: Innovative Applications and Sensor Standards 2016, Proceedings of SPIE—The International Society for Optical Engineering*; Bannon, D.P., Ed.; SPIE: Washington, DC, USA, 2016.
41. Ortega, S.; Callico, G.M.; Plaza, M.L.; Camacho, R.; Fabelo, H.; Sarmiento, R. Hyperspectral database of pathological in-vitro human brain samples to detect carcinogenic tissues. In Proceedings of the International Symposium on Biomedical Imaging, Prague, Czech Republic, 13–16 April 2016.
42. Gat, N. Imaging spectroscopy using tunable filters: A review. In *Wavelet Applications VII, Proceedings of SPIE—The International Society for Optical Engineering*; Szu, H.H., Vetterli, M., Campbell, W.J., Eds.; SPIE: Washington, DC, USA, 2000.
43. Leitner, R.; De Biasio, M.; Arnold, T.; Dinh, C.V.; Loog, M.; Duin, R.P.W. Multi-spectral video endoscopy system for the detection of cancerous tissue. *Pattern Recognit. Lett.* **2013**, *34*, 85–93. [CrossRef]
44. Hagen, N.; Kudenov, M.W. Review of snapshot spectral imaging technologies. *Opt. Eng.* **2013**. [CrossRef]
45. Chen, G.; Qian, S.-E. Denoising of Hyperspectral Imagery Using Principal Component Analysis and Wavelet Shrinkage. *IEEE Trans. Geosci. Remote Sens.* **2011**, *49*, 973–980. [CrossRef]
46. Yuan, Q.; Zhang, L.; Shen, H. Hyperspectral Image Denoising Employing a Spectral-Spatial Adaptive Total Variation Model. *IEEE Trans. Geosci. Remote Sens.* **2012**, *50*, 3660–3677. [CrossRef]
47. Kester, R.T.; Bedard, N.; Gao, L.; Tkaczyk, T.S. Real-time snapshot hyperspectral imaging endoscope. *J. Biomed. Opt.* **2011**, *16*, 56005. [CrossRef] [PubMed]
48. Dai, Q.; Cheng, J.-H.; Sun, D.-W.; Zeng, X.-A. Advances in Feature Selection Methods for Hyperspectral Image Processing in Food Industry Applications: A Review. *Crit. Rev. Food Sci. Nutr.* **2015**, *55*, 1368–1382. [CrossRef] [PubMed]
49. Khodr, J.; Younes, R. Dimensionality reduction on hyperspectral images: A comparative review based on artificial datas. In Proceedings of the 2011 4th International Congress on Image and Signal Processing, Shanghai, China, 15–17 October 2011; Institute of Electrical and Electronics Engineers (IEEE): Piscataway, NJ, USA, 2011.
50. *Pattern Recognition*; Elsevier: Amsterdam, The Netherlands, 2009; ISBN 9781597492720.
51. Bioucas-Dias, J.M.; Plaza, A.; Dobigeon, N.; Parente, M.; Du, Q.; Gader, P.; Chanussot, J. Hyperspectral unmixing overview: Geometrical, statistical, and sparse regression-based approaches. *IEEE J. Sel. Top. Appl. Earth Obs. Remote Sens.* **2012**, *5*, 354–379. [CrossRef]
52. Turvey, C.G.; Mclaurin, M.K. Applicability of the Normalized Difference Vegetation Index (NDVI) in Index-Based Crop Insurance Design. *Weather. Clim. Soc.* **2012**, *4*, 271–284. [CrossRef]
53. Nagaoka, T.; Nakamura, A.; Okutani, H.; Kiyohara, Y.; Sota, T. A possible melanoma discrimination index based on hyperspectral data: A pilot study. *Ski. Res. Technol.* **2012**, *18*, 301–310. [CrossRef]
54. Chang, C.-I. *Hyperspectral data processing: Algorithm design and analysis*; John Wiley & Sons: Hoboken, NJ, USA, 2013.
55. Zuzak, K.J.; Naik, S.C.; Alexandrakis, G.; Hawkins, D.; Behbehani, K.; Livingston, E.H. Characterization of a Near-Infrared Laparoscopic Hyperspectral Imaging System for Minimally Invasive Surgery. *Anal. Chem.* **2007**, *79*, 4709–4715. [CrossRef]
56. Ghamisi, P.; Plaza, J.; Chen, Y.; Li, J.; Plaza, A.J. Advanced Spectral Classifiers for Hyperspectral Images: A review. *IEEE Geosci. Remote Sens. Mag.* **2017**, *5*, 8–32. [CrossRef]
57. Xu, R.; WunschII, D. Survey of Clustering Algorithms. *IEEE Trans. Neural Networks* **2005**, *16*, 645–678. [CrossRef] [PubMed]
58. Fauvel, M.; Tarabalka, Y.; Benediktsson, J.A.; Chanussot, J.; Tilton, J.C. Advances in spectral-spatial classification of hyperspectral images. *Proc. IEEE* **2013**, *101*, 652–675. [CrossRef]
59. Claridge, E.; Hidović-Rowe, D.; Taniere, P.; Ismail, T. Quantifying mucosal blood volume fraction from multispectral images of the colon. In *Medical Imaging 2007: Physiology, Function, and Structure from Medical Images*; Manduca, A., Hu, X.P., Eds.; SPIE: Washington, DC, USA.
60. Hidović-Rowe, D.; Claridge, E.; Ismail, T.; Taniere, P.; Graham, J. Analysis of multispectral images of the colon to reveal histological changes characteristic of cancer. *Med. Image Underst. Anal. MIUA* **2006**, *1*, 66–70.

61. Akbari, H.; Kosugi, Y.; Kojima, K.; Tanaka, N. Wavelet-Based Compression and Segmentation of Hyperspectral Images in Surgery. In *Lecture Notes in Computer Science*; Springer Nature: Berlin, Germany; pp. 142–149.
62. Schols, R.M.; Alic, L.; Beets, G.L.; Breukink, S.O.; Wieringa, F.P.; Stassen, L.P.S. Automated Spectroscopic Tissue Classification in Colorectal Surgery. *Surg. Innov.* **2015**, *22*, 557–567. [CrossRef]
63. Schols, R.M.; Dunias, P.; Wieringa, F.P.; Stassen, L.P.S. Multispectral characterization of tissues encountered during laparoscopic colorectal surgery. *Med. Eng. Phys.* **2013**, *35*, 1044–1050. [CrossRef] [PubMed]
64. Han, Z.; Zhang, A.; Wang, X.; Sun, Z.; Wang, M.D.; Xie, T. In vivo use of hyperspectral imaging to develop a noncontact endoscopic diagnosis support system for malignant colorectal tumors. *J. Biomed. Opt.* **2016**, *21*, 016001. [CrossRef] [PubMed]
65. Wu, I.-C.; Syu, H.-Y.; Jen, C.-P.; Lu, M.-Y.; Chen, Y.-T.; Wu, M.-T.; Kuo, C.-T.; Tsai, Y.-Y.; Wang, H.-C. Early identification of esophageal squamous neoplasm by hyperspectral endoscopic imaging. *Sci. Rep.* **2018**, *8*, 13797. [CrossRef]
66. Beaulieu, R.J.; Goldstein, S.D.; Singh, J.; Safar, B.; Banerjee, A.; Ahuja, N. Automated diagnosis of colon cancer using hyperspectral sensing. *Int. J. Med. Robot. Comput. Assist. Surg.* **2018**, *14*, e1897. [CrossRef]
67. Clancy, N.T.; Arya, S.; Stoyanov, D.; Singh, M.; Hanna, G.B.; Elson, D.S. Intraoperative measurement of bowel oxygen saturation using a multispectral imaging laparoscope. *Biomed. Opt. Express* **2015**, *6*, 4179. [CrossRef]
68. Wirkert, S.J.; Kenngott, H.; Mayer, B.; Mietkowski, P.; Wagner, M.; Sauer, P.; Clancy, N.T.; Elson, D.S.; Maier-Hein, L. Robust near real-time estimation of physiological parameters from megapixel multispectral images with inverse Monte Carlo and random forest regression. *Int. J. Comput. Assist. Radiol. Surg.* **2016**, *11*, 909–917. [CrossRef] [PubMed]
69. Cha, J.; Shademan, A.; Le, H.N.D.; Decker, R.; Kim, P.C.W.; Kang, J.U.; Krieger, A. Multispectral tissue characterization for intestinal anastomosis optimization. *J. Biomed. Opt.* **2015**, *20*, 106001. [CrossRef] [PubMed]
70. Clancy, N.T.; Arya, S.; Stoyanov, D.; Du, X.; Hanna, G.B.; Elson, D.S. Imaging the spectral reflectance properties of bipolar radiofrequency-fused bowel tissue. In Proceedings of the Clinical and Biomedical Spectroscopy and Imaging IV, Munich, Germany, 21–25 June 2015; Volume 9537.
71. Zuzak, K.J.; Naik, S.C.; Alexandrakis, G.; Hawkins, D.; Behbehani, K.; Livingston, E. Intraoperative bile duct visualization using near-infrared hyperspectral video imaging. *Am. J. Surg.* **2008**, *195*, 491–497. [CrossRef] [PubMed]
72. Mitra, K.; Melvin, J.; Chang, S.; Park, K.; Yilmaz, A.; Melvin, S.; Xu, R.X. Indocyanine-green-loaded microballoons for biliary imaging in cholecystectomy. *J. Biomed. Opt.* **2012**, *17*, 116025. [CrossRef] [PubMed]
73. Davies, B. Robotic Surgery—A Personal View of the Past, Present and Future. *Int. J. Adv. Robot. Syst.* **2015**, *12*, 54. [CrossRef]
74. Akbari, H.; Kosugi, Y.; Kojima, K.; Tanaka, N. Detection and analysis of the intestinal ischemia using visible and invisible hyperspectral imaging. *IEEE Trans. Biomed. Eng.* **2010**, *57*, 2011–2017. [CrossRef]
75. Akbari, H.; Uto, K.; Kosugi, Y.; Kojima, K.; Tanaka, N. Cancer detection using infrared hyperspectral imaging. *Cancer Sci.* **2011**, *102*, 852–857. [CrossRef]
76. Gu, X.; Han, Z.; Yao, L.; Zhong, Y.; Shi, Q.; Fu, Y.; Liu, C.; Wang, X.; Xie, T. Image enhancement based on in vivo hyperspectral gastroscopic images: A case study. *J. Biomed. Opt.* **2016**, *21*, 101412. [CrossRef] [PubMed]
77. Ogihara, H.; Hamamoto, Y.; Fujita, Y.; Goto, A.; Nishikawa, J.; Sakaida, I. Development of a Gastric Cancer Diagnostic Support System with a Pattern Recognition Method Using a Hyperspectral Camera. *J. Sens.* **2016**, *2016*, 1–6. [CrossRef]
78. Hohmann, M.; Kanawade, R.; Klämpfl, F.; Douplik, A.; Mudter, J.; Neurath, M.F.; Albrecht, H. *In-vivo* multispectral video endoscopy towards *in-vivo* hyperspectral video endoscopy. *J. Biophotonics* **2017**, *10*, 553–564. [CrossRef] [PubMed]
79. Masood, K.; Rajpoot, N.; Rajpoot, K.; Qureshi, H. Hyperspectral Colon Tissue Classification using Morphological Analysis. In Proceedings of the International Conference on Emerging Technologies, Peshawar, Pakistan, 13–14 November 2006; pp. 735–741.

80. Rajpoot, K.; Rajpoot, N. SVM Optimization for Hyperspectral Colon Tissue Cell Classification. In *Medical Image Computing and Computer-Assisted Intervention (MICCAI) 2004*; Springer Nature: Berlin, Germany, 2004; pp. 829–837.
81. Masood, K.; Rajpoot, N. Texture based classification of hyperspectral colon biopsy samples using CLBP. In *2009 IEEE International Symposium on Biomedical Imaging: From Nano to Macro*; Institute of Electrical and Electronics Engineers (IEEE): Piscataway, NJ, USA, 2009.
82. Zhu, S.; Su, K.; Liu, Y.; Yin, H.; Li, Z.; Huang, F.; Chen, Z.; Chen, W.; Zhang, G.; Chen, Y. Identification of cancerous gastric cells based on common features extracted from hyperspectral microscopic images. *Biomed. Opt. Express* **2015**, *6*, 1135–1145. [CrossRef] [PubMed]
83. Leavesley, S.J.; Walters, M.; Lopez, C.; Baker, T.; Favreau, P.F.; Rich, T.C.; Rider, P.F.; Boudreaux, C.W. Hyperspectral imaging fluorescence excitation scanning for colon cancer detection. *J. Biomed. Opt.* **2016**, *21*, 104003. [CrossRef] [PubMed]
84. Leavesley, S.J.; Deal, J.; Martin, W.A.; Lall, M.; Lopez, C.; Rich, T.C.; Boudreaux, C.W.; Rider, P.F.; Hill, S. Colorectal cancer detection by hyperspectral imaging using fluorescence excitation scanning. In *Optical Biopsy XVI: Toward Real-Time Spectroscopic Imaging and Diagnosis*; Alfano, R.R., Demos, S.G., Eds.; SPIE: Washington, DC, USA, 2018; Volume 10489, p. 19.
85. Deal, J.; Harris, B.; Martin, W.; Lall, M.; Lopez, C.; Boudreaux, C.; Rich, T.; Leavesley, S.; Rider, P. Demystifying autofluorescence with excitation scanning hyperspectral imaging. In *Imaging, Manipulation, and Analysis of Biomolecules, Cells, and Tissues XVI*; Farkas, D.L., Nicolau, D.V., Leif, R.C., Eds.; SPIE: Washington, DC, USA, 2018; Volume 10497, p. 40.
86. Kunhoth, S.; Al Maadeed, S. Building a multispectral image dataset for colorectal tumor biopsy. In Proceedings of the 2017 13th International Wireless Communications and Mobile Computing Conference (IWCMC), Valencia, Spain, 26–30 June 2017.
87. Cassidy, R.J.; Berger, J.; Lee, K.; Maggioni, M.; Coifman, R.R. Analysis of hyperspectral colon tissue images using vocal synthesis models. In Proceedings of the Conference Record of the Thirty-Eighth Asilomar Conference on Signals, Systems and Computers, Pacific Grove, CA, USA, 7–10 November 2004; Institute of Electrical and Electronics Engineers (IEEE): Piscataway, NJ, USA, 2004.
88. Cassidy, R.J.; Berger, J.; Lee, K. Auditory Display of Hyperspectral Colon Tissue Images using Vocal Synthesis Models. In Proceedings of the ICAD 04óTenth Meeting of the International Conference on Auditory Display, Sydney, Australia, 6–9 July 2004.
89. Kiyotoki, S.; Nishikawa, J.; Okamoto, T.; Hamabe, K.; Saito, M.; Goto, A.; Fujita, Y.; Hamamoto, Y.; Takeuchi, Y.; Satori, S.; et al. New method for detection of gastric cancer by hyperspectral imaging: A pilot study. *J. Biomed. Opt.* **2013**, *18*, 26010. [CrossRef] [PubMed]
90. Yuan, X.; Zhang, D.; Wang, C.; Dai, B.; Zhao, M.; Li, B. Hyperspectral Imaging and SPA–LDA Quantitative Analysis for Detection of Colon Cancer Tissue. *J. Appl. Spectrosc.* **2018**, *85*, 307–312. [CrossRef]
91. Kumashiro, R.; Konishi, K.; Chiba, T.; Akahoshi, T.; Nakamura, S.; Murata, M.; Tomikawa, M.; Matsumoto, T.; Maehara, Y.; Hashizume, M. Integrated Endoscopic System Based on Optical Imaging and Hyperspectral Data Analysis for Colorectal Cancer Detection. *Anticancer Res.* **2016**, *36*, 3925–3932.
92. Lim, H.-T.; Murukeshan, V.M. A four-dimensional snapshot hyperspectral video-endoscope for bio-imaging applications. *Sci. Rep.* **2016**, *6*. [CrossRef]
93. Bhutiani, N.; Samykutty, A.; McMasters, K.M.; Egilmez, N.K.; McNally, L.R. In vivo tracking of orally-administered particles within the gastrointestinal tract of murine models using multispectral optoacoustic tomography. *Photoacoustics* **2019**, *13*, 46–52. [CrossRef]
94. Joshi, B.P.; Wang, T.D. Emerging trends in endoscopic imaging. *Nat. Rev. Gastroenterol. Hepatol.* **2016**, *13*, 72–73. [CrossRef]
95. Qiu, Z.; Khondee, S.; Duan, X.; Li, H.; Mandella, M.J.; Joshi, B.P.; Zhou, Q.; Owens, S.R.; Kurabayashi, K.; Oldham, K.R.; et al. Vertical Cross-sectional Imaging of Colonic Dysplasia In Vivo With Multi-spectral Dual Axes Confocal Endomicroscopy. *Gastroenterology* **2014**, *146*, 615–617. [CrossRef]
96. Joshi, B.P.; Miller, S.J.; Lee, C.M.; Seibel, E.J.; Wang, T.D. Multispectral Endoscopic Imaging of Colorectal Dysplasia In Vivo. *Gastroenterology* **2012**, *143*, 1435–1437. [CrossRef]
97. Clancy, N.T.; Lin, J.; Arya, S.; Hanna, G.B.; Elson, D.S. Dual multispectral and 3D structured light laparoscope. In Proceedings of the Multimodal Biomedical Imaging X, San Francisco, CA, USA, 7–12 February 2015; Volume 9316, p. 93160C.

98. Fornasaro, S.; Vicario, A.; De Leo, L.; Bonifacio, A.; Not, T.; Sergo, V. Potential use of MCR-ALS for the identification of coeliac-related biochemical changes in hyperspectral Raman maps from pediatric intestinal biopsies. *Integr. Biol.* **2018**, *10*, 356–363. [CrossRef] [PubMed]
99. Kröger-Lui, N.; Gretz, N.; Haase, K.; Kränzlin, B.; Neudecker, S.; Pucci, A.; Regenscheit, A.; Schönhals, A.; Petrich, W. Rapid identification of goblet cells in unstained colon thin sections by means of quantum cascade laser-based infrared microspectroscopy. *Analyst* **2015**, *140*, 2086–2092. [CrossRef] [PubMed]
100. Petersen, C.R.; Prtljaga, N.; Farries, M.; Ward, J.; Napier, B.; Lloyd, G.R.; Nallala, J.; Stone, N.; Bang, O. Mid-infrared multispectral tissue imaging using a chalcogenide fiber supercontinuum source. *Opt. Lett.* **2018**, *43*, 999. [CrossRef] [PubMed]
101. Iakovidis, D.K.; Sarmiento, R.; Silva, J.S.; Histace, A.; Romain, O.; Koulaouzidis, A.; Dehollain, C.; Pinna, A.; Granado, B.; Dray, X. Towards Intelligent Capsules for Robust Wireless Endoscopic Imaging of the Gut. *IEEE Int. Conf. Imaging Syst. Tech.* **2014**, 95–100.

© 2019 by the authors. Licensee MDPI, Basel, Switzerland. This article is an open access article distributed under the terms and conditions of the Creative Commons Attribution (CC BY) license (http://creativecommons.org/licenses/by/4.0/).

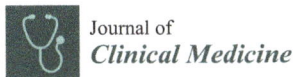

Review

Microbiome—The Missing Link in the Gut-Brain Axis: Focus on Its Role in Gastrointestinal and Mental Health

Karolina Skonieczna-Żydecka [1], Wojciech Marlicz [2,*], Agata Misera [3], Anastasios Koulaouzidis [4] and Igor Łoniewski [1]

1. Department of Biochemistry and Human Nutrition, Pomeranian Medical University in Szczecin, 71-460 Szczecin, Poland; karzyd@pum.edu.pl (K.S.-Z.); igorloniewski@sanum.com.pl (I.L.)
2. Department of Gastroenterology, Pomeranian Medical University, 71-252 Szczecin, Poland
3. Department of Child and Adolescent Psychiatry, Charité Universitätsmedizin, 13353 Berlin, Germany; agata.misera@charite.de
4. Endoscopy Unit, The Royal Infirmary of Edinburgh, EH16 4SA Edinburgh, UK; akoulaouzidis@hotmail.com
* Correspondence: marlicz@hotmail.com; Tel.: +48-(91)-425-32-31

Received: 23 October 2018; Accepted: 5 December 2018; Published: 7 December 2018

Abstract: The central nervous system (CNS) and the human gastrointestinal (GI) tract communicate through the gut-brain axis (GBA). Such communication is bi-directional and involves neuronal, endocrine, and immunological mechanisms. There is mounting data that gut microbiota is the source of a number of neuroactive and immunocompetent substances, which shape the structure and function of brain regions involved in the control of emotions, cognition, and physical activity. Most GI diseases are associated with altered transmission within the GBA that are influenced by both genetic and environmental factors. Current treatment protocols for GI and non-GI disorders may positively or adversely affect the composition of intestinal microbiota with a diverse impact on therapeutic outcome(s). Alterations of gut microbiota have been associated with mood and depressive disorders. Moreover, mental health is frequently affected in GI and non-GI diseases. Deregulation of the GBA may constitute a grip point for the development of diagnostic tools and personalized microbiota-based therapy. For example, next generation sequencing (NGS) offers detailed analysis of microbiome footprints in patients with mental and GI disorders. Elucidating the role of stem cell–host microbiome cross talks in tissues in GBA disorders might lead to the development of next generation diagnostics and therapeutics. Psychobiotics are a new class of beneficial bacteria with documented efficacy for the treatment of GBA disorders. Novel therapies interfering with small molecules involved in adult stem cell trafficking are on the horizon.

Keywords: gut brain axis; microbiota; functional gastrointestinal disorders; inflammatory bowel disease (IBD); adult stem cells

1. Introduction

Recently, a new United Nation's (UN) Commission goals on global mental health and sustainable development has been published [1]. This Commission is in line with other UN General Assembly and High-Level Meeting report and explores the issues of mental health from those with mental disorders to whole populations [2]. Accordingly, good mental health is viewed as fundamental to individual's well-being and overall health. In addition, efforts are being focused on systemic and global changes in order to align mental health across all medical specialties [3,4]. In the context of the previously mentioned documents, the relationship between gut microbiota and mental health seems to be very interesting.

Intestinal microbiota represent one of the richest ecosystems in nature. Professor Rob Knight of the University of California, San Diego [5] reported that more than half of all cells in the human body are microorganisms, which are mainly bacteria as well as fungi and viruses. Until recently, the general belief was that intestinal microbes were mainly involved in digestive processes. With the advent of new molecular techniques and bioinformatics, in-depth research has unraveled the role of intestinal microbiota in a number of physiological processes [6,7]. The topic of global microbial diversity is so crucial and important to human health and wellbeing that scientists from Rutgers University-New Brunswick—In a recent issue of *Science*—Called for the creation of a global microbiota vault to protect humanity's long-term health [8].

The role of the gut microbiome on human health is very diverse and implicated in the pathophysiology of various diseases. Its role in metabolism and obesity development has been clearly documented [9]. More recently, gut microbes have been implicated in the pathogenesis of cancer and microbial contribution in cancer treatment [10]. The pathogenesis and natural history of chronic GI, non-communicable diseases e.g., non-alcoholic steatohepatitis (NASH) [11], functional gastrointestinal disorders (FGIDs) [12], and non-GI disorders e.g., cardiovascular disease (CVD) [13] have been linked to GI tract microbes. The alterations of gut microbiota have been associated with neurodegenerative diseases as well as mood disturbance and depression [14–16]. In fact, mental health alterations are frequently observed in many GI diseases [17–20].

2. Paradigm Changer—Rome IV Criteria and FGIDs

For years, FGIDs were viewed as purely functional disorders with no scientific confirmation of a clear pathogenetic mechanism. According to Rome IV criteria, the phenotype of FGIDs results from an altered transmission of nerve and biochemical signals within the gut-brain-microbiota axis with mechanisms controlled by both genetic and environmental factors [21]. Additionally, few studies conducted in patients suffering from functional dyspepsia (FD) and irritable bowel syndrome (IBS) found alterations in small bowel microbiota. Zhong et al. [22] showed that *Actinomyces*, *Atopobium*, *Leptotrichia*, *Prevotella*, and *Veilonella* counts differ between FD and control patients. The finding was preceded by an observation that, in FD patients, gut barrier integrity is impaired and expressed as lowered transepithelial resistance, diminished expression of proteins of tight junctions, and, lastly, elevated levels of mast cells, eosinophils, and interstitial lymphocytes [23]. Giamarellos-Bourboulis reported a significant reduction in the diversity of small-bowel microbiota and the number of species [24]. Furthermore, Martinez et al. reported that the proportion of dilated junctions and intercellular distance between enterocytes in their apical part was elevated [25]. They also found that higher tryptase mRNA expression leads to overactive bowel movements and looser stool as per Bristol stool scale. Importantly, the degranulation of mast cells was found to positively affect the firing of visceral-nociceptive sensory neurons in IBS [26]. According to the new ROME IV criteria, the following factors contribute to the pathogenesis of FGIDs: (i) motility disturbance, (ii) visceral hypersensitivity, (iii) altered mucosal and immune function, (iv) altered gut microbiota, and (v) altered central nervous system (CNS). All of them are also associated with the concept of the microbiota-gut-brain axis.

The overlap of FGIDs and CNS disorders has been discussed in a few studies. It has been demonstrated that approximately one third of IBS patients suffer from depression [27]. More recently, Batmaz et al. [28] reviewed patients referred either directly to psychiatric clinics or from gastroenterology wards to psychiatrists and concluded that these patients were complaining of both GI and psychiatric symptoms. Furthermore, patients of the latter group complained more frequently of constipation, abdominal pain, and bloating and were more frequently diagnosed with psychotic disorders in comparison to those directly referred to psychiatric clinics. It is estimated that psychiatric symptoms occur in at least 36.5% of FGIDs patients [17]. Stasi et al. found that the highest prevalence of mental or spectrum disorders is in patients with functional constipation (60%) as compared to patients diagnosed with FD (52.4%) and/or functional bloating (47.6%). The most prevalent psychiatric disorder observed in FGIDs were the general anxiety disorder and panic diagnosis [17]. Furthermore,

Wilder-smith et al. [29] identified both GI and CNS symptom profiles secondary to fructose or lactose ingestion.

3. The Emerging Role of the Microbiota-Gut-Brain Axis

Studies in animal models have shown that microbiota play an essential role in shaping the structure and function of the CNS [30]. Using sophisticated strategies for manipulating the microbiome, researchers observed the consequences of these changes one the brain and behavior. For example, it has been found out that the thickness of the myelin sheath, the length of dendrites, and the density of dendritic spines are controlled by microbiota [31,32]. A recent study by Lu et al. [33] conducted in humanized germ-free mice demonstrated that slow-growing mice presented skewed neuron and oligodendrocyte development as well as evident signs of neuro-inflammation. Social competences and repetitive behaviors are, at least in part, a reflection of the composition of intestinal bacteria [34]. These dependencies result directly from the existence of a physical and functional connection between the human digestive tract and the CNS. This concept called the gut-brain axis (GBA) with the participation of neural and biochemical mechanisms can be exploited for the development of new therapies for mental health disorders.

The CNS utilizes neural and endocrine pathways to cooperate with the gut. The sympathetic part of the autonomic nervous system and the hypothalamus-pituitary-adrenal axis (HPA) co-modulate the secretion, motility, and blood flow affecting intestinal permeability and influencing various GI disorders [35]. Gut neural signals are passed through the enteric nervous system (ENS) and the vagus nerve [36]. Biochemical information is carried out by cytokines, chemokines, neurotransmitters, and micro-vesicles [37] as well as directly by-products of gut microbiota metabolic activity, i.e., short chain fatty acids (SCFAs). Eventually, once in the circulation, these molecules influence HPA and GBA [38]. An elevated stress response may impair the psychosomatic well-being [39]. With pioneering work, Sudo et al. [40] demonstrated that gut microbiota is essential to proper stress hormones release and the restoration of intestinal ecosystem may reverse abnormal stress response. More recently, in vivo experimentation has demonstrated that stress mediators and their receptors' expression are reduced in pathogen-free animals [41].

4. How the Gut/Brain Talks to the Brain/Gut

Intestinal microbiota as an integral part of the intestinal barrier controls the transport of antigens through the peri-cellular route to the *lamina propria* where the gut associated lymphoid tissue (GALT) is located [42]. The composition of intestinal microbiota can, therefore, influence intestinal barrier permeability, which guarantees the flow of molecules through the peri-cellular route to blood vessels. Gut microbes permanently train GALT to create immunity against commensal bacteria and food antigens but also to provide defense against pathogenic microorganisms [43]. During dysbiosis, due to GALT activation, effector cells and inflammatory mediators disrupt gut barrier integrity and result in elevated intestinal permeability [44]. The interaction of the intestinal barrier elements, thus, provides a physiologic and selective ability to absorb and secrete specific substances while inhibiting the translocation of microorganisms and the penetration of toxins and other harmful antigens [45,46].

The effects of increased intestinal permeability may manifest locally—In the GI tract—As well as extra-intestinally. For example, the concentration of zonulin—A protein that activates the intracellular signaling pathway leading to tight junctions [47] modulation and a marker of intestinal permeability increases in people with inflammatory and autoimmune diseases [48]. Of importance, the gut barrier resembles in structure and function the blood brain barrier (BBB) [49]. Both barriers are composed of epithelial and endothelial cells laced with lymphatic vessels, macrophages, and cellular tight junctions. It has already been suggested that both IBS and pseudomembranous colitis [50,51] are consequences of microbiota and intestinal barrier dysfunctions and these entities frequently coexist with depression [52,53].

5. Microbiota-Gut-Brain Axis and Susceptibility to Neuropsychiatric and Gastrointestinal Disease and Response to Therapy

The structure of intestinal microbiota is strongly influenced by diet and environmental stressors such as drugs. It seems that these factors dominate over the impact of genotype on the gut flora composition [54]. Consequently, it has been recognized that it may be the optimal marker of susceptibility to express certain clinical phenotypes and, thus, the response to pharmacotherapy [55]. Since the concept of bidirectional signaling between the gut and the brain started to evolve, scientists have made attempts to discover microbial fingerprints in neurology and psychiatry. Emerging research suggested that gut-brain axis dysfunction may be involved in the etiology of depression and anxiety, schizophrenia, addiction, and neurodevelopmental and neurodegenerative diseases as well as age-related cognitive decline [14,56–59]. Major microbiota-related alterations in particular neuropsychiatric conditions are summarized in Table 1.

Table 1. Microbiota and its metabolites alterations in various psychiatric conditions.

The Disease	Microbiota-Related Fingerprint	Reference
Depression	↑ *Bacteroidetes, Proteobacteria, Actinobacteria, Enterobacteriaceae, Alistipes*, propionic, isobutyric, and isovaleric acids ↓ *Faecalibacterium, Bifidobacterium, Lactobacillus*; serotonin, noradrenalin, SCFAs, kynurenic acid, kynurenine	[60–63]
Schizophrenia	↑ *Corinobacteriaceae, Prevotella, Succinivibrio, Collinsella, Megasphaera, Klebsiella, Methanobrevibacter, Clostridium* ↓ *Blautia, Coprococcus, Roseburia,*	[64,65]
Bipolar disorder	↑ *Bacteroides, Actinobacteria, Coriobacteria* ↓ *Faecalibacterium, Roseburia, Alistipes,*	[66,67]
Parkinson's disease	↑ *Bacteroides, Roseburia* ↓ *Blautia, Coprococcus, Dorea, Oscillospira, Akkermansia*	[68]
Autism Spectrum Disorder	↑ *Streptococcus, Clostridiales, Comamonadaceae, Akkermansia, Rhosococcus, Oscillospira, Desulvibrio, Burkholderia, Collinsella, Corynebacterium, Dorea, and Lactobacillus*; acetic and propionic acid, p-cresol, Glutamate, ↓ *Firmicutes, Faecalibacterium, Ruminococcus, Proteobacteria, Fuscobacteria, Verrumicrobia, Bifidobacterium, Neisseria, Alistipes, Bilophila, Dialister, Parabacteroides,* and *Veillonella,* butyric acid, tryptophan, kynurenic acid,	[69–73]
Attention-Deficit Hyperactivity Disorder	↑ *Actinobacteria (Bifidobacterium* genus) ↓ *Firmicutes (Clostridiales* order)	[74]
Alzheimer's disease	↑ *Blautia, Phascolarctobacterium, Gemella, E.coli, Shigella, Ps. aueruginosa* ↓ *Ruminococcaceae, Turicibacteraceae, Peptostreptococcaceae, Clostridiaceae, Mogibacteriaceae,* and the genera *SMB53* (family, *Clostridiaceae) Dialister, Clostridium, Turicibacter,* and cc115 (family *Erysipelotrichaceae)*	[75,76]
Multiple sclerosis	↑ *Akkermansia muciniphila, Acinetobacter calcoaceticus* ↓ *Parabacteroides distasonis*	[77]
Anorexia nervosa	↑ *Methanobrevibacter smithii*	[78]

Nevertheless, uninterrupted stress regulation is pivotal to mental health and altered stress response has been implicated in the origin of psychiatric diseases [58]. Numerous studies conducted in animals and humans have demonstrated that both acute and chronic stress interfere with intestinal barrier integrity and induce adverse alterations in intestinal microbiota composition. This has been confirmed in models of early-life [79] stress and prenatal stress [80]. Yarandi et al. [81] showed that water and ion in the gut might be reduced and elevated, respectively, under stressful conditions. This, in turn, impairs the physical protection of the gut barrier against both pathogenic microorganisms and nociceptive molecules. Furthermore, HPA activation, in particular corticotropin-releasing factor (CRF), showed a causative role in gut integrity disruption [82]. Elevated intestinal permeability was also found to be linked to stress-induced hypersensitivity of the rectum in animals, which were studied by means of partial restraint stress [83]. Winter et al. merged microbiome data from both animals and humans and selected bacterial genera that were either over-represented or appeared in a reduced number following stressor exposure. The first group included: *Desulfovibrio, Eggerthella, Holdemania, Turicibacter, Clostridium, Blautia, Anaerofilum* and *Roseburia* whereas those found in reduced numbers were: *Prevotella, Bacteroides, Mucispirillum, Dialister, Allobaculum, Faecalibacterium, Oscillospira, Ruminococcus, Dorea, Coprococcus,* and *Pseudobytyrivibrio* [84].

Emerging New Concepts in the Development of Neurodegenerative and GI Disease—Gut Microbes, Innate Immunity, and Bone Marrow Stem Cells as Partners in Crime

Mood and psychiatric disorders as well as numerous GI disorders are related to chronic inflammation [85]. For example, post-infectious IBS alters GI tract motility and behavior [86]. A similar effect appears in patients with FD [87]. Behavioral alterations predominate in chronic GI inflammatory disorders [88]. Chronic inflammation of the ENS can easily affect the CNS. However, knowledge on mechanisms behind this phenomenon is still scarce. For decades, inflammation in the brain, which were recently implicated in the pathogenesis of psychiatric diseases, has been considered "sterile." However, recent reports reveal the presence of the gut-vascular barrier (GVB), which, in structure and function, resembles the blood brain barier (BBB) and their communication is mediated via blood and bone marrow systems [89]. GVB controls the dissemination of bacteria from the gut into the bloodstream and the *Salmonella typhimirum* infection has been shown to decrease the Wnt/β catenin-inducible gene Axin2 (a marker of stem cell renewal) in the gut endothelium.

Importantly, the Wnt/β catenin signaling pathway is universally involved in trafficking (mobilization and proliferation) of stem cells deposited in adult tissues [90] including those located in GI tract [91]. Wnt/β catenin system has also been involved in the developmental control of BBB formation [92]. It has been demonstrated that various types of bone marrow-derived stem cells are mobilized into peripheral blood in patients and experimental animals in response to tissue/organ injury [93]. Examples include myocardial infarction [94], stroke [95], deep skin burns [96], and gut inflammation [97]. It has been previously shown that circulating peripheral bone marrow mononuclear cells (PBMNCs) were enriched with cells expressing mRNA of leucine-rich repeat-containing G-protein coupled receptor 5 (lgr-5), Achaete-scute complex homolog 2 (Ascl-2), Doublecortin Like Kinase 1 (Dclk-1), Male-specific lethal 1 homolog (MSL1), and B lymphoma Mo-MLV insertion region 1 homolog (BML-1). These markers are involved in the development of early intestinal lineage [97]. These circulating in PB cells could potentially be involved in reparatory mechanisms of peripheral tissues including the brain [98].

In fact, the release of very small embryonic-like stem cells (VSELs) and more differentiated neural stem cells (NSCs) from bone marrow into the peripheral blood in response to brain injury in rodents [99] and humans [95] has been well documented. Recent research indicates the involvement of other factors such as small bioactive lipids that may direct mobilization and trafficking of stem cells to injured organs [100]. Notably, release of sphingiosine-1-phosphate (S1P) correlates with the activation of the complement cascade and formation of the C5b-C9 membrane attack complex (MAC). Activation of proteolytic and fibrynolitis complement cascades. The release of cleavage fragments (e.g., C5a and desArgC5a fragments) could enhance the mobilization of stem cells from their niche in the bone marrow [101]. Moreover, these stem cells can be attracted from the bone marrow and from the intestinal epithelium in response to tumor or injured tissue derived plasma chemo-atractants such as stromal derived factor-1 (SDF-1), vascular endothelial growth factor (VEGF), zonulin, hepatocyte growth factor (HGF) or shphingosine-1-phosphate (S1P), ceramides, and extracellular nucleotides [102,103]. On the other hand, stem cells may secrete their own growth factors, cytokines, or even membrane-derived micro-vesicles that accelerate the regeneration process [104]. The previously mentioned factors have been frequently implicated in the pathogenesis of gastrointestinal and psychiatric disorders [89,105].

We envision that stem cells together with the GI microbiome are mutually involved in the pathogenesis of disorders of GBA by employing different mechanisms (e.g., autocrine, paracrine, or hormonal effects, immunomodulatory effects, replacement of damaged cells, cytotoxic effects, and neurotoxic effects) in distant tissues and organs. Further studies are needed to assess more accurately the mechanisms of cell-host-microbe interactions (Figure 1). Knowledge around these mechanisms already allows the design of novel treatments targeting GBA. For example, structural analog of S1P —Fingolimod and Ozanimod, functional antagonists of S1P receptors have already been applied in the treatment of relapsing forms of multiple sclerosis [106] as well as ulcerative colitis [107]. Similarly, supplementation with multi-species probiotics (Ecologic® Barrier, Amsterdam, The Netherlands) in a 12-week, placebo-controlled, randomized clinical study, which favorably modified both functional and biochemical markers (e.g., VEGF) of vascular dysfunction in obese postmenopausal women [108].

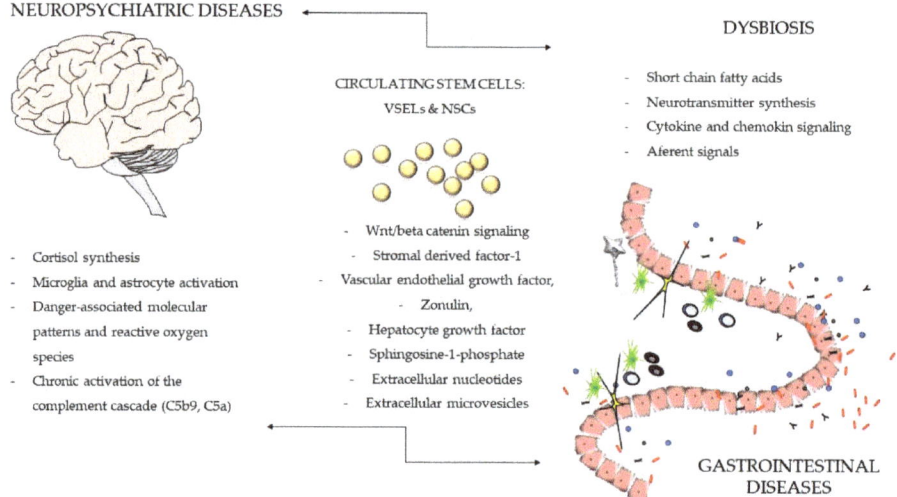

Figure 1. The bidirectional signaling within the GBA with the involvement of sterile inflammation of the brain and actions of microbiota and circulating adult stem cells. For details, see the text.

Emerging scientific data show that rapid changes in diet and lifestyle significantly contribute to the weakening of old evolutionary cell door-keeping mechanisms (e.g., Wnt/β catenin system) in the gut and the brain. The notion that even minor and subclinical stimuli to the gut mucosal and vascular barrier (e.g., infection) can result in significant, though delayed, consequences that may seriously affect the health of an individual is attractive [109], it still requires further detailed studies.

6. Drug-Microbiome Interactions—Still Neglected Problem in Clinical Medicine

Although microbiota alterations play—At least in part—A role in the etiology of neuropsychiatric diseases. Paradoxically, the treatment of these conditions may adversely affect the composition of intestinal microbiota. In fact, multiple drugs were found to be involved in dysbiosis origin [110–112]. Recently, Maier [113] reported that approximately one-fourth of about 10,000 non-antibiotic drugs were found to be able to reduce the in vitro growth of particular bacteria strain. Among these, the psychiatric drugs were predominant. In fact, certain pharmaceuticals utilized in neurology and psychiatry, which are predominantly antidepressants and antipsychotics, were historically characterized for being antibacterial agents. Evidence gathered mostly from animal studies but also in humans suggests that second-generation antipsychotics (SGA), which are mainly olanzapine and risperidone, change the composition of intestinal bacteria toward bacterial species promoting obesity. As demonstrated by several authors, the administration of these psychotropic drugs may increase the *Firmicutes/Bacteroidetes* ratio [114–118] previously found to be a microbiota profile of the obese [119].

The majority of studies aimed to look for the link between antipsychotic-induced metabolic malfunctions and microbiota dysbiosis were in vivo models. In rats treated with olanzapine (OLZ) and mice fed with a high fat diet and administered with OLZ, the microbiome diversity was found to be reduced [115,118]. When treated with another neuroleptic agent, namely risperidone (RIS), fewer operational taxonomy units (OTUs) were found in female mice [117]. Davey et al. demonstrated gender-dependent elevation of *Firmicutes* abundance and a decrease of *Bacteroidetes* [115,116]. Antipsychotic-driven dysbiosis in rodents resulted in decreased counts of beneficial *Actinobacteria* and *Proteobacteria* [115]. The OLZ regimen introduced higher abundance of *Erysipelotrichia* and *Gammaproteobacteria* and lower abundance of *Bacteroidia*. Lastly, OLZ suppressed the growth of anaerobic bacteria [117] and *Escherichia coli* NC101 [118].

In parallel, very few studies in humans explored the alterations of the gut microbiome following SGA treatment. Skewed intestinal microbiota following the psychotropic pharmacotherapy in humans expressed as elevated phylogenetic diversity and evaluated by means of PcoA of unweighted UniFrac distances [120] and reduced Simpson diversity in females [121] have been reported. Chronic use of RIS in children elevated the levels of *Clostridium*, *Lactobacillus*, *Ralstonia*, and *Eubacterium*. This occurred only in patients with a significant gain in BMI [120]. Flowers et al. conducted gut microbiota analyses in adult patients diagnosed with bipolar disorder and demonstrated that psychotropic treatment increased concentration of family *Lachnospiraceae* in the whole cohort of patients treated with SGA and a group of obese subjects. In addition, lowered counts of *Akkermansia* genera were noticed in the whole cohort of patients receiving treatment [121]. Yuan et al. lowered the levels of *Clostridium coccoides* Kaneuchi and *Lactobacillus* spp. and elevated the numbers of *Escherichia coli* Castellani and Chalmers in adult schizophrenia patients since six weeks of RIS treatment, which demonstrated that these variations may have induced body weight gain and increased fasting plasma glucose, homeostasis model assessment of insulin resistance (HOMA-IR), and low density lipoprotein (LDL) cholesterol concentration [122]. As far as metabolic disturbances are concerned, studies by Bahr et al. [120] and Flowers et al. [121] microbiota alteration during psychotropic treatment may correlate with weight gain.

We previously demonstrated that SGA-induced dysbiosis may potentially result in body weight and metabolic disturbances with low-level inflammation and decreased energy expenditure involved in the mechanism. However, since the majority of studies were conducted in rodent models with a high number of unclear risk of bias assessments, these findings need to be considered cautiously and may not be fully replicated in humans [123]. More studies regarding the involvement of psychiatric medications on gut microbiota composition in humans are warranted and, ccurrently, our research team undertook this effort.

The first antidepressant—Iproniazid—Via producing isonicotinoyl radicals may interrupt the bacterial cell cycle and inhibit their growth [124,125]. Tricyclic antidepressants were found to possess anti-plasmid activity and inhibit the growth of *Escherichia coli* Castellani and Chalmers, *Yersinia enterocolitica* Schleifstein & Coleman [126] and *Giardia lamblia* Kofoid & Christiansen [127] by means of decreasing the activity of DNA gyrase [128]. Tricyclic antidepressants are active relative to Plasmodium falciparum [129] and *Leishmania* spp. [130]. Selective serotonin re-uptake inhibitors may inhibit the growth of *Staphylococcus*, *Enterococcus* [131–133], *Citrobacter* spp, *Pseudomonas aeruginosa* Migula, *Klebsiella pneumoniae* Trevisan, *Morganella morganii* Brenner et al., *Clostridium perfringens* Hauduroy et al., and *Clostridium difficile* Prevot [131,134]. Efflux pump inhibition may be involved in these properties [135]. Ketamine may control the growth of *Staphylococcus aureus* Rosenbach, *Staphylococcus epidermidis* Evans, *Entercoccus faecalis* Schleifer and Kilpper-Bälz, *Streptococcus pyogenes* Rosenbach, *Pseudomonas aeruginosa* Migula and *Candida albicans* (C.P.Robin) Berkhout [134,136].

7. Modulation of Microbiota-Gut-Brain Axis as a Promising Tool to Manage Gastrointestinal and Mental Health

Mood disorders and depression are associated frequently with other GI conditions such as liver disease, inflammatory bowel disease (IBD), food intolerance, enteropathies (e.g., celiac disease), and cancer. Recently, Felice and O'Mahony [137] explained the origin of the high coincidence between stress-related psychiatric conditions and GI symptoms. Dysbiotic gut microbiota via synthesizing neuroactive metabolites are able to counteract secretion, motility, and blood flow within the GI tract and, additionally, transfer neural signals through vagus nerve and spinal cord routes. Therefore, the modulation of microbiota-gut-brain pathways opens up new avenues for the management of chronic diseases both of psychiatric and organic origin [12,138–143].

The new treatment avenues could be addressed through the modulation of the microbiota-gut-brain axis by means of prebiotic and probiotic administration. The World Gastroenterology Organization (WGO) recently issued a Global Guideline on Prebiotics and Probiotics use by healthcare professionals [144]. Among probiotics, those are recommended in the management of disorders of gut-brain interaction commonly known as FGIDs: *Lactobacillus plantarum* Bergey et al. 299V, *Bifidobacterium infantis* Reuter 35624, *Bifidobacterium animalis* Scardovi and Trovatelli DN-173 010, and *Saccharomyces boullardii* Henri Boulard CNCM I-745.

Psychobiotics—New Kid on the Block

Psychobiotics are a new class of probiotics which, when ingested, confer mental health benefits through interactions with the microbiota-gut-brain axis [145]. This term should also include prebiotics, which favorably influence the growth of beneficial gut bacteria [146]. Some of the properties of probiotics are prevalent among different strains, e.g., improvement of the intestinal epithelium renewal while the others are strain-specific, e.g., modulation of the CNS function [147]. Misra et al. noted that psychobiotic strains may be involved in the neuroactive substances synthesis, activate directly neural pathways, modulate neurotrophic factors, protect microbiota against stress, and others [148].

The action of psychobiotics was confirmed in mechanistic studies. For example, Ait-Belgnaoui et al. [149] demonstrated that psychobiotics may significantly reduce stress-induced neuronal activation in three brain regions i.e., hypothalamus, amygdala, and hippocampus, and promote the development of dendrites in the cingulate cortex-center of neurogenesis. Another study confirmed that psychobiotics decreased visceral hypersensitivity intensity and such an action correlated with the concentration of stress hormones (noradrenaline, adrenaline, corticosterone) and was possibly regulated by glucocorticoid receptors [150]. In vivo studies also reported that ingestion of psychobiotics improved GI function through the modulation of GBA in animals experiencing maternal separation [151] and *Citrobacter rodentium* infection [152].

Lately, the importance of psychobiotic use in humans has been acknowledged. Diop et al. was the first to demonstrate that probiotic supplementation reduces symptoms of GI disorders caused by stress in healthy people [153]. Messaoudi et al. showed that psychobiotic strains impact positively psychological stress exponents and reduce urinary free cortisol concentration [154]. Steenbergen et al. [155] demonstrated that, after 4 weeks of probiotic supplementation, a statistically significant improvement of aggression and rumination compared to placebo was found. Allen et al. [156] tested the psychobiotic strain to find that it may improve memory and reduce stress while Kato-Katoka [157] who analyzed a group of students during the exam session reported that the incidence of abdominal pain and cold as vegetative stress symptoms was significantly lowered in the group of students receiving probiotics compared to the placebo group. A recent study by Lv et al. [158] summarized that psychobiotics improve the function of the GI tract in patients with schizophrenia.

In addition, meta-analyses have shown that probiotic intervention may positively affect the mood in healthy persons as well as depressive patients [159]. McKean et al. [160] found that probiotic consumption may diminish the symptoms of depression, anxiety, and stress. Surprisingly, the latest meta-analysis concluded that such an intervention may significantly improve the mood of patients with mild to moderate depression but not the mood of healthy individuals [161]. Consequently, psychobiotics and neurobiotics, which are capable of GBA and HPA modulation, could be advocated in the management of patients endangered with iatrogenic complications associated with pharmacotherapy and polypharmacy. However, more studies—Especially of the highest evidence level—Are necessary to elucidate the psychobiotic potential to improve GBA function.

The use of these new probiotic compounds could be of great use in the daily management of stress and depression in FGIDs patients but also with other GI and extra-intestinal complaints associated with mental or mood alterations [162,163]. The data supporting their use are already strong and new studies that shall create even more evidence to medical societies as well as governmental agencies to help them evaluate the microbiota-gut-brain axis therapeutics in the management of stress in contemporary medicine [164,165]. Table 2 includes examples of psychobiotic strains and their clinical applications [144,148,166]. Since a few probiotic strains were found to be effective to counteract mood disorders and FGIDs, there is still limited data in individuals with ASD, Parkinson's disease, and Alzheimer's disease. There is an urgent need for a great investment in clinical trials in these entities [167–171].

Table 2. Probiotics strains with documented efficacy in gut-brain axis disorders [144,148,166,172].

Condition	Strain
Anxiety and depression	*Lactobacillus fermentum* NS8 and NS9, *Lactobacillus casei* Shirota, *Lactobacillus gasseri* OLL2809, *Lactobacillus rhamnosus* JB-1, *Lactobacillus helveticus* Rosell -52, *Lactobacillus acidophilus* W37, *Lactobacillus brevis* W63, *Lactococcus lactis* W19 and W58, *Bifidobacterium longum* Rosell-175, *Bifidobacterium longum* NCC3001, *Bifidobacterium longum* 1714, *Bifidobacterium bifidum* W23, *Bifidobacterium lactis* W52, *Lactobacillus plantarum* 299v
Stress	*Lactobacillus casei* Shirota, *Lactobacillus helveticus* Rosell -52, *Lactobacillus plantarum* PS128, *Bifidobacterium longum* Rosell-175, *Lactobacillus gasseri* CP230 *
FGIDs	*Lactobacillus plantarum* 299v (DSM 9843), *Escherichia coli* DSM17252, *Bifidobacterium animalis* DN-173, *Saccharomyces boulardii* CNCM I-745 *Bifidobacterium infantis* 35624, *Lactobacillus rhamnosus* NCIMB 30174, *Lactobacillus plantarum* NCIMB 30173, *Lactobacillus acidophilus* NCIMB 30175, *Enterococcus faecium* NCIMB 30176

* Para-psychobiotic-heat inactivated strain.

8. Conclusions

Our review suggests some involvements of GBA deregulation in the origin of disorders of the brain and gut. We hypothesize that stem cell-host microbiome cross talk is potentially involved in GBA disorders. Consequently, molecules mediating GBA signaling may constitute a grip point for the development of diagnostic tools and personalized microbiota-based therapies. In addition, novel treatment protocols based on new compounds interfering with gut derived metabolites as well as small molecules and bioactive lipids playing roles in adult stem cell trafficking are awaiting further developments.

Author Contributions: Conceptualization, K.S.-Ż., W.M., I.Ł. Investigation, all. Writing—Original Draft Preparation, K.S.-Ż. Writing—Review, editing, final approval, all. Supervision, W.M. and I.Ł.

Funding: This research received no external funding.

Conflicts of Interest: Igor Łoniewski and Wojciech Marlicz are cofounders and shareholders in the Sanprobi-probiotic manufacturer and marketing company. Karolina Skonieczna-Żydecka received remunerations for speaking engagements from Sanprobi. The content of this study was neither influenced nor constrained by these facts. The other authors have no conflicts of interest to declare.

References

1. World Health Organization. Mental Health Included in the UN Sustainable Development Goals. Available online: http://www.who.int/mental_health/SDGs/en/ (accessed on 25 November 2018).
2. World Health Organization. Third United Nations High-level Meeting on NCDs. Available online: http://www.who.int/ncds/governance/third-un-meeting/en/ (accessed on 25 November 2018).
3. Chandra, P.S.; Chand, P. Towards a new era for mental health. *Lancet* **2018**. [CrossRef]
4. Patel, V.; Saxena, S.; Lund, C.; Thornicroft, G.; Baingana, F.; Bolton, P.; Chisholm, D.; Collins, P.Y.; Cooper, J.L.; Eaton, J.; et al. The Lancet Commission on global mental health and sustainable development. *Lancet* **2018**. [CrossRef]
5. Gallagher, J. More than Half Your Body is not Human. Available online: https://www.bbc.com/news/health-43674270 (accessed on 6 December 2018).
6. Lynch, S.V.; Pedersen, O. The Human Intestinal Microbiome in Health and Disease. *N. Engl. J. Med.* **2016**, *375*, 2369–2379. [CrossRef] [PubMed]
7. Bloomfield, S.F.; Rook, G.A.; Scott, E.A.; Shanahan, F.; Stanwell-Smith, R.; Turner, P. Time to abandon the hygiene hypothesis: New perspectives on allergic disease, the human microbiome, infectious disease prevention and the role of targeted hygiene. *Perspect. Public Health* **2016**, *136*, 213–224. [CrossRef] [PubMed]
8. Bello, M.G.D.; Knight, R.; Gilbert, J.A.; Blaser, M.J. Preserving microbial diversity. *Science* **2018**, *362*, 33–34. [CrossRef] [PubMed]
9. Bretin, A.; Gewirtz, A.T.; Chassaing, B. Microbiota and metabolism: What's new in 2018? *Am. J. Physiol. Endocrinol. Metab.* **2018**, *315*, 1–6. [CrossRef] [PubMed]
10. Rea, D.; Coppola, G.; Palma, G.; Barbieri, A.; Luciano, A.; Del Prete, P.; Rossetti, S.; Berretta, M.; Facchini, G.; Perdonà, S.; et al. Microbiota effects on cancer: From risks to therapies. *Oncotarget* **2018**, *9*, 17915–17927. [CrossRef] [PubMed]
11. Chu, H.; Williams, B.; Schnabl, B. Gut microbiota, fatty liver disease, and hepatocellular carcinoma. *Liver Res.* **2018**, *2*, 43–51. [CrossRef] [PubMed]
12. Marlicz, W.; Yung, D.E.; Skonieczna-Żydecka, K.; Loniewski, I.; van Hemert, S.; Loniewska, B.; Koulaouzidis, A. From clinical uncertainties to precision medicine: The emerging role of the gut barrier and microbiome in small bowel functional diseases. *Expert Rev. Gastroenterol. Hepatol.* **2017**, *11*, 961–978. [CrossRef]
13. Sanduzzi Zamparelli, M.; Compare, D.; Coccoli, P.; Rocco, A.; Nardone, O.M.; Marrone, G.; Gasbarrini, A.; Grieco, A.; Nardone, G.; Miele, L. The metabolic role of gut microbiota in the development of nonalcoholic fatty liver disease and cardiovascular disease. *Int. J. Mol. Sci.* **2016**, *17*, 1225. [CrossRef]
14. Skonieczna-Żydecka, K.; Łoniewski, I.; Maciejewska, D.; Marlicz, W. Mikrobiota jelitowa iskładniki pokarmowe jako determinanty funkcji układu nerwowego. Część I. Mikrobiota przewodu pokarmowego. *Aktualności Neurologiczne* **2017**, *17*, 181–188. (In Polish) [CrossRef]
15. Cenit, M.C.; Sanz, Y.; Codoñer-Franch, P. Influence of gut microbiota on neuropsychiatric disorders. *World J. Gastroenterol.* **2017**, *23*, 5486–5498. [CrossRef] [PubMed]
16. Marizzoni, M.; Provasi, S.; Cattaneo, A.; Frisoni, G.B. Microbiota and neurodegenerative diseases. *Curr. Opin. Neurol.* **2017**, *30*, 630–638. [CrossRef] [PubMed]
17. Stasi, C.; Nisita, C.; Cortopassi, S.; Corretti, G.; Gambaccini, D.; De Bortoli, N.; Fani, B.; Simonetti, N.; Ricchiuti, A.; Dell'Osso, L.; et al. Subthreshold psychiatric psychopathology in functional gastrointestinal disorders: Can it be the bridge between gastroenterology and psychiatry? *Gastroenterol. Res. Pract.* **2017**, *2017*. [CrossRef]
18. Bernstein, C.N.; Hitchon, C.A.; Walld, R.; Bolton, J.M.; Sareen, J.; Walker, J.R.; Graff, L.A.; Patten, S.B.; Singer, A.; Lix, L.M.; et al. Increased burden of psychiatric disorders in inflammatory bowel disease. *Inflamm. Bowel Dis.* **2018**. [CrossRef]
19. Chan, W.; Shim, H.H.; Lim, M.S.; Sawadjaan, F.L.B.; Isaac, S.P.; Chuah, S.W.; Leong, R.; Kong, C. Symptoms of anxiety and depression are independently associated with inflammatory bowel disease-related disability. *Dig. Liver Dis.* **2017**, *49*, 1314–1319. [CrossRef]
20. Frolkis, A.D.; Vallerand, I.A.; Shaheen, A.-A.; Lowerison, M.W.; Swain, M.G.; Barnabe, C.; Patten, S.B.; Kaplan, G.G. Depression increases the risk of inflammatory bowel disease, which may be mitigated by the use of antidepressants in the treatment of depression. *Gut* **2018**. [CrossRef]

21. Drossman, D.A.; Hasler, W.L. Rome IV-functional GI disorders: Disorders of gut-brain interaction. *Gastroenterology* **2016**, *150*, 1257–1261. [CrossRef]
22. Zhong, L.; Shanahan, E.R.; Raj, A.; Koloski, N.A.; Fletcher, L.; Morrison, M.; Walker, M.M.; Talley, N.J.; Holtmann, G. Dyspepsia and the microbiome: Time to focus on the small intestine. *Gut* **2017**, *66*, 1168–1169. [CrossRef]
23. Vanheel, H.; Vicario, M.; Vanuytsel, T.; Van Oudenhove, L.; Martinez, C.; Keita, Å.V.; Pardon, N.; Santos, J.; Söderholm, J.D.; Tack, J.; et al. Impaired duodenal mucosal integrity and low-grade inflammation in functional dyspepsia. *Gut* **2014**, *63*, 262–271. [CrossRef]
24. Giamarellos-Bourboulis, E.; Tang, J.; Pyleris, E.; Pistiki, A.; Barbatzas, C.; Brown, J.; Lee, C.C.; Harkins, T.T.; Kim, G.; Weitsman, S.; et al. Molecular assessment of differences in the duodenal microbiome in subjects with irritable bowel syndrome. *Scand. J. Gastroenterol.* **2015**, *50*, 1076–1087. [CrossRef]
25. Martínez, C.; Lobo, B.; Pigrau, M.; Ramos, L.; González-Castro, A.M.; Alonso, C.; Guilarte, M.; Guilá, M.; de Torres, I.; Azpiroz, F.; et al. Diarrhoea-predominant irritable bowel syndrome: An organic disorder with structural abnormalities in the jejunal epithelial barrier. *Gut* **2013**, *62*, 1160–1168. [CrossRef]
26. Barbara, G.; Wang, B.; Stanghellini, V.; de Giorgio, R.; Cremon, C.; Di Nardo, G.; Trevisani, M.; Campi, B.; Geppetti, P.; Tonini, M.; et al. Mast cell-dependent excitation of visceral-nociceptive sensory neurons in irritable bowel syndrome. *Gastroenterology* **2007**, *132*, 26–37. [CrossRef]
27. Shah, E.; Rezaie, A.; Riddle, M.; Pimentel, M. Psychological disorders in gastrointestinal disease: Epiphenomenon, cause or consequence? *Ann. Gastroenterol.* **2014**, *27*, 224–230.
28. Gastrointestinal Symptoms in Psychiatry: Comparison of Direct Applications and Referrals. Available online: http://www.dusunenadamdergisi.org/ing/fArticledetails.aspx?MkID=1125 (accessed on 19 November 2018).
29. Wilder-Smith, C.H.; Olesen, S.S.; Materna, A.; Drewes, A.M. Fermentable sugar ingestion, gas production, and gastrointestinal and central nervous system symptoms in patients with functional disorders. *Gastroenterology* **2018**, *155*, 1034–1044. [CrossRef]
30. Codagnone, M.G.; Spichak, S.; O'Mahony, S.M.; O'Leary, O.F.; Clarke, G.; Stanton, C.; Dinan, T.G.; Cryan, J.F. Programming bugs: Microbiota and the developmental origins of brain health and disease. *Biol. Psychiatry* **2018**. [CrossRef]
31. Luczynski, P.; Whelan, S.O.; O'Sullivan, C.; Clarke, G.; Shanahan, F.; Dinan, T.G.; Cryan, J.F. Adult microbiota-deficient mice have distinct dendritic morphological changes: Differential effects in the amygdala and hippocampus. *Eur. J. Neurosci.* **2016**, *44*, 2654–2666. [CrossRef]
32. Hoban, A.E.; Stilling, R.M.; Ryan, F.J.; Shanahan, F.; Dinan, T.G.; Claesson, M.J.; Clarke, G.; Cryan, J.F. Regulation of prefrontal cortex myelination by the microbiota. *Transl. Psychiatry* **2016**, *6*, 774. [CrossRef]
33. Lu, J.; Lu, L.; Yu, Y.; Cluette-Brown, J.; Martin, C.R.; Claud, E.C. Effects of intestinal microbiota on brain development in humanized gnotobiotic mice. *Sci. Rep.* **2018**, *8*, 5443. [CrossRef]
34. Desbonnet, L.; Clarke, G.; Shanahan, F.; Dinan, T.G.; Cryan, J.F. Microbiota is essential for social development in the mouse. *Mol. Psychiatry* **2014**, *19*, 146–148. [CrossRef]
35. Marlicz, W.; Poniewierska-Baran, A.; Rzeszotek, S.; Bartoszewski, R.; Skonieczna-Żydecka, K.; Starzyńska, T.; Ratajczak, M.Z. A novel potential role of pituitary gonadotropins in the pathogenesis of human colorectal cancer. *PLoS ONE* **2018**, *13*, e0189337. [CrossRef]
36. Kaelberer, M.M.; Buchanan, K.L.; Klein, M.E.; Barth, B.B.; Montoya, M.M.; Shen, X.; Bohórquez, D.V. A gut-brain neural circuit for nutrient sensory transduction. *Science* **2018**, *361*. [CrossRef]
37. Paolicelli, R.C.; Bergamini, G.; Rajendran, L. Cell-to-cell communication by extracellular vesicles: Focus on microglia. *Neuroscience* **2018**. [CrossRef]
38. Kavvadia, M.; Santis, G.L.D.; Cascapera, S.; Lorenzo, A.D. Psychobiotics as integrative therapy for neuropsychiatric disorders with special emphasis on the microbiota-gut-brain axis. *Biomed. Prev.* **2017**, *2*, 8. [CrossRef]
39. Riboni, F.V.; Belzung, C. Stress and psychiatric disorders: From categorical to dimensional approaches. *Curr. Opin. Behav. Sci.* **2017**, *14*, 72–77. [CrossRef]
40. Sudo, N.; Chida, Y.; Aiba, Y.; Sonoda, J.; Oyama, N.; Yu, X.-N.; Kubo, C.; Koga, Y. Postnatal microbial colonization programs the hypothalamic-pituitary-adrenal system for stress response in mice. *J. Physiol. (Lond.)* **2004**, *558*, 263–275. [CrossRef]

41. Crumeyrolle-Arias, M.; Jaglin, M.; Bruneau, A.; Vancassel, S.; Cardona, A.; Daugé, V.; Naudon, L.; Rabot, S. Absence of the gut microbiota enhances anxiety-like behavior and neuroendocrine response to acute stress in rats. *Psychoneuroendocrinology* **2014**, *42*, 207–217. [CrossRef]
42. König, J.; Wells, J.; Cani, P.D.; García-Ródenas, C.L.; MacDonald, T.; Mercenier, A.; Whyte, J.; Troost, F.; Brummer, R.-J. Human intestinal barrier function in health and disease. *Clin. Transl. Gastroenterol.* **2016**, *7*, 196. [CrossRef]
43. Fond, G.; Boukouaci, W.; Chevalier, G.; Regnault, A.; Eberl, G.; Hamdani, N.; Dickerson, F.; Macgregor, A.; Boyer, L.; Dargel, A.; et al. The "psychomicrobiotic": Targeting microbiota in major psychiatric disorders: A systematic review. *Pathol. Biol.* **2015**, *63*, 35–42. [CrossRef]
44. Spadoni, I.; Zagato, E.; Bertocchi, A.; Paolinelli, R.; Hot, E.; Di Sabatino, A.; Caprioli, F.; Bottiglieri, L.; Oldani, A.; Viale, G.; et al. A gut-vascular barrier controls the systemic dissemination of bacteria. *Science* **2015**, *350*, 830–834. [CrossRef]
45. Brown, E.M.; Sadarangani, M.; Finlay, B.B. The role of the immune system in governing host-microbe interactions in the intestine. *Nat. Immunol.* **2013**, *14*, 660–667. [CrossRef]
46. Groschwitz, K.R.; Hogan, S.P. Intestinal barrier function: Molecular regulation and disease pathogenesis. *J. Allergy Clin. Immunol.* **2009**, *124*, 3–20. [CrossRef]
47. Tripathi, A.; Lammers, K.M.; Goldblum, S.; Shea-Donohue, T.; Netzel-Arnett, S.; Buzza, M.S.; Antalis, T.M.; Vogel, S.N.; Zhao, A.; Yang, S.; et al. Identification of human zonulin, a physiological modulator of tight junctions, as prehaptoglobin-2. *Proc. Natl. Acad. Sci. USA* **2009**, *106*, 16799–16804. [CrossRef]
48. Fasano, A. Zonulin and its regulation of intestinal barrier function: The biological door to inflammation, autoimmunity, and cancer. *Physiol. Rev.* **2011**, *91*, 151–175. [CrossRef]
49. Sharon, G.; Sampson, T.R.; Geschwind, D.H.; Mazmanian, S.K. The central nervous system and the gut microbiome. *Cell.* **2016**, *167*, 915–932. [CrossRef]
50. Al-Asmakh, M.; Anuar, F.; Zadjali, F.; Rafter, J.; Pettersson, S. Gut microbial communities modulating brain development and function. *Gut Microbes* **2012**, *3*, 366–373. [CrossRef]
51. Daneman, R.; Rescigno, M. The gut immune barrier and the blood-brain barrier: Are they so different? *Immunity* **2009**, *31*, 722–735. [CrossRef]
52. Mayer, E.A.; Craske, M.; Naliboff, B.D. Depression, anxiety, and the gastrointestinal system. *J. Clin. Psychiatry* **2001**, *62* (Suppl. 8), 28–37.
53. Carding, S.; Verbeke, K.; Vipond, D.T.; Corfe, B.M.; Owen, L.J. Dysbiosis of the gut microbiota in disease. *Microb. Ecol. Health Dis.* **2015**, *26*, 26191. [CrossRef]
54. Rothschild, D.; Weissbrod, O.; Barkan, E.; Kurilshikov, A.; Korem, T.; Zeevi, D.; Costea, P.I.; Godneva, A.; Kalka, I.N.; Bar, N.; et al. Environment dominates over host genetics in shaping human gut microbiota. *Nature* **2018**, *555*, 210–215. [CrossRef]
55. Foster, J.A.; Neufeld, K.-A.M. Gut-brain axis: How the microbiome influences anxiety and depression. *Trends Neurosci.* **2013**, *36*, 305–312. [CrossRef]
56. Sherwin, E.; Dinan, T.G.; Cryan, J.F. Recent developments in understanding the role of the gut microbiota in brain health and disease. *Ann. N. Y. Acad. Sci.* **2018**, *1420*, 5–25. [CrossRef]
57. Rogers, G.B.; Keating, D.J.; Young, R.L.; Wong, M.-L.; Licinio, J.; Wesselingh, S. From gut dysbiosis to altered brain function and mental illness: Mechanisms and pathways. *Mol. Psychiatry* **2016**, *21*, 738–748. [CrossRef]
58. Bastiaanssen, T.F.S.; Cowan, C.S.M.; Claesson, M.J.; Dinan, T.G.; Cryan, J.F. Making sense of ... the microbiome in psychiatry. *Int. J. Neuropsychopharmacol.* **2018**. [CrossRef]
59. Grochowska, M.; Wojnar, M.; Radkowski, M. The gut microbiota in neuropsychiatric disorders. *Acta Neurobiol. Exp.* **2018**, *78*, 69–81. [CrossRef]
60. Aizawa, E.; Tsuji, H.; Asahara, T.; Takahashi, T.; Teraishi, T.; Yoshida, S.; Ota, M.; Koga, N.; Hattori, K.; Kunugi, H. Possible association of Bifidobacterium and Lactobacillus in the gut microbiota of patients with major depressive disorder. *J. Affect. Disord.* **2016**, *202*, 254–257. [CrossRef]
61. Jiang, H.; Ling, Z.; Zhang, Y.; Mao, H.; Ma, Z.; Yin, Y.; Wang, W.; Tang, W.; Tan, Z.; Shi, J.; et al. Altered fecal microbiota composition in patients with major depressive disorder. *Brain Behav. Immun.* **2015**, *48*, 186–194. [CrossRef]
62. Szczesniak, O.; Hestad, K.A.; Hanssen, J.F.; Rudi, K. Isovaleric acid in stool correlates with human depression. *Nutr. Neurosci.* **2016**, *19*, 279–283. [CrossRef]

63. Ogyu, K.; Kubo, K.; Noda, Y.; Iwata, Y.; Tsugawa, S.; Omura, Y.; Wada, M.; Tarumi, R.; Plitman, E.; Moriguchi, S.; et al. Kynurenine pathway in depression: A systematic review and meta-analysis. *Neurosci. Biobehav. Rev.* **2018**, *90*, 16–25. [CrossRef]
64. Schwarz, E.; Maukonen, J.; Hyytiäinen, T.; Kieseppä, T.; Orešič, M.; Sabunciyan, S.; Mantere, O.; Saarela, M.; Yolken, R.; Suvisaari, J. Analysis of microbiota in first episode psychosis identifies preliminary associations with symptom severity and treatment response. *Schizophr. Res.* **2018**, *192*, 398–403. [CrossRef]
65. Shen, Y.; Xu, J.; Li, Z.; Huang, Y.; Yuan, Y.; Wang, J.; Zhang, M.; Hu, S.; Liang, Y. Analysis of gut microbiota diversity and auxiliary diagnosis as a biomarker in patients with schizophrenia: A cross-sectional study. *Schizophr. Res.* **2018**. [CrossRef]
66. Evans, S.J.; Bassis, C.M.; Hein, R.; Assari, S.; Flowers, S.A.; Kelly, M.B.; Young, V.B.; Ellingrod, V.E.; McInnis, M.G. The gut microbiome composition associates with bipolar disorder and illness severity. *J. Psychiatr. Res.* **2017**, *87*, 23–29. [CrossRef]
67. Painold, A.; Mörkl, S.; Kashofer, K.; Halwachs, B.; Dalkner, N.; Bengesser, S.; Birner, A.; Fellendorf, F.; Platzer, M.; Queissner, R.; et al. A step ahead: Exploring the gut microbiota in inpatients with bipolar disorder during a depressive episode. *Bipolar Disord.* **2018**. [CrossRef]
68. Keshavarzian, A.; Green, S.J.; Engen, P.A.; Voigt, R.M.; Naqib, A.; Forsyth, C.B.; Mutlu, E.; Shannon, K.M. Colonic bacterial composition in Parkinson's disease. *Mov. Disord.* **2015**, *30*, 1351–1360. [CrossRef]
69. De Angelis, M.; Francavilla, R.; Piccolo, M.; De Giacomo, A.; Gobbetti, M. Autism spectrum disorders and intestinal microbiota. *Gut Microbes* **2015**, *6*, 207–213. [CrossRef]
70. Kushak, R.I.; Winter, H.S.; Buie, T.M.; Cox, S.B.; Phillips, C.D.; Ward, N.L. Analysis of the Duodenal Microbiome in Autistic Individuals: Association With Carbohydrate Digestion. *J. Pediatr. Gastroenterol. Nutr.* **2017**, *64*, 110–116. [CrossRef]
71. Lee, Y.; Park, J.-Y.; Lee, E.-H.; Yang, J.; Jeong, B.-R.; Kim, Y.-K.; Seoh, J.-Y.; Lee, S.; Han, P.-L.; Kim, E.-J. Rapid assessment of microbiota changes in individuals with autism spectrum disorder using bacteria-derived membrane vesicles in urine. *Exp. Neurobiol.* **2017**, *26*, 307–317. [CrossRef]
72. Strati, F.; Cavalieri, D.; Albanese, D.; De Felice, C.; Donati, C.; Hayek, J.; Jousson, O.; Leoncini, S.; Renzi, D.; Calabrò, A.; et al. New evidences on the altered gut microbiota in autism spectrum disorders. *Microbiome* **2017**, *5*, 24. [CrossRef]
73. Bryn, V.; Verkerk, R.; Skjeldal, O.H.; Saugstad, O.D.; Ormstad, H. Kynurenine pathway in autism spectrum disorders in children. *Neuropsychobiology* **2017**, *76*, 82–88. [CrossRef]
74. Aarts, E.; Ederveen, T.H.A.; Naaijen, J.; Zwiers, M.P.; Boekhorst, J.; Timmerman, H.M.; Smeekens, S.P.; Netea, M.G.; Buitelaar, J.K.; Franke, B.; et al. Gut microbiome in ADHD and its relation to neural reward anticipation. *PLoS ONE* **2017**, *12*, e0183509. [CrossRef]
75. Cattaneo, A.; Cattane, N.; Galluzzi, S.; Provasi, S.; Lopizzo, N.; Festari, C.; Ferrari, C.; Guerra, U.P.; Paghera, B.; Muscio, C.; et al. Association of brain amyloidosis with pro-inflammatory gut bacterial taxa and peripheral inflammation markers in cognitively impaired elderly. *Neurobiol. Aging* **2017**, *49*, 60–68. [CrossRef]
76. Vogt, N.M.; Kerby, R.L.; Dill-McFarland, K.A.; Harding, S.J.; Merluzzi, A.P.; Johnson, S.C.; Carlsson, C.M.; Asthana, S.; Zetterberg, H.; Blennow, K.; et al. Gut microbiome alterations in Alzheimer's disease. *Sci Rep.* **2017**, *7*, 13537. [CrossRef]
77. Cekanaviciute, E.; Yoo, B.B.; Runia, T.F.; Debelius, J.W.; Singh, S.; Nelson, C.A.; Kanner, R.; Bencosme, Y.; Lee, Y.K.; Hauser, S.L.; et al. Gut bacteria from multiple sclerosis patients modulate human T cells and exacerbate symptoms in mouse models. *Proc. Natl. Acad. Sci. USA* **2017**, *114*, 10713–10718. [CrossRef]
78. Schwensen, H.F.; Kan, C.; Treasure, J.; Høiby, N.; Sjögren, M. A systematic review of studies on the faecal microbiota in anorexia nervosa: Future research may need to include microbiota from the small intestine. *Eat. Weight Disord.* **2018**, *23*, 399–418. [CrossRef]
79. Bailey, M.T.; Dowd, S.E.; Galley, J.D.; Hufnagle, A.R.; Allen, R.G.; Lyte, M. Exposure to a social stressor alters the structure of the intestinal microbiota: Implications for stressor-induced immunomodulation. *Brain Behav. Immun.* **2011**, *25*, 397–407. [CrossRef]
80. Zijlmans, M.A.C.; Korpela, K.; Riksen-Walraven, J.M.; de Vos, W.M.; de Weerth, C. Maternal prenatal stress is associated with the infant intestinal microbiota. *Psychoneuroendocrinology* **2015**, *53*, 233–245. [CrossRef]
81. Yarandi, S.S.; Peterson, D.A.; Treisman, G.J.; Moran, T.H.; Pasricha, P.J. modulatory effects of gut microbiota on the central nervous system: how gut could play a role in neuropsychiatric health and diseases. *J. Neurogastroenterol. Motil.* **2016**, *22*, 201–212. [CrossRef]

82. Kelly, J.R.; Kennedy, P.J.; Cryan, J.F.; Dinan, T.G.; Clarke, G.; Hyland, N.P. Breaking down the barriers: The gut microbiome, intestinal permeability and stress-related psychiatric disorders. *Front. Cell. Neurosci.* **2015**, *9*, 392. [CrossRef]
83. Ait-Belgnaoui, A.; Bradesi, S.; Fioramonti, J.; Theodorou, V.; Bueno, L. Acute stress-induced hypersensitivity to colonic distension depends upon increase in paracellular permeability: Role of myosin light chain kinase. *Pain* **2005**, *113*, 141–147. [CrossRef]
84. Winter, G.; Hart, R.A.; Charlesworth, R.P.G.; Sharpley, C.F. Gut microbiome and depression: What we know and what we need to know. *Rev. Neurosci.* **2018**, *29*, 629–643. [CrossRef]
85. Bauer, M.E.; Teixeira, A.L. Inflammation in psychiatric disorders: What comes first? *Ann. N. Y. Acad. Sci.* **2018**. [CrossRef]
86. Spiller, R.; Lam, C. An Update on Post-infectious Irritable Bowel Syndrome: Role of Genetics, Immune Activation, Serotonin and Altered Microbiome. *J. Neurogastroenterol. Motil.* **2012**, *18*, 258–268. [CrossRef]
87. Futagami, S.; Itoh, T.; Sakamoto, C. Systematic review with meta-analysis: Post-infectious functional dyspepsia. *Aliment. Pharmacol. Ther.* **2015**, *41*, 177–188. [CrossRef]
88. Neuendorf, R.; Harding, A.; Stello, N.; Hanes, D.; Wahbeh, H. Depression and anxiety in patients with Inflammatory Bowel Disease: A systematic review. *J. Psychosom. Res.* **2016**, *87*, 70–80. [CrossRef]
89. Ratajczak, M.Z.; Pedziwiatr, D.; Cymer, M.; Kucia, M.; Kucharska-Mazur, J.; Samochowiec, J. Sterile inflammation of brain, due to activation of innate immunity, as a culprit in psychiatric disorders. *Front. Psychiatry* **2018**, *9*. [CrossRef]
90. Kahn, M. Wnt signaling in stem cells and cancer stem cells: A tale of two coactivators. *Prog. Mol. Biol. Transl. Sci.* **2018**, *153*, 209–244. [CrossRef]
91. Kabiri, Z.; Greicius, G.; Zaribafzadeh, H.; Hemmerich, A.; Counter, C.M.; Virshup, D.M. Wnt signaling suppresses MAPK-driven proliferation of intestinal stem cells. *J. Clin. Invest.* **2018**, *128*, 3806–3812. [CrossRef]
92. Xing, L.; Anbarchian, T.; Tsai, J.M.; Plant, G.W.; Nusse, R. Wnt/β-catenin signaling regulates ependymal cell development and adult homeostasis. *Proc. Natl. Acad. Sci. USA* **2018**, *115*, 5954–5962. [CrossRef]
93. Ratajczak, M.Z.; Liu, R.; Marlicz, W.; Blogowski, W.; Starzynska, T.; Wojakowski, W.; Zuba-Surma, E. Identification of very small embryonic/epiblast-like stem cells (VSELs) circulating in peripheral blood during organ/tissue injuries. *Methods Cell. Biol.* **2011**, *103*, 31–54. [CrossRef]
94. Wojakowski, W.; Tendera, M.; Kucia, M.; Zuba-Surma, E.; Paczkowska, E.; Ciosek, J.; Hałasa, M.; Król, M.; Kazmierski, M.; Buszman, P.; et al. Mobilization of bone marrow-derived Oct-4+ SSEA-4+ very small embryonic-like stem cells in patients with acute myocardial infarction. *J. Am. Coll. Cardiol.* **2009**, *53*, 1–9. [CrossRef]
95. Paczkowska, E.; Kucia, M.; Koziarska, D.; Halasa, M.; Safranow, K.; Masiuk, M.; Karbicka, A.; Nowik, M.; Nowacki, P.; Ratajczak, M.Z.; et al. Clinical evidence that very small embryonic-like stem cells are mobilized into peripheral blood in patients after stroke. *Stroke* **2009**, *40*, 1237–1244. [CrossRef]
96. Drukała, J.; Paczkowska, E.; Kucia, M.; Młyńska, E.; Krajewski, A.; Machaliński, B.; Madeja, Z.; Ratajczak, M.Z. Stem cells, including a population of very small embryonic-like stem cells, are mobilized into peripheral blood in patients after skin burn injury. *Stem Cell. Rev.* **2012**, *8*, 184–194. [CrossRef]
97. Marlicz, W.; Zuba-Surma, E.; Kucia, M.; Blogowski, W.; Starzynska, T.; Ratajczak, M.Z. Various types of stem cells, including a population of very small embryonic-like stem cells, are mobilized into peripheral blood in patients with Crohn's disease. *Inflamm. Bowel Dis.* **2012**, *18*, 1711–1722. [CrossRef]
98. Stonesifer, C.; Corey, S.; Ghanekar, S.; Diamandis, Z.; Acosta, S.A.; Borlongan, C.V. Stem cell therapy for abrogating stroke-induced neuroinflammation and relevant secondary cell death mechanisms. *Prog. Neurobiol.* **2017**, *158*, 94–131. [CrossRef]
99. Ratajczak, J.; Zuba-Surma, E.; Paczkowska, E.; Kucia, M.; Nowacki, P.; Ratajczak, M.Z. Stem cells for neural regeneration—A potential application of very small embryonic-like stem cells. *J. Physiol. Pharmacol.* **2011**, *62*, 3–12.
100. Kim, C.; Schneider, G.; Abdel-Latif, A.; Mierzejewska, K.; Sunkara, M.; Borkowska, S.; Ratajczak, J.; Morris, A.J.; Kucia, M.; Ratajczak, M.Z. Ceramide-1-phosphate regulates migration of multipotent stromal cells and endothelial progenitor cells–implications for tissue regeneration. *Stem Cells* **2013**, *31*, 500–510. [CrossRef]
101. Jabłoński, M.; Mazur, J.K.; Tarnowski, M.; Dołęgowska, B.; Pędziwiatr, D.; Kubiś, E.; Budkowska, M.; Sałata, D.; Wysiecka, J.P.; Kazimierczak, A.; et al. Mobilization of peripheral blood stem cells and changes in the concentration of plasma factors influencing their movement in patients with panic disorder. *Stem Cell. Rev.* **2017**, *13*, 217–225. [CrossRef]

102. Adamiak, M.; Bujko, K.; Cymer, M.; Plonka, M.; Glaser, T.; Kucia, M.; Ratajczak, J.; Ulrich, H.; Abdel-Latif, A.; Ratajczak, M.Z. Novel evidence that extracellular nucleotides and purinergic signaling induce innate immunity-mediated mobilization of hematopoietic stem/progenitor cells. *Leukemia* **2018**, *32*, 1920–1931. [CrossRef]
103. Ratajczak, M.Z.; Kim, C.; Ratajczak, J.; Janowska-Wieczorek, A. Innate immunity as orchestrator of bone marrow homing for hematopoietic stem/progenitor cells. *Adv. Exp. Med. Biol.* **2013**, *735*, 219–232.
104. Ratajczak, M.Z.; Ratajczak, J. extracellular microvesicles as game changers in better understanding the complexity of cellular interactions-from bench to clinical applications. *Am. J. Med. Sci.* **2017**, *354*, 449–452. [CrossRef]
105. Kucharska-Mazur, J.; Tarnowski, M.; Dołęgowska, B.; Budkowska, M.; Pędziwiatr, D.; Jabłoński, M.; Pełka-Wysiecka, J.; Kazimierczak, A.; Ratajczak, M.Z.; Samochowiec, J. Novel evidence for enhanced stem cell trafficking in antipsychotic-naïve subjects during their first psychotic episode. *J. Psychiatr. Res.* **2014**, *49*, 18–24. [CrossRef]
106. Hunter, S.F.; Bowen, J.D.; Reder, A.T. The direct effects of fingolimod in the central nervous system: Implications for relapsing multiple sclerosis. *CNS Drugs* **2016**, *30*, 135–147. [CrossRef]
107. Mutneja, H.R.; Arora, S.; Vij, A. Ozanimod treatment for ulcerative colitis. *N. Engl. J. Med.* **2016**, *375*, e17. [CrossRef]
108. Szulińska, M.; Łoniewski, I.; van Hemert, S.; Sobieska, M.; Bogdański, P. Dose-dependent effects of multispecies probiotic supplementation on the lipopolysaccharide (LPS) level and cardiometabolic profile in obese postmenopausal women: A 12-week randomized clinical trial. *Nutrients* **2018**, *10*, 773. [CrossRef]
109. Marlicz, W.; Loniewski, I.; Grimes, D.S.; Quigley, E.M. Nonsteroidal anti-inflammatory drugs, proton pump inhibitors, and gastrointestinal injury: Contrasting interactions in the stomach and small intestine. *Mayo Clin. Proc.* **2014**, *89*, 1699–1709. [CrossRef]
110. Le Bastard, Q.; Al-Ghalith, G.A.; Grégoire, M.; Chapelet, G.; Javaudin, F.; Dailly, E.; Batard, E.; Knights, D.; Montassier, E. Systematic review: Human gut dysbiosis induced by non-antibiotic prescription medications. *Aliment. Pharmacol. Ther.* **2018**, *47*, 332–345. [CrossRef]
111. Utzeri, E.; Usai, P. Role of non-steroidal anti-inflammatory drugs on intestinal permeability and nonalcoholic fatty liver disease. *World J. Gastroenterol.* **2017**, *23*, 3954–3963. [CrossRef]
112. Wallace, J.L.; Syer, S.; Denou, E.; de Palma, G.; Vong, L.; McKnight, W.; Jury, J.; Bolla, M.; Bercik, P.; Collins, S.M.; et al. Proton pump inhibitors exacerbate NSAID-induced small intestinal injury by inducing dysbiosis. *Gastroenterology* **2011**, *141*. [CrossRef]
113. Maier, L.; Pruteanu, M.; Kuhn, M.; Zeller, G.; Telzerow, A.; Anderson, E.E.; Brochado, A.R.; Fernandez, K.C.; Dose, H.; Mori, H.; et al. Extensive impact of non-antibiotic drugs on human gut bacteria. *Nature* **2018**, *555*, 623–628. [CrossRef]
114. Koliada, A.; Syzenko, G.; Moseiko, V.; Budovska, L.; Puchkov, K.; Perederiy, V.; Gavalko, Y.; Dorofeyev, A.; Romanenko, M.; Tkach, S.; et al. Association between body mass index and Firmicutes/Bacteroidetes ratio in an adult Ukrainian population. *BMC Microbiol.* **2017**, *17*. [CrossRef]
115. Davey, K.J.; O'Mahony, S.M.; Schellekens, H.; O'Sullivan, O.; Bienenstock, J.; Cotter, P.D.; Dinan, T.G.; Cryan, J.F. Gender-dependent consequences of chronic olanzapine in the rat: Effects on body weight, inflammatory, metabolic and microbiota parameters. *Psychopharmacology (Berl.)* **2012**, *221*, 155–169. [CrossRef]
116. Davey, K.J.; Cotter, P.D.; O'Sullivan, O.; Crispie, F.; Dinan, T.G.; Cryan, J.F.; O'Mahony, S.M. Antipsychotics and the gut microbiome: Olanzapine-induced metabolic dysfunction is attenuated by antibiotic administration in the rat. *Transl. Psychiatry* **2013**, *3*, 309. [CrossRef]
117. Bahr, S.M.; Weidemann, B.J.; Castro, A.N.; Walsh, J.W.; deLeon, O.; Burnett, C.M.L.; Pearson, N.A.; Murry, D.J.; Grobe, J.L.; Kirby, J.R. Risperidone-induced weight gain is mediated through shifts in the gut microbiome and suppression of energy expenditure. *EBioMedicine* **2015**, *2*, 1725–1734. [CrossRef]
118. Morgan, A.P.; Crowley, J.J.; Nonneman, R.J.; Quackenbush, C.R.; Miller, C.N.; Ryan, A.K.; Bogue, M.A.; Paredes, S.H.; Yourstone, S.; Carroll, I.M.; et al. The antipsychotic olanzapine interacts with the gut microbiome to cause weight gain in mouse. *PLoS ONE* **2014**, *9*, e115225. [CrossRef]
119. Castaner, O.; Goday, A.; Park, Y.-M.; Lee, S.-H.; Magkos, F.; Shiow, S.-A.T.E.; Schröder, H. The Gut Microbiome Profile in Obesity: A Systematic Review. Available online: https://www.hindawi.com/journals/ije/2018/4095789/ (accessed on 8 October 2018).

120. Bahr, S.M.; Tyler, B.C.; Wooldridge, N.; Butcher, B.D.; Burns, T.L.; Teesch, L.M.; Oltman, C.L.; Azcarate-Peril, M.A.; Kirby, J.R.; Calarge, C.A. Use of the second-generation antipsychotic, risperidone, and secondary weight gain are associated with an altered gut microbiota in children. *Transl. Psychiatry* **2015**, *5*, 652. [CrossRef]
121. Flowers, S.A.; Evans, S.J.; Ward, K.M.; McInnis, M.G.; Ellingrod, V.L. Interaction between atypical antipsychotics and the gut microbiome in a bipolar disease cohort. *Pharmacotherapy* **2017**, *37*, 261–267. [CrossRef]
122. Yuan, X.; Zhang, P.; Wang, Y.; Liu, Y.; Li, X.; Kumar, B.U.; Hei, G.; Lv, L.; Huang, X.-F.; Fan, X.; et al. Changes in metabolism and microbiota after 24-week risperidone treatment in drug naïve, normal weight patients with first episode schizophrenia. *Schizophr. Res.* **2018**. [CrossRef]
123. Skonieczna-Żydecka, K.; Łoniewski, I.; Misera, A.; Stachowska, E.; Maciejewska, D.; Marlicz, W.; Galling, B. Second-generation antipsychotics and metabolism alterations: A systematic review of the role of the gut microbiome. *Psychopharmacology* **2018**. [CrossRef]
124. Lei, B.; Wei, C.J.; Tu, S.C. Action mechanism of antitubercular isoniazid activation by *Mycobacterium tuberculosis* KatG, isolation, and characterization of inha inhibitor. *J. Biol. Chem.* **2000**, *275*, 2520–2526. [CrossRef]
125. Jena, L.; Waghmare, P.; Kashikar, S.; Kumar, S.; Harinath, B.C. Computational approach to understanding the mechanism of action of isoniazid, an anti-TB drug. *Int. J. Mycobacteriol.* **2014**, *3*, 276–282. [CrossRef]
126. Csiszar, K.; Molnar, J. Mechanism of action of tricyclic drugs on *Escherichia coli* and *Yersinia enterocolitica* plasmid maintenance and replication. *Anticancer Res.* **1992**, *12*, 2267–2272.
127. Binding of Tricyclic Antidepressant Drugs to Trophozoites of Giardia Lamblia. Available online: http://jglobal.jst.go.jp/en/public/20090422/200902093831082291 (accessed on 29 September 2018).
128. Antiplasmid Activity of Tricyclic Compounds. Available online: https://www.ncbi.nlm.nih.gov/pubmed/3047509 (accessed on 29 September 2018).
129. Bitonti, A.J.; Sjoerdsma, A.; McCann, P.P.; Kyle, D.E.; Oduola, A.M.; Rossan, R.N.; Milhous, W.K.; Davidson, D.E. Reversal of chloroquine resistance in malaria parasite Plasmodium falciparum by desipramine. *Science* **1988**, *242*, 1301–1303. [CrossRef]
130. Antidepressants Cause Lethal Disruption of Membrane Function in the Human Protozoan Parasite Leishmania. Available online: http://science.sciencemag.org/content/226/4677/977 (accessed on 29 September 2018).
131. Munoz-Bellido, J.L.; Munoz-Criado, S.; Garcìa-Rodrìguez, J.A. Antimicrobial activity of psychotropic drugs: Selective serotonin reuptake inhibitors. *Int. J. Antimicrob. Agents* **2000**, *14*, 177–180. [CrossRef]
132. Ayaz, M.; Subhan, F.; Ahmed, J.; Khan, A.-U.; Ullah, F.; Ullah, I.; Ali, G.; Syed, N.-I.-H.; Hussain, S. Sertraline enhances the activity of antimicrobial agents against pathogens of clinical relevance. *J. Biol. Res. (Thessalon)* **2015**, *22*, 4. [CrossRef]
133. Coban, A.Y.; Tanriverdi Cayci, Y.; Keleş Uludağ, S.; Durupinar, B. Investigation of antibacterial activity of sertralin. *Mikrobiyol. Bul.* **2009**, *43*, 651–656.
134. Kruszewska, H.; Zareba, T.; Tyski, S. Examination of antimicrobial activity of selected non-antibiotic medicinal preparations. *Acta Pol. Pharm.* **2012**, *69*, 1368–1371.
135. Bohnert, J.A.; Szymaniak-Vits, M.; Schuster, S.; Kern, W.V. Efflux inhibition by selective serotonin reuptake inhibitors in Escherichia coli. *J. Antimicrob. Chemother.* **2011**, *66*, 2057–2060. [CrossRef]
136. Begec, Z.; Yucel, A.; Yakupogullari, Y.; Erdogan, M.A.; Duman, Y.; Durmus, M.; Ersoy, M.O. The antimicrobial effects of ketamine combined with propofol: An in vitro study. *Braz J. Anesthesiol.* **2013**, *63*, 461–465. [CrossRef]
137. Felice, V.D.; O'Mahony, S.M. The microbiome and disorders of the central nervous system. *Pharmacol. Biochem. Behav.* **2017**, *160*, 1–13. [CrossRef]
138. Mörkl, S.; Wagner-Skacel, J.; Lahousen, T.; Lackner, S.; Holasek, S.J.; Bengesser, S.A.; Painold, A.; Holl, A.K.; Reininghaus, E. The role of nutrition and the gut-brain axis in psychiatry: A review of the literature. *Neuropsychobiology* **2018**, 1–9. [CrossRef]
139. Liang, S.; Wu, X.; Jin, F. Gut-Brain Psychology: Rethinking psychology from the microbiota–gut–brain axis. *Front. Integr. Neurosci.* **2018**, *12*. [CrossRef]
140. Tilg, H.; Schmiderer, A.; Djanani, A. Gut microbiome-immune crosstalk affects progression of cancer. *Transl. Gastroenterol. Hepatol.* **2018**, *3*. [CrossRef]

141. Tilg, H.; Grander, C. Microbiota and diabetes: An increasingly relevant association. *Pol. Arch. Int. Med.* **2018**, *128*, 333–335. [CrossRef]
142. Adolph, T.E.; Grander, C.; Moschen, A.R.; Tilg, H. Liver–microbiome axis in health and disease. *Trends Immunol.* **2018**, *39*, 712–723. [CrossRef]
143. Quigley, E.M.M. Prebiotics and probiotics in digestive health. *Clin. Gastroenterol. Hepatol.* **2018**. [CrossRef]
144. WGO Practice Guideline —Probiotics and Prebiotics. Available online: http://www.worldgastroenterology.org/guidelines/global-guidelines/probiotics-and-prebiotics (accessed on 5 October 2018).
145. Dinan, T.G.; Stanton, C.; Cryan, J.F. Psychobiotics: A novel class of psychotropic. *Biol. Psychiatry* **2013**, *74*, 720–726. [CrossRef]
146. Sarkar, A.; Lehto, S.M.; Harty, S.; Dinan, T.G.; Cryan, J.F.; Burnet, P.W.J. Psychobiotics and the manipulation of bacteria-gut-brain signals. *Trends Neurosci.* **2016**, *39*, 763–781. [CrossRef]
147. Hill, C.; Guarner, F.; Reid, G.; Gibson, G.R.; Merenstein, D.J.; Pot, B.; Morelli, L.; Canani, R.B.; Flint, H.J.; Salminen, S.; et al. Expert consensus document: The International Scientific Association for Probiotics and Prebiotics consensus statement on the scope and appropriate use of the term probiotic. *Nat. Rev. Gastroenterol. Hepatol.* **2014**, *11*, 506–514. [CrossRef]
148. Misra, S.; Mohanty, D. Psychobiotics: A new approach for treating mental illness? *Crit. Rev. Food Sci. Nutr.* **2017**, 1–7. [CrossRef]
149. Ait-Belgnaoui, A.; Colom, A.; Braniste, V.; Ramalho, L.; Marrot, A.; Cartier, C.; Houdeau, E.; Theodorou, V.; Tompkins, T. Probiotic gut effect prevents the chronic psychological stress-induced brain activity abnormality in mice. *Neurogastroenterol. Motil.* **2014**, *26*, 510–520. [CrossRef]
150. Ait-Belgnaoui, A.; Payard, I.; Rolland, C.; Harkat, C.; Braniste, V.; Théodorou, V.; Tompkins, T.A. *Bifidobacterium longum* and *Lactobacillus helveticus* synergistically suppress stress-related visceral hypersensitivity through hypothalamic-pituitary-adrenal axis modulation. *J. Neurogastroenterol. Motil.* **2018**, *24*, 138–146. [CrossRef]
151. Gareau, M.G.; Jury, J.; MacQueen, G.; Sherman, P.M.; Perdue, M.H. Probiotic treatment of rat pups normalises corticosterone release and ameliorates colonic dysfunction induced by maternal separation. *Gut* **2007**, *56*, 1522–1528. [CrossRef]
152. Gareau, M.G.; Wine, E.; Reardon, C.; Sherman, P.M. Probiotics prevent death caused by citrobacter rodentium infection in neonatal mice. *J. Infect. Dis.* **2010**, *201*, 81–91. [CrossRef]
153. Diop, L.; Guillou, S.; Durand, H. Probiotic food supplement reduces stress-induced gastrointestinal symptoms in volunteers: A double-blind, placebo-controlled, randomized trial. *Nutr. Res.* **2008**, *28*, 1–5. [CrossRef]
154. Messaoudi, M.; Lalonde, R.; Violle, N.; Javelot, H.; Desor, D.; Nejdi, A.; Bisson, J.-F.; Rougeot, C.; Pichelin, M.; Cazaubiel, M.; et al. Assessment of psychotropic-like properties of a probiotic formulation (*Lactobacillus helveticus* R0052 and *Bifidobacterium longum* R0175) in rats and human subjects. *Br. J. Nutr.* **2011**, *105*, 755–764. [CrossRef]
155. Steenbergen, L.; Sellaro, R.; van Hemert, S.; Bosch, J.A.; Colzato, L.S. A randomized controlled trial to test the effect of multispecies probiotics on cognitive reactivity to sad mood. *Brain Behav. Immun.* **2015**, *48*, 258–264. [CrossRef]
156. Allen, A.P.; Hutch, W.; Borre, Y.E.; Kennedy, P.J.; Temko, A.; Boylan, G.; Murphy, E.; Cryan, J.F.; Dinan, T.G.; Clarke, G. Bifidobacterium longum 1714 as a translational psychobiotic: Modulation of stress, electrophysiology and neurocognition in healthy volunteers. *Transl. Psychiatry* **2016**, *6*, 939. [CrossRef]
157. Kato-Kataoka, A.; Nishida, K.; Takada, M.; Kawai, M.; Kikuchi-Hayakawa, H.; Suda, K.; Ishikawa, H.; Gondo, Y.; Shimizu, K.; Matsuki, T.; et al. Fermented milk containing *Lactobacillus casei* strain shirota preserves the diversity of the gut microbiota and relieves abdominal dysfunction in healthy medical students exposed to academic stress. *Appl. Environ. Microbiol.* **2016**, *82*, 3649–3658. [CrossRef]
158. Lv, F.; Chen, S.; Wang, L.; Jiang, R.; Tian, H.; Li, J.; Yao, Y.; Zhuo, C. The role of microbiota in the pathogenesis of schizophrenia and major depressive disorder and the possibility of targeting microbiota as a treatment option. *Oncotarget* **2017**, *8*, 100899–100907. [CrossRef]
159. Huang, R.; Wang, K.; Hu, J. Effect of probiotics on depression: A systematic review and meta-analysis of randomized controlled trials. *Nutrients* **2016**, *8*, 483. [CrossRef]

160. McKean, J.; Naug, H.; Nikbakht, E.; Amiet, B.; Colson, N. Probiotics and subclinical psychological symptoms in healthy participants: a systematic review and meta-analysis. *J. Altern Complement. Med.* **2017**, *23*, 249–258. [CrossRef]
161. Ng, Q.X.; Peters, C.; Ho, C.Y.X.; Lim, D.Y.; Yeo, W.-S. A meta-analysis of the use of probiotics to alleviate depressive symptoms. *J. Affect. Disord.* **2018**, *228*, 13–19. [CrossRef]
162. Kazemi, A.; Noorbala, A.A.; Azam, K.; Eskandari, M.H.; Djafarian, K. Effect of probiotic and prebiotic vs placebo on psychological outcomes in patients with major depressive disorder: A randomized clinical trial. *Clin. Nutr.* **2018**. [CrossRef]
163. Reininghaus, E.Z.; Wetzlmair, L.-C.; Fellendorf, F.T.; Platzer, M.; Queissner, R.; Birner, A.; Pilz, R.; Hamm, C.; Maget, A.; Koidl, C.; et al. The impact of probiotic supplements on cognitive parameters in euthymic individuals with bipolar disorder: A pilot study. *Neuropsychobiology* **2018**, 1–8. [CrossRef]
164. Citi, S. Intestinal barriers protect against disease. *Science* **2018**, *359*, 1097–1098. [CrossRef]
165. Zhou, L.; Foster, J.A. Psychobiotics and the gut-brain axis: In the pursuit of happiness. *Neuropsychiatr Dis. Treat.* **2015**, *11*, 715–723. [CrossRef]
166. Nishida, K.; Sawada, D.; Kawai, T.; Kuwano, Y.; Fujiwara, S.; Rokutan, K. Para-psychobiotic *Lactobacillus gasseri* CP2305 ameliorates stress-related symptoms and sleep quality. *J. Appl. Microbiol.* **2017**, *123*, 1561–1570. [CrossRef]
167. Barichella, M.; Pacchetti, C.; Bolliri, C.; Cassani, E.; Iorio, L.; Pusani, C.; Pinelli, G.; Privitera, G.; Cesari, I.; Faierman, S.A.; et al. Probiotics and prebiotic fiber for constipation associated with Parkinson disease: An RCT. *Neurology* **2016**, *87*, 1274–1280. [CrossRef]
168. Tamtaji, O.R.; Taghizadeh, M.; Daneshvar Kakhaki, R.; Kouchaki, E.; Bahmani, F.; Borzabadi, S.; Oryan, S.; Mafi, A.; Asemi, Z. Clinical and metabolic response to probiotic administration in people with Parkinson's disease: A randomized, double-blind, placebo-controlled trial. *Clin. Nutr.* **2018**. [CrossRef]
169. Ticinesi, A.; Tana, C.; Nouvenne, A.; Prati, B.; Lauretani, F.; Meschi, T. Gut microbiota, cognitive frailty and dementia in older individuals: A systematic review. *Clin. Interv. Aging* **2018**, *13*, 1497–1511. [CrossRef]
170. Agahi, A.; Hamidi, G.A.; Daneshvar, R.; Hamdieh, M.; Soheili, M.; Alinaghipour, A.; Esmaeili Taba, S.M.; Salami, M. Does severity of Alzheimer's disease contribute to its responsiveness to modifying gut microbiota? A double blind clinical trial. *Front. Neurol.* **2018**, *9*, 662. [CrossRef]
171. Patusco, R.; Ziegler, J. Role of probiotics in managing gastrointestinal dysfunction in children with autism spectrum disorder: An update for practitioners. *Adv. Nutr.* **2018**, *9*, 637–650. [CrossRef]
172. Rudzki, L.; Ostrowska, L.; Pawlak, D.; Małus, A.; Pawlak, K.; Waszkiewicz, N.; Szulc, A. Probiotic *Lactobacillus plantarum* 299v decreases kynurenine concentration and improves cognitive functions in patients with major depression: A double-blind, randomized, placebo controlled study. *Psychoneuroendocrinology* **2018**, *100*, 213–222. [CrossRef]

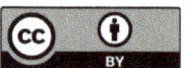

© 2018 by the authors. Licensee MDPI, Basel, Switzerland. This article is an open access article distributed under the terms and conditions of the Creative Commons Attribution (CC BY) license (http://creativecommons.org/licenses/by/4.0/).

MDPI
St. Alban-Anlage 66
4052 Basel
Switzerland
Tel. +41 61 683 77 34
Fax +41 61 302 89 18
www.mdpi.com

Journal of Clinical Medicine Editorial Office
E-mail: jcm@mdpi.com
www.mdpi.com/journal/jcm

www.ingramcontent.com/pod-product-compliance
Lightning Source LLC
LaVergne TN
LVHW070606100526
838202LV00012B/579